Clinical Information Systems

Bruce I. Blum

Clinical Information Systems

With 104 Figures

Springer Science+Business Media, LLC

Bruce I. Blum
Applied Physics Laboratory
The Johns Hopkins University
Laurel, Maryland 20707
U.S.A.

Library of Congress Cataloging-in-Publication Data
Blum, Bruce I.
Clinical Information systems.
Bibliography: p.
Includes index.
1. Information storage and retrieval systems—
Medicine. 2. Medicine—Data processing. I. Title.
R858.B578 1986 610'.28'5 85-26084

Originally published by Springer-Verlag New York Inc in 1986.
Softcover reprint of the hardcover 1st edition 1986

Typeset by World Composition Services, Inc., Leesburg, Virginia.

9 8 7 6 5 4 3 2 1

ISBN 978-3-540-96190-1 ISBN 978-3-662-26537-6 (eBook)
DOI 10.1007/978-3-662-26537-6

to Harriet

Contents

Introduction

As its name implies, this book deals with clinical information systems. The clinical information system (or CIS) is an automated system with a long term database containing clinical information used for patient care. This definition excludes business systems (no clinical data), physiological monitoring systems (no long term database), and many research systems (not used in patient care). The theses of this book are (a) that CIS technology is mature, (b) that the CIS will have a major impact upon patient care and the health delivery system, and (c) that the number of commercial systems which now offer these potential benefits is very small. The objective of this book is to establish the above theses and thereby (a) inform both users and developers, (b) increase the demand for more sophisticated products, and finally, (c) provide marketplace incentives to advance the state of the art.

The CIS is an application of computer technology for a specific class of problems. Its development requires a knowledge of the technology with an understanding of the application area. As with any tool-based application, the scope of the product will be limited by the capability of the tool. In the case of the CIS, reliable computers with comprehensive database facilities became commercially available in the early 1970s. By the mid 1970s there was a maturation of the literature, and evaluations of 5-years' use began to appear. As will be shown, there have been surprisingly few new ideas introduced since the 1970s. The major effort has been one of integrating older ideas with the new technology. Progress has been made through the engineering of more effective solutions.

The greatest change over the past decade has come in the scope and cost of the computer equipment available to support a CIS. The personal computer has impacted public awareness in all areas; application to health care is no exception. This can be seen by examining the interest in medical computing conferences. The largest American conference is the Symposium on Computer Applications in Medical Care (SCAMC). Its first meeting, in 1977, was attended by under 200; within 5 years the annual attendance routinely exceeded 2,000. While many participants are professional workers in medical informatics, many others are one-time attendees with a desire for "computer literacy" or an interest in sharing their personal computing interests.

As I appraise the field in the mid 1980s, I see a large body of information available about the CIS and its benefits. The material is broadly scattered, of uneven quality, and sometimes associated with obsolescent technology. It is difficult for the naive user to locate and assimilate. In fact, it also is frequently ignored by the professional user. For example, consider what one of Shortliffe's students reported after an extensive literature review of medical data base systems.

Medical system implementors don't read (presumably because they "know what they want"). An enormous duplication of effort, both good and bad takes place. Bibliographies are typically incomplete, and fundamental issues are almost always overlooked. When reading is done, it is done incestuously.*

Modern computers—and in particular personal computers—are now so powerful that an inexperienced user can produce very impressive results. This was brought home to me at a recent SCAMC meeting when one physician opened his talk on medical decision-making tools with the statement that 2 years ago he knew nothing about computers. Clearly, this is a reflection of the facility of modern computer systems. Yet, that presenter would hardly preface a paper in a neurology conference with a comparable statement about brain surgery.

One fear I have is that seduction by the personal computer will result in large numbers of impressive toy systems, distorted views of the development process, and frustrations with the limitations of computer technology. It is now possible to do in months with thousands of dollars what previously took years and tens of thousands of dollars. The question is, are we doing it better? The wheel is such a marvelous invention, we get great pleasure each time we invent it. Only by learning from past experience will we build better systems.

In what follows I have attempted to extract what I consider to be the most useful information for persons interested in clinical information systems. In doing this, I had several problems. First, who was the audience? Since the primary objective of the CIS is to improve care, the book had to be directed at health care providers: physicians, nurses, etc. However, since the CIS also impacts the delivery system, it should also include material for administrators and other professionals who might use (or help select) such systems. Finally, because system implementors require this knowledge, this book is intended for their use as well.

In addition to the problem of a broad audience, there is a concern with respect to the readers' background and interest. A text in calculus, for example, assumes a prior knowledge of algebra and presents a well-defined subject; its goal is to provide a skill to be used in subsequent studies. In the case of the CIS, however, there are two issues. Firstly, the field is too young, and I do not know what facts or calculus-like skills to teach. Secondly, readers come with different

* E. H. Shortliffe, The Science of Biomedical Computing, in J. Anderson, F. Gremy, A. Levy, and J. C. Pages, *Information Science and Medical Education*, North Holland, 1983. Also reprinted in *Medical Informatics* (9, 3/4) 1984, p 191.

backgrounds and interests. Some know nothing of computer technology, others know nothing of the application area.

As a result, I have organized the book into three major parts. Part I is an introduction. It contains an historical introduction to modern computers and a summary of computer applications in medicine. Part II is concerned with computer systems: hardware, software, and implementation. Finally, Part III discusses clinical information systems in hospitals, ambulatory care, and medical decision making. In each case the chapters are written as more-or-less self contained essays. I have tried to emphasize the historical context, suggest issues for research, and identify facts. I have been very free with my opinions, and the casual reader should have no difficulty in separating my editorial judgments from the scientific results.

As a by-product of this organization, there are some difficulties with the book. Each chapter has been written so that both a novice and experienced reader can benefit from it. For the novice there is a general structuring and introduction; for the experienced reader there are suggestions of new ways to look at familiar objects. In particular, I would hope that the chapters on computer systems will be of interest to computer professionals while those on clinical applications would be useful to specialists in medical informatics. However, the novice reader may not have a background which enables him to understand fully a chapter at first reading. My only suggestion is to be pragmatic and skip over what cannot be absorbed easily; return to the chapter as your understanding (or need to know) grows.

Another problem with the book's orientation is the way in which I have dealt with references. Each chapter has a section containing suggestions for further reading plus footnotes for citations. I believe that this is satisfactory for Parts I and II; the topics covered have too vast a literature to be adequately covered in this survey. However, this is not true for Part III. At first I attempted to embed the references in the text, but I found that my treatment of the topics was illustrative rather than comprehensive. Thus, many references either would not appear, or the text would have to be altered to include artificial references. I therefore decided to include a Selected Readings section following the Glossary. In all cases, the interested reader can identify documents by the author's name. This is—to me—an unsatisfactory compromise, but I believe it makes the text a little more readable.

Finally, there is a concern about the level of detail. Many issues are too complex to be treated adequately in a book of this breadth. Therefore, I have simplified; what is presented is accurate but not necessarily complete. Also, I have been somewhat casual with my use of words. Many terms are used differently by different people. Where there is no preferred usage, I tend to use these terms interchangeably. The glossary of computer terminology should clarify any ambiguity.

The book is intended to be used as either a general introduction or a text in a medical computing class. In part it is based upon a course I taught at Johns

Hopkins. In this case there were lectures, outside readings, and a single class project. Probably a better course organization would be to combine this text with lectures and a hands-on programming activity. The former would present the broader concepts, while the latter would provide a concrete realization of some of the issues. I also believe that the book can be a useful supplementary text in any course on computer applications.

The preparation of this book has greatly benefitted from the support and encouragement of many friends and colleagues. In particular, I am deeply grateful to Dr. Carl Bostrom and the Applied Physics Laboratory for the financial support to write the book. I also wish to thank those who read drafts and corrected errors. They are (alphabetically) C. Bitterli, M. Collen, R. Gardner, B. Hamill, E. Hammond, C. McDonald, J. Reggia, R. Rich, A. Shapiro, E. Shortliffe, and V. Sigillito. Of course, I am responsible for the errors in fact or judgment which remain. One cannot appreciate the contribution of Elsie Cote without first seeing a sample of my handwriting. She transformed scribbles into grammatical, properly spelled text which could be edited and reviewed; thank you. Finally, I want to acknowledge Harriet's help. She supplied the appropriate measures of support, encouragement, and goading over a period which was longer than either of us had anticipated. And she made it all seem like fun.

Part I. Background and Introduction

1 History of Computers

1.1. Introduction

We are in the midst of a revolution in technology and in the way we process information. The computer is at the heart of this revolution. Where it will take us is unknown, but we do know that events are moving rapidly. In fact, virtually everything related to digital computers took place in my generation's adult lifetime. And I am not old.

Because the impact of computers is so new, the rules for their use are still being formulated. There is a broad diversity of users. Some, like myself, have 20 or more years experience in the field; others are facing their first encounter. For those with a long history of involvement, the initial concepts were formulated in an era of now obsolete technology. Much of what we learned no longer has relevance. Yet the roots of computer science are tied to the history of the past 30 years. Today's solutions are structured in the context of yesterday's problems.

For those first learning about computers, on the other hand, there are entirely different perceptions. The technology of the past (for example, the 80-column punch card) is an anachronism; personal computers have made interaction and user friendliness the norm. Programming—the preparation of instructions for the computer to process—is no longer a profession to be learned on the job; it is a skill soon to be acquired by all.

The purpose of this chapter is to help put this revolution in some perspective. One's view of the technology is partially determined by when and how he or she was first exposed. Today, a large portion of the professional community is deeply committed to programming languages and computer concepts that are over 20 years old. Meanwhile, others who are first learning to apply the technology have no comprehension of alternative approaches. Although we cannot predict what the future will bring, we do know that we cannot understand where we are without some insight into the forces that brought us here.

This chapter is divided into three sections. The first reviews the early history of computation. It provides a basis for understanding the intellectual impact of the early computers. The second section discusses the first generations of digital computers from which the foundations of computer science were established. The final section traces the developments in technology over the past two decades.

1.2. The Early Foundations

Counting is universal to all societies. The bases vary from 10 to 60; concepts range from precision to generic wholes such as "many," "hrair," and "infinity." In most early societies, counting and adding relied on physical markers or tokens, a principle identical to that used in the abacus. Columns or squares were drawn on a counting surface, and markers were used to record values for each column. When the markers exceeded the space available in one column, they were removed and a "carry" marker was added to the next column.

This separation between computation and transcription allowed the Romans to use a cumbersome number representation that was effective for communication but not arithmetic. The use of columns with differing bases also allowed England to flourish with a monetary system in which 12 pence made a shilling and 20 shillings made a pound. Indeed, Great Britain's Chancellor of the Exchequer, the minister responsible for the treasury, still takes his name from the counting table used by his predecessors. In 1971, however, the pressures of modern computation forced Great Britain to adopt a decimal currency.

1.2.1. Napier's Bones

One of the earliest computational tools for multiplication can be traced back to John Napier (1550-1617) who published the first book of logarithms in 1614. To help him carry out the computation for these tables, he developed several mechanical devices. As he wrote in 1617:

> The difficulty and prolixity of calculation, the weariness of which is so apt to deter from the study of mathematics, I have always, with what little powers and little genius I possess, laboured to eradicate. And with that end in view, I have published of late years the Cannon of Logarithms. . . . For the sake of those who prefer to work with the natural numbers as they stand, I have excogitated three other compendious modes of calculation, of which the first is by means of numbering rods and these I have called Rabdologia. Another, by far the most expeditious of all for multiplication, and which on that account I have not inaptly called the Promptuary of Multiplication, is by means of little plates of metal disposed in a box. And lastly, a third method, namely Local Arithmetic performed upon a chessboard. (Reprinted with permission from M. R. Williams: *The use of Napier's bones in calculating instruments. Ann Hist Comp* (5,3) July, 1983, p.280. © 1983 AFIPS, reprinted by permission.)

The most popular of these devices was the Rabdologia, better known as Napier's bones because bone, horn, and ivory were used to construct them. The bones were simply recordings of the multiplication tables arranged to facilitate computation. To understand how they were used, it is helpful first to know how

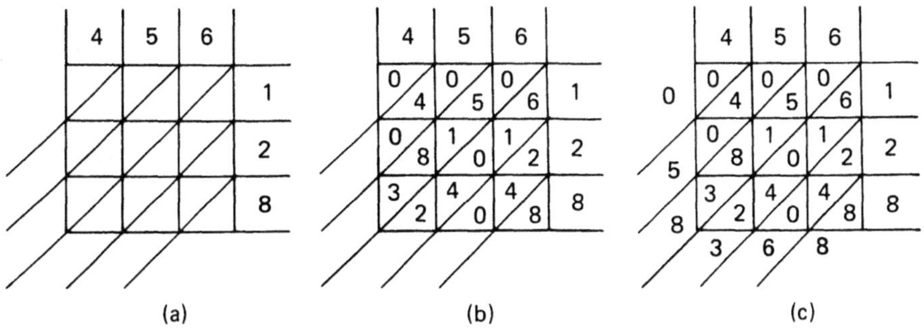

FIGURE 1.1. The Gelosia Method of Multiplication.

multiplication was manually performed at that time. The technique was called the Gelosia Method, and it involved first drawing a grid and placing the digits in the multiplier in the columns at the top and the digits in multiplicand in the rows at the right (Fig. 1.1a). Each element in the grid was divided with a diagonal and the product of the digits was written with the 10s to the left of the diagonal and the units to the right (Fig. 1.1b). Finally, the diagonals were summed to produce the product (Fig. 1.1c).

There were 10 numbering rods or bones as shown in Fig. 1.2. Each contained 10 sections with the digit at the top and the multiplication table written in the diagonal format. To perform a multiplication, the rods for the multiplicand were arranged in order and the product for each digit of the multiplier was computed, recorded, and later added to provide the final product. For example, to perform the computation in Fig. 1.1, the 4, 5, and 6 rods would be placed side by side and the diagonals of the partial products in the 1, 2, and 8 rows would be summed. There were also rods used for computing the square root and cube root. Again, the rods served only as reminding and guiding devices; the final computation involved recording and addition or subtraction.

The use of the bones spread rapidly, and their use in China was recorded only a few years after their introduction to Europe. The Promptuary of Multiplication was a two-dimensional projection of the numbering rods that sought to avoid the recording and addition of the partial products. Housed in a large box, it consisted of sets of strips for the multiplier and multiplicand digits. Although it did not use any mechanical action, it was difficult (and expensive) to manufacture and thus had limited popularity.

Although the contribution of Napier's bones pales in comparison with that of the logarithm, it does offer some interesting insights into how technology advances. The numbering rods mechanized the Gelosia Method of multiplication; they probably would never have been conceived in this form if another multiplication method had been used. The tool was developed out of a need to support a computation intensive activity; its form was an extension of a manual procedure.

It would be some 13 years before William Oughtred (1575-1660) thought of

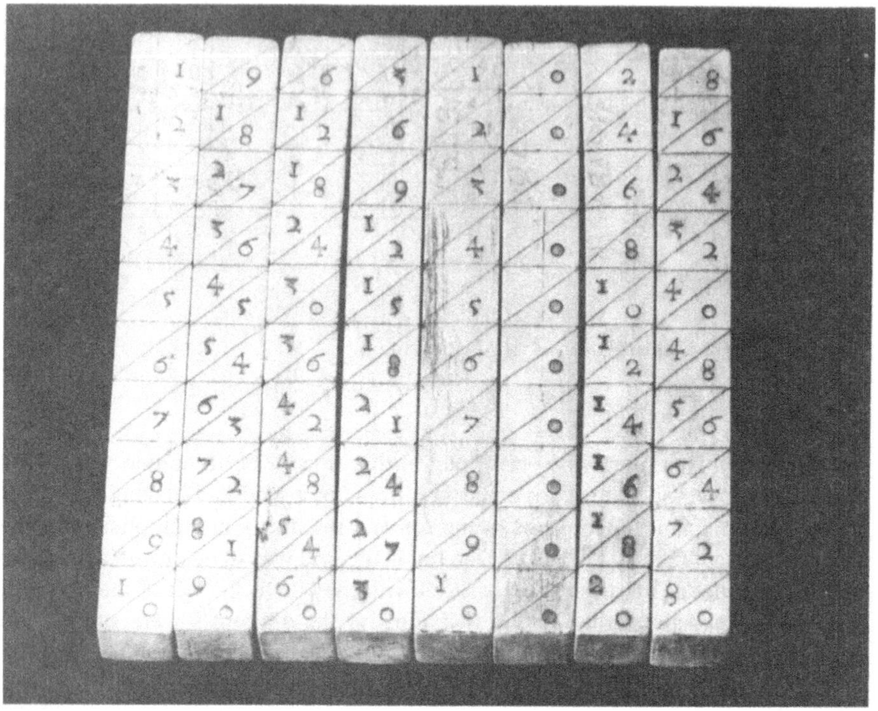

FIGURE 1.2. Napier's Bones. (Smithsonian Institution Print 58996E, reprinted by permission.)

inscribing logarithmic scales on long rods to produce the first slide rule. Thus we go from multiplication with digital precision to multiplication as an approximation formed by adding logarithms.

1.2.2. Some Early Calculators

When discussing mechanical calculators, it is common to begin with the work of Blaise Pascal (1623-1662). A child prodigy, Pascal had a brief but exceptionally productive life. He is credited with founding the modern theory of probability and establishing the basis for the integral calculus. In physics, his experiments contributed to our knowledge of atmospheric pressure and the equilibrium of fluids. In 1645 Pascal converted to Jansenism—a religious movement that asserted the irreducible freedom of the individual soul under God. The *Provincial Letters,* written in support of a leading Jansenist, have been identified as the beginning of French classical literature. His posthumous religious writings, *Penseés,* were a major philosophic statement. From this rich and varied existence, we shall discuss only how he constructed the first adding machine in 1642.

At an early age, Pascal was working as a clerk for his father, a tax collector

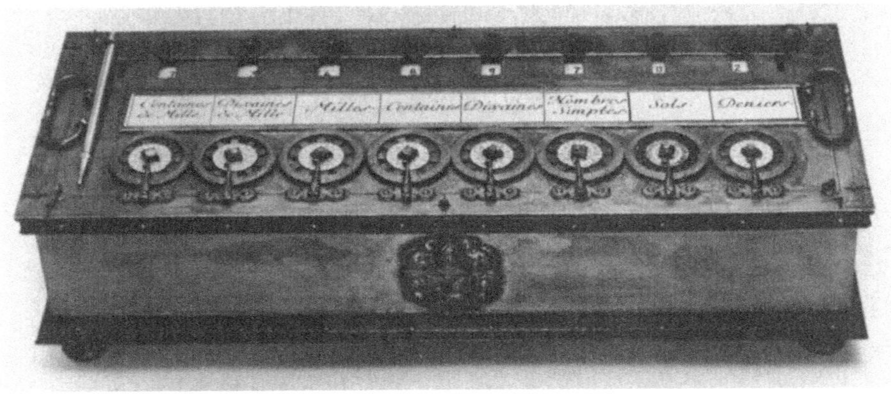

FIGURE 1.3. Pascal's Arithmetic Engine. (The Computer Museum, Boston, MA, reprinted by permission.)

in Rouen. To help with the totaling of accounts, he developed an adding machine. It was a small box with a series of eight revolving wheels—similar to a telephone dial—each connected to a drum containing the digits 0, 1, . . . 9. As a wheel was turned, the drum rotated, making one of the numerals on the drum visible through a register window (see Fig. 1.3). Addition was performed by "dialing" in the addend. The fundamental innovation was the implementation of a ratchet linkage to transfer the "carry" to the next highest drum. This ratchet linkage *(sautier)* was an independent reinvention of a concept documented by Hero of Alexandria in the third century A.D.

The first operating model was constructed in 1642 and publicly presented in 1645. It performed addition and subtraction directly; it multiplied and divided by use of repeated addition and subtraction. Only some 50 units were built, and the adding machine had a limited impact on computation.

The modification of Pascal's calculator to perform multiplication was done by Gottfried Wilhelm von Leibniz (1646-1716). He too was a mathematician, scientist, and philosopher whose accomplishments make this contribution simply an item of historic interest. Leibniz added a movable carriage that operated on wheels utilizing an active and inactive pin principle with a delayed carry mechanism. In this way, the calculator could perform repeated additions and subtractions without requiring the operator to follow an algorithm. Unfortunately, the concepts were beyond the technology of the time, and the calculators of both Pascal and Leibniz proved to be neither reliable nor practical.

1.2.3. The Analytical Engine

No history of modern computers would be complete without a discussion of the contributions of Charles Babbage (1791-1871). In a preelectronic era, he worked out many of the concepts of automatic computation that we find in today's digital computers. His success was limited by the state of engineering and his temper-

TABLE 1.1. Difference for a table of squares.

Number	Square	First difference	Second difference
1	1		
2	4	3	
3	9	5	2
4	16	7	2
5	25	9	2
6	36	11	2

ament. Nevertheless, his writings and thoughts provided inspiration to some of the early innovators in electronic computing.

The initial impetus for his work was a desire to eliminate the many errors he found in the printed tables of logarithms, astronomical data, and insurance information. While pursuing graduate studies in mathematics, he surveyed the available calculators and found none that matched his needs.

> I considered that a machine to execute the mere isolated operations of arithmetic would be comparatively of little value, unless it were very easily set to do its work, and unless it executed not only accurately, but with great rapidity, whatever it was required to do. . . . To insure accuracy in the printed tables, it was necessary that the machine which computed tables should also set them up in type, or else supply a mould in which stereotype plates of those tables could be cast.[1]

The method he selected was that of differences. Since the output would be a table, one needed only to establish the differences between table rows. Given this difference, one could compute the next table row by a simple addition of the difference. Of course, not all tables could be computed using a single difference; some required two or more differences. A simple illustration will help.

Assume we wish to compute a table of integers and their squares. We compute the first difference as the difference between successive squares. We then compute the second difference between successive first differences. The result is a constant value (2) and we are finished (see Table 1.1). Other tables might require sixth or seventh differences before arriving at a constant value.

Babbage's Difference Engine was a calculator designed to produce tables by adding differences. In the table of squares example, it would be initiated with a 1 on the number column, a 3 on the first difference column, and a 2 on the second difference column. By use of gears, a turn of the wheel would add the first difference column to the number column and the second difference column to the first difference column. It would also print, or set in a mold, the number in the first column. (There were no automatic typesetting machines at this time, so this technology would also have to be developed.)

Babbage received a grant through the Royal Society to build a Difference Engine that would calculate to six orders of difference and 20 places of accuracy

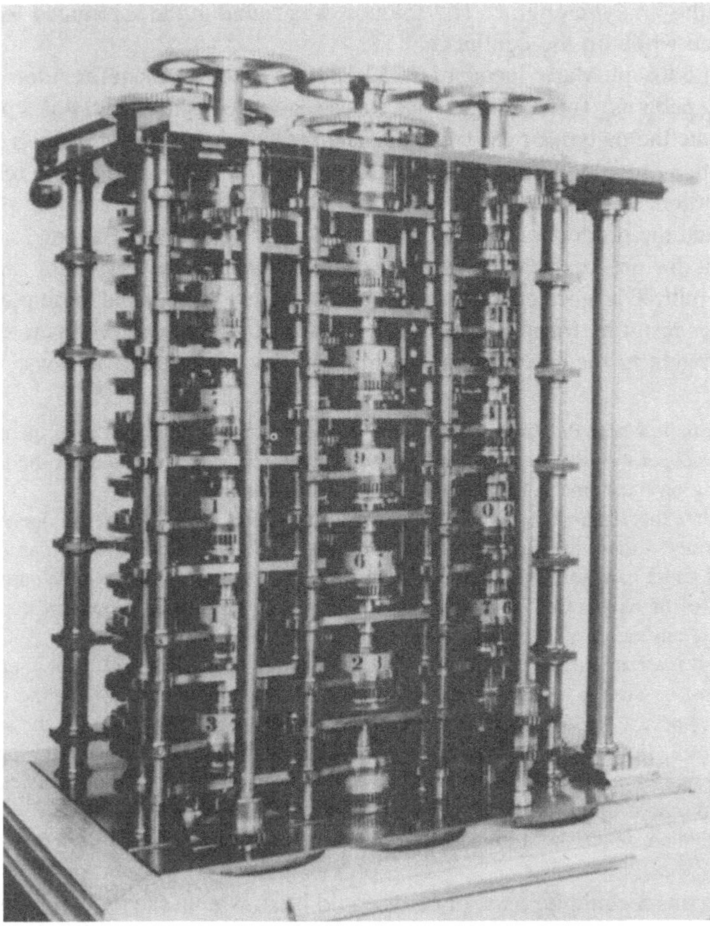

FIGURE 1.4. Part of Babbage's Difference Engine. (Smithsonian Institution Print 53190, reprinted by permission.)

(Fig. 1.4). The funds were limited, the wording of the agreement vague, the technical difficulties enormous, and the attention of Babbage easily distracted. In 1827 Babbage lost his father, two of his children, and his wife. He took a year off from his labors, and visited the continent. When he returned to the Difference Engine, he found progress slow and expectations great. Although some additional money for the Difference Engine was finally approved, disputes with his engineer effectively terminated the project in 1833.

By now, however, Babbage had even more ambitious ideas. What if, instead of arranging the engine in a line, it was organized around a central shaft. With this orientation, output could become input, or, as he put it, the engine could bite its own tail and control itself. There remained only the problem of how to control this analytic engine. The solution was found in the automated looms he examined while on the continent.

In 1806 Joseph Marie Jacquard (1752-1834) perfected a loom for automatically weaving patterns. The driving device was a sequence of cards with holes punched to indicate the pattern or use of color. The presence of a hole allowed a hooked wire with a thread to be inserted into the pattern; the absence of a hole restricted the insertion. In this way, the pattern could be abstracted as a set of punched cards, and the production of the cloth could be programmed. Babbage now had the basis for an Analytical Engine design. It consisted of two parts: the store and the mill. The store contained all the variables to be operated upon plus those quantities resulting from previous operations. The quantities to be operated upon were brought to the second part, the mill. It was described as follows:

> Every formula which the Analytical Engine can be required to compute consists of certain algebraical operations to be performed upon given letters, and of certain other modification depending on the numerical value assigned to those letters.
>
> There are therefore two sets of cards, the first to direct the nature of the operations to be performed—these are called operation cards: the other to direct the particular variables on which those cards are required to operate—these latter are called variable cards. Now the symbol of each variable or constant is placed at the top of a column capable of containing any required number of digits.
>
> Under this arrangement, when any formula is required to be computed, a set of operation cards must be strung together, which contains the series of operations in the order in which they occur. Another set of cards must then be strung together, to call in the variables into the mill, in the order in which they are required to be acted upon. Each operation card will require three other cards, two to represent the variables and constants and their numerical values upon which the previous operation card is to act, and one to indicate the variable on which the arithmetical result of this operation is to be placed.[2]

Using this technique, a set of cards could be drawn up (and reused) for every formula. Where a formula was required but not present, the engine would ring a bell and stop until an attendant fetched and loaded the formula. If the wrong formula was entered, a louder bell would ring. As Ada, Countess of Lovelace, put it, "We may say most aptly that the Analytical Engine weaves algebraic patterns just as the Jacquard-loom weaves flowers and leaves."

Because of his lack of success with the Difference Engine, Babbage was forced to use his own money to produce his Analytical Engine. It sought to express each number to 50 digits of accuracy and manage a store of 1,000 numbers. (To this day, the term store is used for memory in Great Britain.) Lord Byron's daughter, Ada, was a gifted mathematician who was attracted to Babbage's work. She translated some of his papers, helped organize some of his notes, and wrote some of the earliest punched card programs. As the result of this activity, she is credited as being the first programmer.

The production of the Analytic Engine was too ambitious for its time and creator. There was, however, a successful implementation of the Difference Engine. Developed by George and Edward Scheutz of Sweden, the device computed four orders of differences to 14 places and automatically printed the results. The device was brought to England in 1854 and a copy was later brought to the United States to print astronomical tables. Perhaps a more disciplined approach might have produced a less ambitious gear-driven, stored program calculator. In any event, we must acknowledge Babbage's genius and early contribution.

1.2.4. Foundations for the Computer Age

The contributions that we have examined were all precursors to modern computational machines. Although each clearly demonstrated great insight, each was beyond the engineering of its period, and each found little practical use. Yet, starting in the mid-19th century the ability to engineer mass produced machines improved. Commerce flourished, and the need to manage information grew.

Keyboards today are common. The Pascal calculator, however, used a dial device. One of the first of the key-driven adding machines was patented in 1850 by D. D. Parmelee. It transferred the energy of pushing down a key to a ratchet-toothed bar. The length of the key was a function of the digit, e.g., the "9" key was nine times longer than the "1" key. Unfortunately, there was no mechanism for overcoming the momentum imparted by the initial key stroke, and the ratchet-toothed numerical bar frequently would overshoot. Further, since there was only one set of keys, each column had to be added separately.

In 1857 Thomas Hill got a patent on a multiple-order key driven machine. As one of his contemporaries commented, it had the same deficiencies as Parmelee's design.

> The functions of the Hill mechanism would, perhaps, be practical if it were not for the physical law that bodies set in motion tend to remain in motion. . . . The feature lacking was a means for controlling the action of the mechanism under the tremendously increased speed produced by the use of depressible keys as an activating means. . . . Imagine the sudden whirl his numeral wheel would receive on a quick depression of a key and then consider that he provided no means for stopping these wheels.[3]

It would be some 30 years before effective multiple-order key driven machines would be available. The first successful device, the Comptometer, was invented by Dorr E. Felt (Fig. 1.5). He recognized the deficiencies of contemporary machines and the need to perform addition faster than the unaided average expert.

> The construction of such a complicated machine from metal, as I had schemed up, was not within my reach from a monetary standpoint, so I decided to put my ideas into wood.
>
> It was near Thanksgiving Day of 1884, and I decided to use the holiday in the construction of the wooden model. I went to the grocer's and selected a box which seemed to me to be about the right size for the casing. It was a macaroni box, so I have always called it the macaroni box model. For keys I procured some meat skewers from the butcher around the corner and some staples from a hardware store for the key guides and an assortment of elastic bands to be used for springs. When Thanksgiving day came I got up early and went to work with a few tools, principally a jackknife.
>
> I soon discovered that there were some parts which would require better tools than I

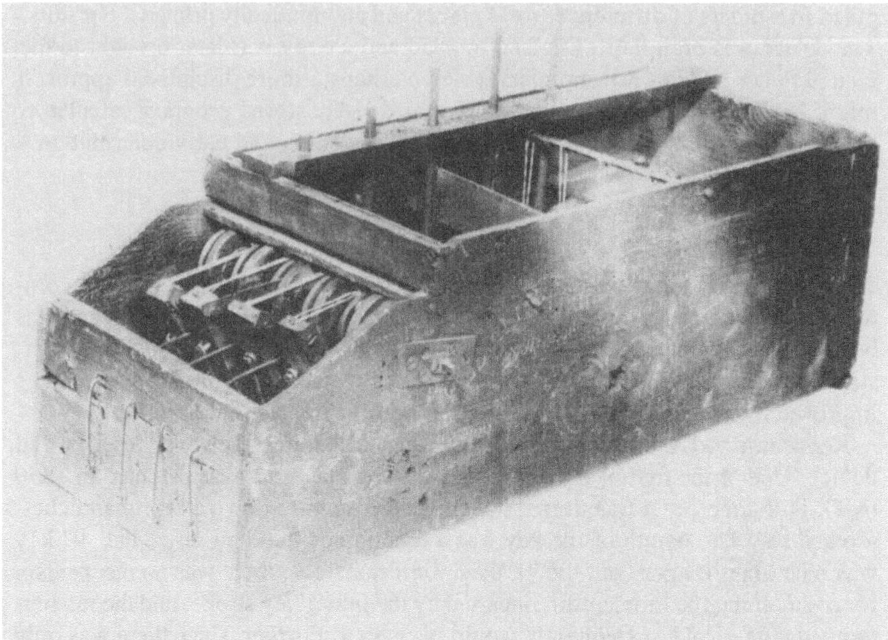

FIGURE 1.5. Felt's Macaroni Box Comptometer. (Smithsonian Institution Print 3284A, reprinted by permission.)

> had at hand for the purpose, and when night came I found that the model I had expected to construct in a day was a long way from being complete or in working order. I finally had some of the parts made out of metal, and finished the model soon after New Year's day, 1885.[4]

The resultant calculator was both effective and reliable. Felt also supplied his customers with detailed instructions for the four basic arithmetic operations, square and cube roots, interest, etc. The Comptometer became a practical tool and preempted the market for some 15 years.

The next step was to add printing. Felt added a recorder to go with his calculator. The paper was advanced by a lever that set a spring for the printing device, and each figure was printed as the key was depressed. The stage was now set for the development of the cash register.

The idea for a cash register is generally credited to James Ritty. A restaurant owner, he got the idea for a transaction recorder while watching a gauge that counted propeller revolutions. His first model had a large clock-like dial with two hands: one for dollars and the other for cents. A later model was called Ritty's Incorruptible Cashier. Recording of the transaction was crude. It consisted of punching a hole in a paper tape: one column for each key. At the end of the day, the proprietor would count the holes and multiply by the value of the column.

Ritty's machine sold poorly and he sold the business to Jacob H. Eckert who, in 1882, organized the National Manufacturing Company. The next owner, John H. Patterson, changed the name to the National Cash Register (NCR) Company. Patterson recognized the need to help the customer understand and solve the problems of his business. By emphasizing sales procedures and training, Patterson was able to build NCR into one of the largest builders of general business equipment.

Calculators and cash registers soon led to bookkeeping machines. The first was patented by Leon Bollée in 1889. Keyboards were also extended to include letters. The first successful commercial typewriter was marketed by Remington in 1874. It produced only capital letters. By 1878 a shift key had been introduced, but this feature was not included with all manufacturer's machines. Since the typewriter was a new device, there were questions about how the keys should be arranged.

Some keyboards opted for putting the letters T, H, and E near one another. The World typewriter grouped A, N, and D together, whereas the Edison Mimeograph had groupings of T, H, and E; A, N, and D; O and F; and I, N, and G. Although the shift key had been known since 1875, some manufacturers of the 1890s found it too complicated or tiring for the operator. Their machines had dual sets of keys: one for uppercase, the other for lowercase. The arrangement of the keys varied from eight rows on the Yost machine to one very long row on the Saturn keyboard.

This lack of standards produced obvious problems in training. One design that began to attract attention was called the Ideal keyboard. The layout was based on the fact that more than 70% of all English words are made up of the letters D H I A T E N S O R. Consequently, placing all these keys in one row should make typing more efficient. Although some manufacturers adopted the Ideal keyboard, it was the Universal keyboard with its familiar top row of Q W E R T Y U I O P that finally won out. The key positions were selected to slow down the operators; it was feared that, if they typed too fast, the mechanism would jam. The success of the Universal keyboard, therefore, is a tribute to man's ability to overcome designed adversity; it was not until the 1930s that the psychologist August Dvorak began to develop the efficient keyboard layout that now bears his name.

By 1909 noiseless typewriters were on the market, and an electric typewriter was available. The first wave of office automation was underway. Another major innovation was the use of the punched card. Although the roots of punched cards clearly go back to Jacquard's looms and Babbage's Analytical Engine, their use in data processing are all derived from the work of Herman Hollerith. His foundation patents in the field gave him a virtual monopoly in punched-card data processing from 1890 to World War I.

Hollerith was graduated from Columbia in 1879 and took a job with the Census. He became the protégé of John Shaw Billings, an army surgeon, who was then serving as the director of the division for vital statistics. Billings was an innovator. He designed the Johns Hopkins Hospital and had a keen interest in the use of

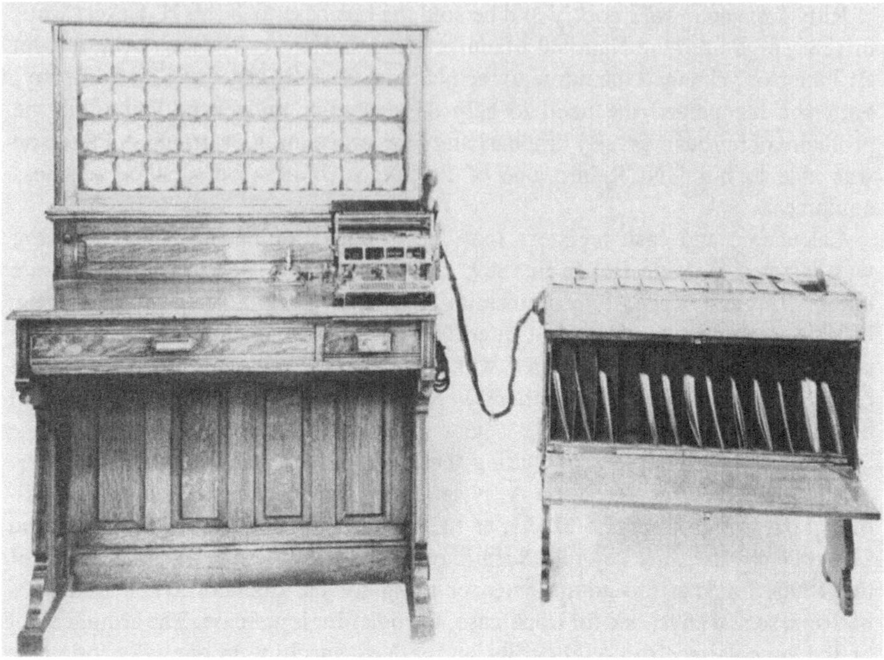

FIGURE 1.6. The Hollerith Tabulating Machine. (Smithsonian Institution Print 64563, reprinted by permission.)

mechanical tabulating tools. One of his ideas was to use cards with each containing the description of an individual punched into it. Hollerith studied the idea and found it feasible.

Hollerith left the Census to go to M.I.T. in 1882. There he discovered that his true vocation was invention. He went to the Patent Office, and then set up shop as a "Solicitor and Expert on Patents." Soon he had the first of his foundation patents. By 1889 he had developed a system used by the Army Surgeon General's office to process medical statistics. A description of this system was accepted as a doctoral dissertation, and in 1890 Columbia awarded him a Ph.D. degree.

The early work of Hollerith is most closely associated with the Census of 1890. As the population of the United States grew, the compilation of the decennial census became more and more burdensome. The 1880 census took over 5 years to process, and one could foresee that future censuses might require 10 or more years of compilation before the results could be published. In 1889 a committee was appointed to consider how to tabulate the coming census. Three systems were considered; Hollerith's was clearly the superior and he was awarded the contract. It was a good choice. Tabulation was reduced from the 7.5 year estimate for manual processing to a mere 2 months of machine supported activity.

Hollerith now sought to mass produce his machines (see Fig. 1.6). He subcontracted the keypunch to Pratt & Whitney and the tabulator to Western Electric. After some years of experimentation with player piano-like rolls of paper, he settled on the use of manila cards. The card size was based on the size of dollar bills because it was economical to buy cabinets and drawers with those subdivisions. He described his system as follows:

> Data cards were punched with holes on spots indicating particular information, such as employment. To obtain the total number of men working in factories, for example, the data cards were placed one by one over mercury-filled cups. The machine dropped rows of telescoping pins onto the surface of the card. Wherever there was a hole, a pin dropped through the hole into the mercury, thus completing an electrical circuit and activating a switch. The closing switch caused a needle on a dial to jump one or more spaces, depending on the information on the card. When all of the cards were passed through the machine, the desired answer showed directly on the dial.[5]

Processing of a card rang a bell; when the bell did not sound, the operator pulled out the card for examination.

In 1900 Hollerith began to develop a second generation of equipment. The card design was modified so that numeric information was arranged in columns. This allowed the development of a simple keypunch, an automatic-feed card sorter and an automatic-feed tabulator of vastly improved performance. Many of these innovations directly resulted in the data processing standards of the mid-20th century.

For the 1910 census, the bureau decided to establish its own facilities. New machines were to be designed. The developer, James Powers, was to retain the patent rights for his contributions. In 1911 he formed the Powers Accounting Machine Company, which in 1927 became the Tabulating Machines Division of the Remington-Rand Corporation. Hollerith had also organized a company in 1896: the Tabulating Machine Company. In 1912 he sold his patent and property rights to a holding company, Computing-Tabulating-Recording Company (CTR). Management of the company was soon assumed by Thomas J. Watson, a former NCR executive. There was a conflict between Watson's commercial goals and Hollerith's devotion to purely inventive objectives. Watson prevailed and, in 1924, formed the International Business Machine Corporation.

By 1934 the electric typewriter was commercially available, machines were used to collect and tabulate data, mechanical calculators were reliable, and there were many large corporations that could manufacture, market, and maintain these systems. Everything was in place for the next level of sophistication. It was only the economic depression that limited experimentation.

1.3. Early Electronic Computers

Computers are divided into two classes: analog computers and digital computers. Analog computers use some continuous quantity (such as electric current) in performing calculations. Some examples are the odometer, which continuously displays the tenths of a mile; the slide rule, which allows the user to select a

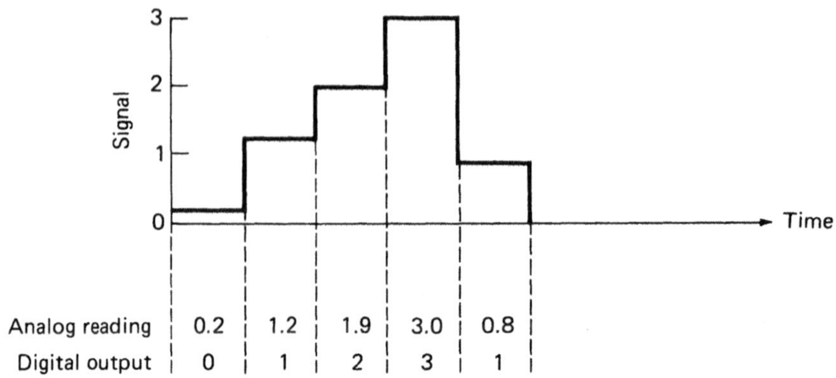

FIGURE 1.7. Comparison of analog and digital interpretation of a signal.

point on a continuous scale, and the classical chronometer, which uses pointers on a continuous dial to indicate time.

The digital computer, on the other hand, uses discrete units. A value is either a 0 or a 1; nothing in between. In the case of decimal machines—such as the early calculators—the values were the digits, 0, 1, . . . 9 with no intermediate values. The advantage of a digital system is its precision and repeatability. For example, if a counting device converts a voltage into a value, small changes in the current will affect the output. However, if the range of outputs is sequenced as discrete steps, then minor changes in the voltage will have no effect on the result. This is illustrated in Fig. 1.7.

1.3.1. Electromechanical Calculators

Some of the earliest computers were analog. Many used electronic circuits to model a network, solve heat transfer problems, process systems of ordinary differential equations, and so on. The relative accuracy of the solution was traded off against the speed of solution, the ease in formulating the problem, or the degree of exactness required. As digital computers became more powerful and inexpensive, the use of analog computers became less common. In some cases hybrid computers were used that merged the capabilities of both systems. This chapter will consider only digital computers.

The first digital computers used telephone relays. In 1937 George Stibitz of Bell Telephone Laboratory produced a type of digital computer to help him in his calculations. The device converted decimal digits to binary numbers (i.e., either 0 or 1; see Chapter 3). He had worked out the basis for an adder, and his Complex Number Computer was the first program-controlled electrical digital calculator. It could do a nine-digit division in 30 to 40 seconds.

At about the same time, Howard Aiken, while still a graduate student at Harvard, approached IBM with a proposal for a large-scale calculator to be built using relays. Work started in 1939 and 5 years later the Automatic Sequence

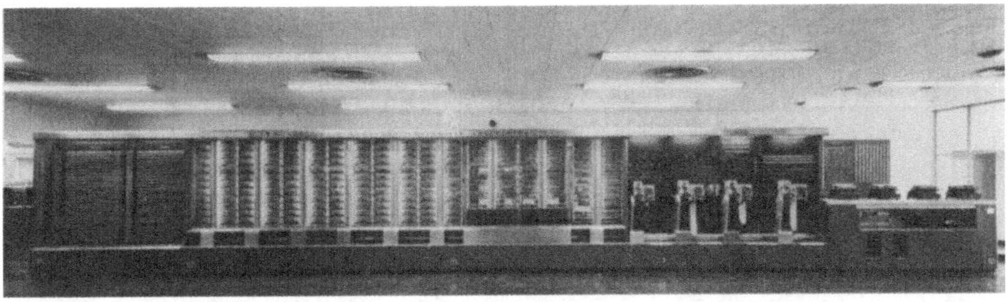

FIGURE 1.8. The Automatic Sequence Controlled Calculator—Mark I. (Courtesy of Cruff Photo Lab, Harvard University. Photographer: Paul Donaldson.)

Controlled Calculator, or Mark I (Fig. 1.8) was presented to Harvard. It was during this period that Aiken discovered Babbage's writings and admitted that he had learned "more about computation from Babbage than any other individual." In fact, he declared the Mark I was "Babbage's dream come true."

The calculator was 51 feet long and 8 feet high. It contained 760,000 parts and 500 miles of wire. Internally, it consisted largely of standard Hollerith counters modified with automatic tape sequence control for directing the operation of the machine. All numbers were 23 decimal digits long plus a sign. It could add, subtract, multiply, divide, or reference tables of results already computed. There were 60 registers for constants and 72 adding registers. Processing was controlled by instructions read from a punched paper tape. Each instruction was of the form: "Take the number out of unit A, deliver it to B, and start operation in C." All instructions were executed sequentially and there was no branching logic.

The Mark I could perform a multiplication in about 3 seconds; it could direct its answers to punched cards or an electric typewriter. It was flexible and reliable and was used for over 15 years to produce large mathematical tables. It was followed by a Mark II (1946), Mark III (1950), and Mark IV (1952). The Mark II, 12 times faster than its predecessor, was introduced at a 4-day scientific symposium that brought together 250 experts. Thus, although the use of relays was soon abandoned, the work of Aikin and the Harvard Computation Laboratory had a major impact on the development of digital computing.

1.3.2. The Early Vacuum Tube Machines

Events had combined, in the late 1930s and early 1940s, to foster the concept of electronic computing. Several independent activities were underway. At Iowa State College, John Vincent Atanasoff sought ways to increase the computational capabilities available to him. Working with a graduate student, Clifford Berry, he built a prototype computer in 1939. He was unable to generate interest in it, and the scope of his work was largely unknown until it was brought to light in a 1973 patent-infringement lawsuit.

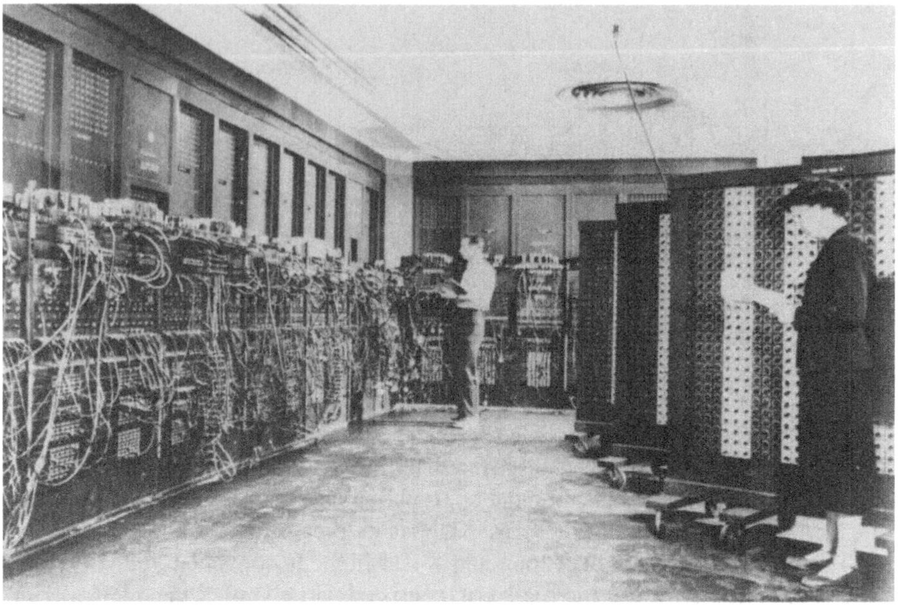

FIGURE 1.9. The Electronic Numerical Integrator and Calculator—ENIAC. (Smithsonian Institution Print 53192, reprinted by permission.)

Other work during this period was conducted by the German Konrad Zuse. His first effort, the Z1, was begun in his living room. Most of his work was carried out independently with no knowledge of what others were doing. At about the same time, in England, development started on a programmable device designed to break German machine ciphers. Clouded in secrecy even to this day, there was little transfer of knowledge from that project. Nevertheless, it did have a profound effect on those involved in the project.

There was one system, however, that served to focus interest on electronic computation. This was the ENIAC developed by John W. Mauchly and J. Presper Eckert (Fig. 1.9). It was early in World War II and the Aberdeen Proving Ground needed firing and bombing tables with related control data. Productivity was enhanced through use of an analog device—the Bush differential analyzer—and by electromechanical calculators. Mauchly, who had come to the Moore School of the University of Pennsylvania to study the differential analyzer, recognized the potential for replacing the relays with vacuum tubes. Working with the younger Eckert, he prepared an internal memo proposing the construction of an electronic calculator. The memo lay buried for almost a year, but in 1943 they were given the go-ahead.

Mauchly was the innovator, Eckert the chief engineer. Together they produced the Electronic Numerical Integrator and Computer, or ENIAC. It occupied a space of 30 by 50 feet, consisted of 30 separate units (plus power supply and cooling), and contained 18,000 vacuum tubes, 70,000 resistors, 10,000 capacitors, and 6,000 switches. Through careful engineering they were able to construct simple, binary circuit combinations that allowed the vacuum tubes to operate at levels below their normal ratings. The ENIAC could perform 5,000 additions or 300 multiplications per second—far superior to any electromechanical device. It was in production use for almost 10 years and processed 80,223 hours of work.

New concepts were crystalizing, and Mauchly and Eckert's work provided a baseline. ENIAC had shown what could be done. But it was large, expensive, and clumsy to program. It did not have the flexibility of the Mark I that read instructions from punched paper tape which could be easily programmed or arranged in endless loops for sections of a program. Instead, it required that hundred of plugs and switches be set—an operation that took several hours. Nevertheless, its formal dedication in February, 1946 ushered in the modern era of computers. The concept had been demonstrated; now a series of one-of-a-kind computers would contribute further to our understanding. One of the most important of these next machines was the Electronic Discrete Variable Automatic Computer (EDVAC) which was begun in 1946 by Eckert and Mauchly with John von Neumann. The EDVAC was not completed until 1950; and by this time Eckert and Mauchly had formed their own company to produce computers commercially.

The EDVAC was the first computer designed to use an internally stored program. It also used a binary representation for numbers. In this way, all numbers could be expressed as strings of 1s and 0s, rather than in the form of the 10-decimal digits. Although this use of the base 2 is unnatural for people, it is the most efficient representation for electronic circuits that have only two states: on and off.

The EDVAC established a prototype for the modern computer. Yet each new machine of the era added new insights. Table 1.2 lists the names and some of the characteristics of these early computers. By today's microcomputer standards, they were all very small in capacity. At the time, however, the ability to store 1,000 numbers generally was an upper bound.

One method of storage was the cathode-ray tube (CRT). A beam, written as on or off, created a charge on the surface of the tube that could be read (and fed back) by using an electrode on the surface of the screen. This Williams Tube Memory was able to store thirty two 32-bit numbers.

Another storage approach was to use ultrasonic delay lines. In this case, an electronic signal was converted to a sequence of sonic pulses sent through a column of mercury, and then amplified and demodulated as an electronic signal. Because propagation through the mercury was relatively slow, this technique provided a means of storing a sequence of pulses in the tube. The mercury tubes were usually organized in sets of 32 and were from 0.5 to 1.5 meters long. It was this technique that was used to provide 1,024 words of memory for the EDVAC.

Both the Williams tube and ultrasonic delay lines were slow, expensive, and

TABLE 1.2. Some characteristics of the early computers.

Computer	Decimal or binary	Word length	Clock frequency KH	Memory Types*	Memory No. of words	Input output	No. of tubes
EDVAC	B	44 bits	1,000	Mercury	1,024	Paper tape	3,600
UNIVAC	D	12 characters	2,250	Mercury	1,000	Magnetic tape	5,600
IAS	B	40 Bits	Asynch.	Williams	1,024	Cards	2,300
EDSAC	B	35 bits	500	Mercury	512	Paper tape	3,800
Ferranti I	B	40 bits	100	Williams	256	Paper tape	3,800
Pilot ACE	B	32 bits	1,000	Mercury	360	Cards	800
SEAC	B	45 bits	1,000	Mercury	512	Paper tape	1,300
SWAC	B	36 bits	125	Williams	256	Paper tape; cards	2,300
Whirlwind I	B	16 bits	1,000	Core	256	Paper tape	6,800
Harvard Mark III	D	16 decimals	28	Drum*	4,000	Magnetic tape	5,000
Burroughs	D	9 decimals	125	Drum	800	Paper tape	3,271
ERA 1101	B	24 bits	400	Drum	16,384	Paper tape	2,200

*The Mercury delay line, Williams tube, and core memory were described in the text. The drum contained a large magnetic recording surface on the outside of a drum. It was a forerunner of the modern disk. From A. Ralston and E. D. Reilly (eds), *Encyclopedia of Computer Science and Engineering*, 1983.[6]

subject to failure. Data were organized as two-dimensional arrays; a third dimension would provide access to the individual bits and thereby speed processing. Jay Forrester of MIT began thinking about the problem in 1947. His solution was the magnetic core which became the standard storage medium until its replacement by solid state electronic memory.

Having conceptualized the solution in 1947, the problem lay dormant until 1949 when an event triggered a more detailed examination..

I remember very clearly how it happened. I was reading a technical journal one evening, just leafing through the advertisements in the magazine *Electrical Engineering*, when I saw an advertisement for a material called Deltamax, which had a very rectangular hysteresis loop. It had been developed for magnetic amplifiers. . . . When I saw this nonlinear rectangular magnetic hysteresis loop, I asked, "Can we use it as a computer memory? Is there some way to fit it into a three-dimensional array for information storage?" The idea immediately began to dominate my thinking, and for the next two evenings I went out after dinner and walked the streets in the dark thinking about it, turning over various configurations and control methods in my mind until I began to see a configuration in which we could use a magnetic element with a rectangular hysteresis loop in a three-dimensional array, and where in principle one could get access to the interior part of the structure through the control of voltages on the *x, y,* and, *z* coordinate axes. As a result, my notebook entries of that spring of 1949 are complete in almost every detail in which magnetic-core memory is being used today.[7] (Copyright The Trustees of the Science Museum, South Kensington, London, England, reprinted by permission.)

The first implementation in a computer was in 1953 in the Whirlwind I. The core memory doubled the operating speed, quadrupled the input data rate, and reduced maintenance time for the storage row from 4 hours a day to 2 hours a week. Reliability of the vacuum tubes, however, continued to be a problem. For example, ILLIAC, at the University of Illinois, was programmed to do all its calculations three times; the final result was determined by majority vote. It required the (then) world's largest air conditioner and was supported by two undergraduates who constantly roamed about inside the computer with shopping carts full of replacement tubes. Despite these difficulties, the ability to do thousands of calculations per second made the electronic computer a valuable resource.

1.3.3. The Intellectual Foundation of Computing

By 1950 the principal concepts of electronic computing had been established. Although new technology would dramatically alter capability and functionality, virtually all that followed in the next three decades has its roots in the 1940s. It is useful, therefore, to understand these foundations.

One must begin by at least mentioning George Boole (1815-1864). This self-educated Englishman was the founder of modern symbolic logic. By expressing logical concepts in mathematical form, he reduced logic to a propositional calculus—now called Boolean algebra. His work has had a major impact on the theory of probability, the geometry of sets, information theory, and the design of electronic computers and switching circuits.

Alan Turing (1912-1954) had a more direct impact on modern computing. He became interested in mathematical logic in 1935 and published a classic paper in 1937 on computable numbers in which he introduced the concepts of the Turing machine. This paper showed that a machine was capable of solving any computation that a human could solve as long as the solution was laid out as a sequence of explicit instructions. In effect, Turing proposed that one could take a function and break its evaluation down into simple repetitive operations. This was the formalization of the algorithm.

The Turing machine had an alphabet and a finite set of states. The machine read the cells of a tape of infinite length. Each cell contained a symbol from the alphabet that instructed the machine to read a symbol, change it to another symbol, or enter into a new state. Thus, well before computers were being developed, Turing was building a concept of finite automata that would lead to the modern stored program.

The Turing machine was an abstraction. But the new computer had the ability to sequence through a finite set of instructions. Von Neumann recognized that by storing this sequence as a program, the computer would have almost unlimited flexibility. He wrote:

> Since the orders that exercise the entire control are in the memory, a higher degree of flexibility is achieved than in any previous mode of control. Indeed, the machine, under control of its orders, can extract numbers (or orders) from the memory, process them (as numbers!), and return them to the memory (to the same or other locations); i.e., it can change the contents of the memory—indeed this is its normal *modus operandi*. Hence it can, in particular, change the orders (since these are in the memory!)—the very orders that control its actions. Thus all sorts of sophisticated order-systems become possible, which keep successively modifying themselves and hence also the computational processes that are likewise under their control. . . . Although all of this may sound farfetched and complicated, such methods are widely used and very important in recent machine-computing—or, rather, computation-planning practice.[8]

Because the computer was able to process so rapidly, the question was asked: Does it contain intelligence? The early computers were referred to by the press as "giant brains." Later, manufacturers would try to quell customer fears of an anthropomorphic machine by reinforcing the idea that computers were stupid but very fast; they did only what they were instructed to do. Research in robotics and expert systems is leading us to reconsider that simplistic view.

During this early period, reference was made to biological models. For example, Turing stated that a machine would contain intelligence if it could meet the following criteria. Place a test person in a room connected to a communication device. At the other end of the device are another person and a computer; either may be connected to the test person. The machine would be considered intelligent if the test person could not determine if he was communicating with a person or a computer. This definition is still repeated when artificial intelligence (AI) is discussed.

Von Neumann used a biological model for computer architecture. His analysis was as follows:

> The natural componentry [the brain] favours automata with more but slower organs. Hence it is to be expected that an efficiently organized large automaton (like the human nervous system) will tend to pick up as many logical (or informational) items as possible simultaneously, and process them simultaneously, while an efficiently organized large artificial automaton (like a large modern computing machine) will be more likely to do things successively—one thing at a time, or at any rate not so many things at a time; that is, large and efficient natural automata are likely to be highly *parallel*, while large and efficient artificial automata will tend to be less so, and rather to be *serial*.[9]

As a consequence of this view, virtually all machines were designed with a processor, a memory, and a *serial* link between the two. As computers have become fast and more powerful, this serial link has become known as the von Neumann bottleneck. The Japanese Fifth generation computers targeted for the 1990s are designed to be highly *parallel;* their target application is artificial intelligence. As the technology advances, new assumptions are formulated. Nevertheless, the accomplishments in computer technology of the 1980s are firmly rooted in the ideas of the 1940s and 1950s.

1.3.4. The Early Commercial Computers

In 1947, Eckert and Mauchly left the University of Pennsylvania to form their own company. Their second product was the UNIVersal Automatic Computer (UNIVAC I), the first of which was installed in the Census Bureau in 1951. It contained 5,000 vacuum tubes, could add two numbers within 2 microseconds (2 millionths of a second), and employed magnetic tape to speed the input of data. It was the most advanced system of its kind—and remained so for several years.

Financial problems forced Eckert-Mauchly Computer Corporation to sell their company to Remington Rand, which also acquired other leading and complementary engineering firms. These acquisitions provided Remington Rand with early technical superiority over their competitors but did not lead to commercial success. Why?

From the beginning, the UNIVAC I sales effort was insufficient, unaggressive, and unimaginative. The Eckert-Mauchly personnel, for the most part, had a scientific rather than a business orientation. They realized the limitations of their machine and tended to dampen the enthusiasm of prospective customers who came to them with prophetic visions of the potential of electronic data processing. They knew that these visions would become reality only with a later generation of computers, and they did not encourage the very expensive experimentation which would almost invariably prove them to have been right. Most of this experimentation was eventually carried out on competitor's equipment, spurred on by promises made by salesmen who often understood little or nothing about the capabilities of the equipment they were selling. (From S. Rosen: Electronic Computers: a historical survey. *Comput Surv* (1,1), p 11, 1969. Copyright 1969, Association for Computing Machinery, Inc., reprinted by permission.)

As we know, it was IBM that rose to a position of dominance. We have seen something of their history with punch card machines and the Mark I calculator. Their product line of the late 1940s included electronic multipliers, an Electronic Calculating Punch, and the Card Programmed Calculator. But it was not until the Korean War stimulated defense spending that IBM announced its first true computer. Delivered in 1953, the Defense Calculator (IBM 701) contained 2,048 words of memory and was much faster than the UNIVAC I. As we shall see, good engineering, effective marketing, and a commitment to its customers allowed IBM to grow rapidly from this relatively late start.

Just as the first vacuum-tube computers were being built, the basis for a competitive technology was being developed. Although the vacuum tube had great advantages over the relay, its demands for power, generation of heat, and limited life all presented problems. The solution was the transistor (for transfer resistor). Developed at Bell Labs in 1947 from semiconducting materials (initially germanium, later silicon and now germanium again), the transistor could serve as an on/off switch. By 1954, the Philco Corporation had developed transistors suitable for use in high speed computers. Thus in 1958, when IBM was ready to introduce the vacuum tube based 709, its technology was obsolete.

The transistor ushered in a new generation of computers. Smaller, faster, more reliable, this second-generation computer had a dramatic impact on the commercial, scientific, and industrial world. This was the first wave of the revolution. The number of products and vendors grew too rapidly to be cataloged here. We shall limit our discussion to one major product: the IBM 7090. In its time, it represented the top of the scientific computer line. It had the computing power of today's personal computer.

In 1958, the Ballistic Missile Early Warning System required very fast computers for data analysis and general computation. IBM won the contract by offering to deliver the 709 vacuum-tube computer for program development and promising a transistorized version, the 7090, for operational use. The next year, two 7090s were delivered on schedule. But they were rough prototypes, and scores of engineers went with them to make them work. This shaky start angered IBM users and encouraged competitors. Eventually, however, the bugs were worked out, and hundreds of IBM 7090s (and later 7094s) were sold.

The price of a 7090 was about $3 million. It contained 32,768 words of memory with each word 36 bits in length. Because both the card-input device and the printers were relatively slow, each system contained a second, smaller system (generally an IBM 1401 business computer). The smaller system copied the card images onto magnetic tape and/or printed the magnetic tape's contents onto paper. The 7090 "talked" only to the magnetic tape device. (Disk and large drum storage devices were not yet common commercial products.)

The system, therefore, consisted of a very fast 7090 processor with a bank of magnetic tapes. There was an operator's console with lights to display the contents of important words in the processor's memory. The system completed one job at a time. Computer operators were needed to mount and unmount tapes and to load cards into card readers. All programs and data had to be punched onto 80 column cards before they could be read into the machines. The computer printer was limited to reports with 120 or 132 characters per line.

The computer had become an essential part of our society. The space program would be impossible without it; large corporations could not manage their operations without it. The initial reaction to punch-cards—which one should not "bend, spindle, or mutilate"—gave way to a respect for this new technology. Two generations of computers had been tested and accepted. There could be no turning back from the information processing revolution.

1.4. The Modern Computer

The third generation of computers grew out of both a new technology and a desire to correct earlier design limitations. The change in technology came in two steps. First, the use of wires between components was eliminated by printing the connections on a board and then mounting the components to the board (thus, the printed circuit). Then it became possible to etch transistors with their connectors on a chip of silicon. By combining the printing of connections and the etching of transistors, one obtained an integrated circuit (IC). (With advances in manufacturing techniques, the number of components that could be etched on a chip grew. We now speak of large-scale integration, LSI, and very large scale integration, VLSI.)

Lower-cost integrated circuits led to larger and more powerful computers and provided new design opportunities. Second-generation computers typically supported only uppercase letters; it was necessary to change the design of the basic word size and the magnetic tape formats to provide both upper- and lowercase outputs. Second-generation computers addressed either words (e.g., the 7090) or characters (e.g., the 1401). The next-generation machine accessed both. Second-generation computers could process only one job at a time, the next generation, many. A new generation of computers was coming; so much had been learned in so short a time that this next generation would represent a break with the past.

1.4.1. The Third Generation

In 1964, IBM announced their third generation System/360 computers offered in six compatible models. These computers were intended as replacements for existing IBM computer models but were quite different from them. Consequently, the movement of data and programs from the old machines to the new ones was difficult and costly, and customers suffered from the conversion process and resented it. One heritage of this negative experience is that IBM has maintained some degree of compatibility between the System/360 computer and all of its succeeding computer generations. Computer companies with large installed customer bases must evaluate decisions to introduce new technologies by "how they will impact their existing customer base." The reality is that the social investment in computing dampens the rate of technologic change. A corollary to this principal is that the smaller the existing customer base, the bolder the innovation. (This partly explains the success of the microcomputer systems.)

We return to the third-generation computer. The problems faced by Eckert and Mauchly were solved. Speed, reliability, and capacity were available. This success led to new and different problems: How were the stored programs to be managed? As previously noted, the IBM 7090 had 32K words of storage (K stands for 1,024, which is 2^{10}. Properties of powers of 2 make them convenient units for computers). The larger computers in the 360-line could contain millions of words of storage (written M for 2^{20} or 1,048,576). Clearly, this was enough storage to hold many programs in memory at once. This raises the question of how to manage the execution of many different programs concurrently.

1.4.1.1. Software and Programming Languages

Hardware is, as its name implies, those parts of a computer system that are composed of manufactured equipment. Hardware is a potential that requires stored programs to actuate. Software is the program (and associated documentation) that causes the hardware to accomplish a desired goal. The earliest programs were wired into plug boards or punched onto paper tape. As computers grew larger and faster, the programs grew in size and complexity. For small programs, it was sufficient to write the instructions just as they would be processed by the computer. A hole in the paper tape would be a "1," no hole a "0." Certain strings of 0s and 1s represented instructions (for example, 001 might be the instruction to add two numbers and 010 might be an instruction to multiply them). A series of such instructions constituted a program. But these were difficult programs to write and debug because the meaning of these instructions was obscured by the codes.

Better ways had to be found. The first step was to use mnemonics to represent the binary digit (bit) configurations. Thus, if "001" meant "add" to the computer, the programmer could write "ADD" instead of "001" and could use names (e.g., "AVERAGE") to identify the memory locations referenced by his program. The first programming language maintained a one-to-one correspondence between the mnemonic and the machine hardware instructions, but it enabled the programmer to use names (or symbols) for the values he wished to process, e.g., X, Y, SPEED. The language was called "assembly language" (or symbolic assembly language) because the process of converting the mnemonic instructions into machine code was called "assembly." Later versions of assembly language allowed the programmer to define a single "instruction" that represented a series of many machine-language instructions. These "larger" instructions are called macros; any assembly language that can accept these is called a macro-assembly language.

Although assembly languages were a vast improvement over the use of bits, they still left the process of coding at the engineering level. What was necessary was a language that would more naturally express the problems to be solved. In the late 1950s three such high order languages (HOL) were developed. They continue to be the three most widely used languages today. They are:

FORTRAN: For mathematical and engineering applications
COBOL: For business applications
LISP: For artificial intelligence applications.

These and other programming languages will be discussed in further detail in Chapter 4. It is sufficient now to note that their availability opened the door to new applications and a new class of programmers. Users could view the computer as a tool without fully understanding how it worked. As the developers of second-generation computers found ways to improve productivity through high-order languages, they raised a new series of problems.

- The instructions written in assembly language had to be converted to machine code. (The program to do this is called the assembler.)
- The instructions written in FORTRAN, for example, had to be converted to machine code. (The process is called compilation and it is done by a program called a compiler. Earlier compilers produced assembly-language outputs for input to an assembler).
- For some large applications, it was necessary to produce programs composed of more than one separately compiled assembly program. These individual programs had to be linked together and then loaded to run. This is managed by a link loader.
- Application programmers had to be provided with instructions to inform the computer what they wished done with an application, e.g., use these data with this program, compile the program, or do both. Thus, the need for a command language (or control language, or job control language, JCL).
- The input card images on magnetic tape had to be processed, and the material to be listed had to be written onto magnetic tape. Also, the other magnetic tape units had to be managed.

- And when things went wrong? Well, there was nothing else to do but find out why. The standard approach was to list the contents of all the memory locations used by the program. Called a "dump," this listing had a numeric representation of each bit in memory (i.e, the 1s and 0s listed in an octal or hexadecimal representation.)

As can be readily seen, that is a lot to manage—even in a second-generation computer where only one job was being processed at a time. Certainly, a tool was needed to manage all of these activities; it was called the operating system.

1.4.1.2. System Architecture for a Third Generation

Now to return to our chronology. By the early 1960s, we had new manufacturing techniques that allowed the production of computers 10,000 times larger in capacity than those of the 1940s. There were also high-order languages with growing numbers of users who knew and cared little about the computer's inner workings. And finally, there were experiments with operating systems intended to bring the users and hardware together. The question was: How can such large machines be used economically? The answer lay in logically dividing one large machine into many smaller ones.

As we have seen, some computer processes are slower than others. Techniques were constantly employed to avoid slowing down the fastest by off-loading the slowest. Thus, magnetic tape was used so that the arithmetic processor would not be delayed by the relatively slow card reader or printer. By the time of the third-generation computers, the arithmetic processor had become very fast; so fast, in fact, that even reading a magnetic tape or disk would slow it down. For example, the processor sent a command to the tape to start reading some data. Because the tape had mechanical delays, it could not transmit the data to the processor unit as fast as the processor unit could accept it. And so, thousands of instruction cycles could be wasted while the computer took the time to wind the tape to the location of the desired data and transmit the data to the central processing unit. However, now that the computer memory could contain a million or more words of storage, there was a way to avoid this waste. The computer could keep more than one program in memory at a time. When one program had to get data from a magnetic tape, the central processing unit could serve another program that was ready to compute. In this way, computation (i.e., central processing unit activity) could be balanced with reading and writing (i.e., input and output). On the average, the mix of programs residing in core would complement each other, and the net amount of computer work (throughput) would increase. There was an overhead cost, of course, for the operating system management.

With the third-generation computers came a new wave of architectural concepts. There was multiprogramming: the use of a single computer to process more than one job (task) at one time (i.e., to run concurrently) as well as multiprocessing: the use of more than one central processor unit linked to a single computer system (this redundancy was for graceful failure [fault tolerance] and better throughput). Finally, there was time-sharing (interactive use of a computer using multiprogramming). Although the interactive use of computers was explored as early as the late 1950s it was not until the third-generation computers were developed that it became economical. Time-sharing also was integrated with remote access to a computer that might be miles away, and for the first time users could lease computer time as a utility.

By the mid-1960s, the third generation of computers had been accepted. New applications were proliferating. The professions of systems analyst and programmer were created. Computers were becoming inexpensive and ubiquitous. Time-sharing allowed users to rent only the computer time they needed. A decade of learning and progress was about to begin.

1.4.2. The Fourth Generation

When the industry—mainly IBM—advanced from the second- to the third-generation computers, there was a major trauma. The programs and data were not transportable, the new operating systems were complex, the human interfaces had changed. If there had been no investment in the older technology, everyone would have approved the improvements. But, even though computers were still in only their second decade, there already was an investment in obsolescence. The result was that the industry vowed never again to subject its users to a dramatic change. Consequently, there is no dividing line between the third- and fourth-generation computers. The fourth-generation computers are smaller, faster, and cheaper. If they were designed to be compatible with an existing computer line, then the changes are transparent to the software. In this way, IBM's 360 was able to evolve to the 370 and then to the 33XX/43XX computers without unduly impacting their users.

Yet new product lines were introduced: the minicomputer and, later, the microcomputer. The Digital Equipment Corporation was the first to establish itself in the minicomputer market. Starting with the PDP-5 (1963) and PDP-8 (1965), Digital produced a line of small computers that could become an integral part of some larger system. Initially used as process-control devices or communication managers, the first minicomputers brought the power of digital computers to a new range of products. As part of a larger system, the computer often was embedded in the system's design. Normally, these embedded computers were limited to external sensors to which they had to respond in "real-time," i.e., without delays. Examples of such products and devices include the computerized axial tomography (CAT) scanner and military weapon systems. (This use of computers in military systems led to advances in miniaturization and ultimately to the microcomputer.)

Although the first minicomputers were used for data collection and processing, it was not long before operating systems were developed and minicomputers became general-purpose, multiuser computers. As manufacturing techniques improved, minicomputers grew more sophisticated while mainframe computers became more compact. By the mid-1970s, the label was meaningless; within the price-performance overlap, there was really no distinction.

The next major breakthrough came when it was recognized that not only could individual circuits be etched in miniature on a silicon chip, but an entire central processing unit (CPU) could be implemented on a chip. In 1971, Ted Hoff of Intel Corporation produced the first "computer on a chip," and now the process went in two directions. Manufacturers, such as Texas Instruments, developed circuits that would have mass markets. They produced hand-held calculators, digital watches, and sophisticated toys using a chip developed and programmed for a specific set of functions. The motivation was the economics implicit in large scale production.

The other direction for innovation took advantage of the general flexibility of the new devices. New functions could be produced with new programs. The first to exploit the power of the microprocessor was a small New Mexico company that began marketing the Altair to the hobbyist market. The name of the computer was derived from the name of a planet on the popular TV series Star Trek. The computer sold for $621 ($395 in kit form), but its absence of programs, poor documentation, and ineffective design limited interest to all but the highly motivated.

The Altair was not a success. But, its appearance as a cover story in the January 1975 issue of *Popular Electronics* magazine generated considerable interest. New vendors appeared with add-ons and fix-it kits. By September 1975 *Byte* magazine was founded specifically for the microcomputer community. The technology was now available for wide dissemination. But most of the companies were too small to have any impact beyond the electronic hobby market.

To reach the lay person, it was necessary to have a complete product, useful software, effective documentation, and a broad marketing base that could support advertising, sales, and distribution. In 1977 two companies with these qualifications entered the field. Commodore, a manufacturer of hand-held calculators, announced a personal computer it called the Pet. Soon after, the Tandy Company announced that its Radio Shack chain would also offer a microcomputer, the TRS-80.

The success of these initial offerings opened a whole new era in computing. Soon new companies, such as Apple Computer, grew up, while established companies, such as IBM, adjusted to meet the new demand. By 1980, some two dozen firms produced 724,000 personal computers with a value of $1.8 billion; the next year there were 20 more firms in the marketplace and the sales were almost $3 billion. A recent study now projects that by 1986 the value of personal computer shipments in the United States will exceed the value of mainframe shipments; they expect 20 million personal computers with a value of over $67 billion.

1.4.3. The Next Generations

Each decade, the progress in computer technology has exceeded what was anticipated at the start of the decade. Thus, it would be foolish to project where computers will take us by the end of the decade. Nevertheless, the accomplishments of the next few years will rely on products currently under development.

Thus, it seems fitting to close this chronology with a brief review of the state-of-the-art.

Semiconductor devices are likely to continue improving at their current rate through the end of the century. This implies that multichip 32-bit processors will be replaced by one-chip processors of 32-bits or with 64-bit multichip processors. Thus, the computational power previously reserved only for large computers will be available at a cost of about $25. Similar trends will produce larger and faster memories at reduced costs. Finally the technologies used for mass storage will continue to improve in capability/price. As the physical limits of electromechanical magnetic devices are reached, new technologies—such as laser beam recording—will be available to produce even more capability for a fixed price.

This new technology will be applied in several ways. New supercomputers will be developed to process calculations beyond the capability of today's largest machines. The supercomputers will avoid the von Neumann bottleneck by using more than one processor in parallel. At the other end of the spectrum, the fourth-generation computer will shrink to the size of a microcomputer; telecommunications and networking will blur the distinctions among a local workstation, a computer, and a system.

One particular activity has taken the Fifth Generation Computer as its name. This is a Japanese sponsored cooperative venture to produce a generation of computers built upon a new theoretical foundation. Following a study initiated in 1979, the Japanese government determined that, as a nation with limited material resources, its economic survival would be closely linked to its ability to export the products of its knowledge. They therefore organized the Fifth Generation Computer System Project in 1982 with the objective of producing a prototype by 1990. This system would unify achievements in

- Knowledge-based expert systems, a branch of artificial intelligence (see Chapters 2 and 9)
- New, more powerful programming languages (see Chapter 4)
- Decentralized computing (see Chapter 3)
- Advances in VLSI technology (as briefly noted above).

The result would be systems capable of processing natural languages such as English or Japanese in the form of either text or voice; expert consultation; access to data bases for decision making, etc. The project is very ambitious and will probably not achieve complete success. Nevertheless, it clearly points to a new direction for computers.

1.5. Concluding Remarks

In less than four decades there has been a revolution in information processing. Some of what we do is based on a sound understanding of the technology; much of what we do still is embedded in style and folklore. Moreover, it is not clear which is which. In the remainder of this book I shall address how the technology can be applied to the delivery of health care. I will always try to separate the fact from the folklore. Of course, I may not always be able to distinguish between the two.

By way of conclusion, I warn the reader to be aware that the technology is moving very rapidly. Just as few in 1970 could predict the microcomputer impact, it is clear that there will be advances in the 1990s that we cannot anticipate now. Nevertheless, there should be few surprises in the next few years. What we do in clinical information systems in the remainder of this decade will be firmly embedded in today's technology. The objective of this book is to illustrate how that technology can be applied to improve care.

For Further Reading

The computer age is sufficiently mature to have fostered an interest in recording its history. The materials in this chapter have been assembled from a variety of sources. *The Encyclopedia of Computer Science and Engineering*, 2nd edit., edited by Anthony Ralston and Edwin D. Reilly, Jr., Van Nostrand Reinhold, 1983, is a very useful source with overview sections and biographies. A hard to find, but very readable, popular introduction is available in M. Harmon, *Stretching Man's Mind: A History of Data Processing*, by Mason Charter, New York, 1975; the discussion of computers, however, is dated. Paul Freiberger and Michael Swaine, *Fire in the Valley: The Making of the Personal Computer*, Osborne/McGraw-Hill, 1984, is one of several very readable modern histories. K. D. Fishman, *The Computer Establishment*, McGraw-Hill, 1981 contains an interesting review of the business aspects of the industry. *Information Systems in the 80's*, by Ulric Weil, Prentice Hall, 1982, looks at the areas of greatest growth in this decade. Finally, I note that some new history texts—which I have not reviewed—are in progress or recently published; rich and up to date reading resources should be available soon.

For persons interested in researching the history of computing, B. Randell has selected an outstanding collection of source materials in *The Origins of Digital Computers*, third edit, Springer-Verlag, 1982. A second collection of papers has been edited by N. Metropolis, J. Howlett and G. Rota in *A History of Computing in the Twentieth Century*, Academic Press, 1981. Finally, J. W. Cortada has compiled *An Annotated Bibliography on the History of Data Processing*, Greenwood Press, 1983. Among the more popular current works that deal with a limited area are Tracy Kidder, *The Soul of a New Machine*, Little, Brown and Co., 1981, and S. Levy, *Hackers: Heroes of the Computer Revolution*, Doubleday & Co., 1984.

Papers and articles dealing with the history of computing appear from time to time. AFIPS publishes a journal, the *Annals of the History of Computing*, and the ACM has sponsored R. L. Wexelblat (ed) *A History of Programming Languages*, Academic Press, 1981. Among the more accessible review papers are S. Rosen, Electronic Computers: A Historical Survey, *ACM Computer Surveys*

(1,1), 1969; the January 3, 1983 issue of *Time* which made the computer the Machine of the Year, the October 1982 issue of the *National Geographic* which was devoted to the chip and the September, 1984 issue of *Scientific America* dedicated to computer software. Biographical articles periodically appear in magazines such as *Scientific American* and *Datamation*.

References

1. Cited in Margaret Harmon, *Stretching Man's Mind: A History of Data Processing*, Mason Charter, New York, 1975, p66, reprinted by permission. All rights reserved.
2. Cited in Harmon, *Op cit*, p74.
3. Cited in Harmon, *Op cit*, p85.
4. Cited in Harmon, *Op cit*, p87.
5. Cited in Harmon, *Op cit*, p103.
6. Adapted from S. Rosen, Digital Computers: History in Anthony Ralston, Edwin D. Reilly, Jr. (eds), *Encyclopedia of Computer Science and Engineering*, Second Edition, Van Nostrand Reinhold Co., New York, 1983, pp538-9.
7. Conversation: Jay W. Forrester, Interviewed by Christopher Evans, *Annals of the History of Computing* (5,3) July 1983, pp298-299.
8. John von Neumann, *The Computer and the Brain*, Yale University Press, 1958, Cited in J. Bernstein, *The Analytical Engine*, Random House, N.Y. 1966, p62, reprinted by permission.
9. *Ibid* p87.

2
Computers and Health Care

2.1. Historical Overview

The history of medical computing has been closely tied to the growing capability of computers. In general, there has been a lag of 5 years between a technical advance in the computer field and its use in medical computing. It is convenient, therefore, to divide computer development into phases by decade and medical applications into 10-year phases that span the decades. By following this convention, it is possible to describe the state-of-the-art in medical computing in the context of the computer technology available to support it. It is also possible to project—based on current trends in computer technology—what the next phase of medical computing may bring.

2.1.1. Phases in Computer Development

Table 2.1 identifies four phases in computer development. As we have seen, the computer technology of the 1950s was characterized by a transition from vacuum tubes to the more reliable transistors. Computers remained large, required considerable support in both maintenance and environmental control, and were generally limited to running one job at a time. Operating systems were developed to facilitate the use of the computer by programmers and operators. Tools to write programs grew from assembly languages to high-order languages such as COBOL and FORTRAN. In the larger facilities, computers were linked to isolate the slower operations (such as card reading and printing of output) by relegating them to smaller, less expensive computers; transfer between machines was normally by magnetic tape.

This first phase of computer system use was characterized by a high cost for equipment, restricted availability of computer time, and a heuristic approach to problem-solving. The applications were limited to those of computational complexity or the routine processing of high volume data. (Of course, the term Electronic Data Processing during this phase also included punch card sorters

TABLE 2.1. Phases in computer development.

1950s	A new technology
1960s	Foundations and export
1970s	Revolution in technology
1980s	An ubiquitous tool

and plug board printers.) There was a very limited community of developers, and most training came on the job.

The 1960s saw two major parallel developments: the use of integrated circuits and the growth of computer science. One result was the manufacture of large, reliable computers that were too powerful to justify dedication to a single task. Consequently, multiprogramming operating systems were developed that allowed a single computer to execute several tasks concurrently. This same technology provided an environment for interactive applications.

In addition to these larger computers, smaller computers (minicomputers) also were manufactured. Generally considered special purpose or process control devices, few had much support by way of operating systems and languages. In many cases, smaller devices were electronically linked to larger mainframe computers. The cost of equipment still was high, but the range of applications had grown dramatically. The cost of program preparation was becoming a significant factor in the total cost of a system. Computer science established itself as a formal discipline; it provided an intellectual foundation for the development and evaluation of computer tools and systems. Academic programs were established to train both programmers and scientists.

The 1970s witnessed an unanticipated revolution in very large scale integration (VLSI) which produced computers of great reliability, small size, and low cost. The principal mainframe computers remained functionally the same; but their increased availability and reduced prices resulted in proliferation. Previously impractical applications were now cost-effective.

During this phase it was clear that the greatest cost component in a system had become the cost of software development. Whereas the upgrading of hardware easily could be accomplished by the direct replacement of components with identical interfaces, modifications to the software development process were more difficult. The field of software engineering was introduced to address these problems and refine the methodologies for implementation. Although development tools still were deficient, a framework for improvement had been established. Yet social and economic factors inhibited the rate of change. Maintenance absorbed about half the life cycle cost of an application, and massive investments in obsolescent training and products limited the rate of change.

Although we are just in the middle of the 1980s, some of the characteristics of this phase are obvious. First, computers are no longer confined to the computer room; they are integral components of watches, cameras, and kitchen appliances. It is now possible for the hobbyist to own the equivalent computer power of the largest systems of the 1950s, packaged as microcomputers (personal computers). Because of the lowered cost and smaller packaging, computer architectures also are undergoing change. Networks allow the integration of multiple systems, and the Japanese are involved in a major effort to produce a fifth generation computer for artificial intelligence applications.

As the cost of hardware falls, the relative cost of software development continues to grow. Yet, on the other hand, computer literacy also is growing. In just two decades, we have gone from the slogan "do not bend, fold, or mutilate" to a population that uses computer terminals at work, in the bank, and even in the supermarket. Programming now is a skill taught in third grade; virtually every college student is routinely exposed to more computer science than was available in the early 1960s. Every new engineer and scientist is also a programmer.

2.1.2. Phases in Medical Computing

In reviewing the accomplishments of medical computing, it is convenient to group the applications according to the objects they process. There are three types of objects:

Data. These are the uninterpreted elements that are given to the problem solver (the Latin word *datum* means "the given"). Examples are a patient's name, a test result, or a diagnosis. Most mathematical computation operates only on data. The use of a formula to compute the body surface area from the patient's height and weight is a simple example of an application that operates only on data.

Information. This is a collection of data that contains meaning. The processing of data usually ends with a display of information. For this definition, however, we insist that the data (and information) be stored in a permanent, accessible database. An example of information in this context is an online patient medical record that includes the name, laboratory results, and diagnosis.

Knowledge. This is the formalization of the relationships among elements of information and data. The formulation may be descriptive—as in the case of a textbook—or it may be computer processible. In the second case, the knowledge may be expressed as a formula (as in the case of the body surface area problem) or as a collection of rules. The use of knowledge generally suggests the ability to infer data or information from that already present.

This categorization of processing objects is artificial; there are no clear boundaries among the three. Nevertheless, the structuring does provide a useful way to approach the phases of medical computing. This is shown in Table 2.2.

The first phase of medical computing spanned the period from 1955 to 1965. The emphasis was on experimentation and an understanding of the technology. Few practical applications were implemented. The technology could not reliably and economically support the concepts of the visionaries. Although the tendency to overpromise and underdeliver led to a period of general rejection and skep-

TABLE 2.2. Phases in medical computing.

1955–65	Experimentation and orientation
1965–75	Data processing success
1975–85	Information processing success
1985–	Knowledge processing success

ticism, this phase did produce a rethinking of needs and an orientation to the new technology.

The next phase, from the mid 1960s to the mid 1970s, was primarily characterized by accomplishments in the processing of medical data. The ability of the computer to provide reliable, rapid computation produced a new environment for the collection and analysis of data. The results were a growth in the biomedical engineering disciplines and experimentation with embedded computers in devices such as the CAT scanner. This emphasis was (and continues to be) reflected in the table of contents in the leading computer-oriented biomedical journals.

Successes in information processing during this phase were limited. For example, in the late 1960s, Lockheed tried to apply space age analysis to develop a comprehensive information system for hospitals. After losing millions of dollars, they sold their prototype to Technicon, which used it as a foundation for their Medical Information System. A more sobering appraisal of the complexity of clinical information systems followed. Although simple business systems and special process control applications (such as a laboratory system) were within the state-of-the-art, most attempts to implement information systems met with limited success. The half life of a system during this phase was roughly equal to the publication cycle, and many documented systems were no longer operational by the time they were reported.

By the third phase—from mid 1975 to date—computer technology was able to support the information processing requirements of the medical community. Consequently 1975 presented a watershed in the scientific literature. Reports were now available that evaluated 5 years' operational experience with systems. Although most applications required some outside funding, systems now were produced that were fully supported by operational revenues. Families of transportable systems were being developed, and medical information systems had become a billion dollar industry.

We are about to enter into the next phase of medical computing. As will be seen in Chapter 9, we have made many advances in understanding how to apply knowledge to medical decision making. Although much of this currently is limited to research settings, there are some operational systems in use. Moreover, advances in technology and a renewed interest in artificial intelligence suggest that the years between 1985 and 1995 will see the successful installation of knowledge-based systems for patient care.

And so, the growth of computer applications to medical care has been almost as dramatic as the growth of computers. In phase 1 (1955-1965) we considered how we might use computers to process data in the clinical laboratory, and in phase 2 (1965-1975) we were able to implement these systems. By phase 3 (1975-1985) we were able to integrate these data with other information needed for patient care. Soon, we shall be able to apply our knowledge of disease process and patient care to suggest diagnosis, therapy, and maintenance.

The following three sections present a brief overview of the use of computers in medicine. The material is organized by the objects processed: data, information and knowledge. A final section looks at medical informatics—the discipline concerned with the management and application of medical information and knowledge.

2.2. Data Oriented Applications

Systems that I categorize as data oriented applications are in their third generation. The first generation of applications were those for which the computers were designed: mathematical computations. Input data were prepared in the form of punched cards, magnetic tape, or paper tape; the outputs were either printed or saved in one of the above media. FORTRAN became the primary language for mathematical and engineering programming. The emphasis was on the formalization of knowledge as FORTRAN programs to provide solutions to computational problems.

Once the power of the computer had been demonstrated, the next generation of applications branched in two directions. The first was a direct extension of the previous work. Using and building on program libraries, more and more complex problems were considered. The computer provided a tool to perform computations rapidly and accurately. Problems beyond the scope of pencil and paper solutions could now be formulated and solved. In the medical area, this was reflected in the growth of bioengineering, the modeling of biological systems, and a more quantified approach to physiology.

The second type of application took advantage of the computer's ability to repeat simple processes routinely and accurately. In this context, the computer was used to automate clerical tasks and identify new applications that otherwise would be impossible due to the clerical burden. These types of applications gradually merged with the first to produce systems for statistical analysis, searching, and graphics.

The current generation of data-oriented applications includes extensions of the problems addressed in the previous generation. The new applications also take advantage of advances in computer technology such as microprocessors and imaging devices. The microprocessors allow the designer to embed the computer as an integral part of the system. Thus the user is unaware that a computer is being used. Controls manage the device and not the computers; changes to the computer programs are not allowed. Closely linked to the use of embedded computers is the use of imaging devices.

In the remainder of this section, we shall sample some of the more common uses of computers in patient care that process data. The intent is to display the range of "data oriented" medical systems available today; references for further reading are provided.

2.2.1. Business Data Processing

It may seem strange to start a discussion of computer systems for patient care with a description of their use by the business office. Nevertheless, in the context of impact, this is probably the correct place to begin. Virtually all hospitals of 100 beds and larger rely on some form of automated support for their financial management. The use of automated billing systems or services also is growing for ambulatory care. As third-party payors require forms or automated records, the use of computers is seen as a cost-saving tool. In the case of large hospitals with their many statutory reporting functions, they are essential.

As a result of the computer's ability to perform data processing, most large health care facilities have accepted automation. But the tools installed are narrowly focused on the financial needs of the organization. They do not address the clinical needs of the institution, nor can they be made to do so. The users, programmers, and vendors have insights into the administrative aspects of health care delivery; few are qualified to consider the application of computers in the care process.

The consequence is that the greatest computer expertise at a large institution is dedicated to nonclinical data processing applications. Yet these people also are asked to select, administer, or develop clinical systems. By identifying this application first, I intend to suggest that it is as technically different from clinical information systems as each of the systems that follows. But the administrative and clinical systems use the same patient data base, frequently the same computer, and often share the same management. That is one reason why we have systems that can send computer printed bills to the patient that identify each drug and procedure and at the same time have no automated tools that tell the provider the status of the current orders or the results of the latest tests.

2.2.2. The Clinical Laboratory

The clinical laboratory provides an example of how data processing capabilities can accommodate great volume increases through the use of rapid data acquisition and workload management. In a tightly closed loop, this is normally called process control: that is, certain features of the process are continuously measured and—based on the results of these measurements—modifications to the process are initiated. In the clinical laboratory there are both closed loops within instruments, and loosely coupled loops that involve human interaction. This discussion will be limited to the data processing performed in the clinical laboratory; the processing of the clinical information generated by the laboratory will be considered in Chapter 7.

Although one speaks of the clinical laboratory, it is far more realistic to speak of various laboratories: hematology, clinical chemistry, clinical microbiology, etc. Each processes different materials, using different techniques and tools, supported by varying degrees of automation. Clinical chemistry is generally the most automated of the laboratories, and we shall limit our review to this.

The most frequently ordered tests are for blood serum chemistries. The serum is obtained by centrifuging a blood sample that has been allowed to clot. Without going into any discussion of how the data are to be interpreted clinically, it is sufficient to identify the types of data analyzed.

- *Electrolytes*. Tabulations of the concentrations of sodium, potassium, calcium, phosphorus, chlorine, and magnesium are the most commonly requested.
- *Low-molecular-weight organic substances*. This includes both nutrients and waste products. Most commonly measured substances are the carbohydrates (e.g., glucose), fats (e.g., cholesterol), nitrogen-containing substances, (e.g., creatinine), and bile pigment, (e.g., bilirubin).
- *Enzymes*. In tissue damage, certain enzymes are liberated from the cells and can be detected in the blood. The most commonly reported enzymes are SGOT, LDH, SGPT, and CPK.

Approximately 75% of all serum chemistries are ordered for some of the above data.

Most of the wet chemistry tests are quite simple to perform. A reagent is mixed with the sample and the reaction brings about a change in the mixture. The change is normally visible as a color change, i.e., a change in the way light is transmitted through the substance. The change is proportional to the amount of the chemistry being measured, and the result is determined by matching the change against a standardized set of changes. Of course, the same method is used for other specimens such as whole blood, urine, cerebrospinal fluid, etc.

In 1957 Skeggs described a method for automating the process just described. It was implemented as the Auto Analyzer by Technicon Instruments, and it remains the most commonly applied technique to this day. The samples are placed in cups in a sampler; manual work lists link samples with specimens (and patient identification). Carefully measured samples are extracted from the cups and entered into a long coiled plastic tube with air bubbles used to separate the samples. Under continuous flow, the samples are moved through the coil from module to module. Within a module, reagents are mixed with the sample, the resultant color intensity is measured by a colormeter, and the result is displayed on a strip chart recorder. Using this technology, most of the commonly requested wet-chemical tests can be performed rapidly and inexpensively. To process different tests, one only has to vary the reagent, modify the environment (e.g., heat the sample), or use alternative methods for measuring the reaction (e.g., flame photometry, fluorometry).

Processing time was improved further with the introduction of the Sequential Multiple Analyzer (SMA) in 1964. Additional channels were added so that 6 (SMA 6) or 12 (SMA 12/60) tests could be completed using a single patient specimen. The manual testing of reagent reactions was no longer a limiting factor; the processing of samples and the determination of results from strip chart reactions was becoming the critical path. This led to the development of the SMAC which used a computer to link printout, request, and sample; monitor the processing; transform the intermediate analysis signals to calibrated results; and perform continuous self-monitoring procedures. One consequence of devices such as the SMAC was that they allowed the clinical laboratory to increase dramatically the number of tests it could process. For example, Mount Sinai Hospital in New York performed 260,000 tests in the entire year of 1965. Once the SMAC was installed, the chemistry department was performing 8-10,000 tests per day. Moreover, the results were available sooner.

Here we have an example of how the data processing function of a computer was able to increase productivity, improve response time, and support a growing demand. That is, the computer served as an enabling device—it enabled the clinical laboratory to perform as many tests as the clinicians thought necessary. In the process, the cost per test also fell. But it would be misleading to consider the role of the computer here to be one of cost reduction. The limiting factor was never the cost; it was the ability to process a sufficient number of tests within a reasonable time frame. The breakthrough of automation allowed the demand to grow and the cost to fall. The lowered cost and improved responsiveness, in turn, increased demand.

The use of computers in autoanalyzers now is a common application for the clinical laboratory. Moreover, management of the clinical laboratory also has become subject to automated support. The laboratory is viewed as an organization that receives requests and specimens and returns results. Some of its processing is automated; other tests are manual. Some functions may be performed on an immediate (stat) basis with the results reported by telephone; others—such as the growth and testing of cultures—may take weeks to complete. Thus, the management of a clinical laboratory involves the management of large volumes of data. Consequently, it represents another application area well suited to data processing.

Two figures illustrate the operational complexity of a laboratory. Table 2.3 summarizes the types and volumes of tests a large clinical laboratory must support,[1] and Fig. 2.1 provides an overview of the processing flow within the laboratory from the initial receipt of the request to the delivery of the result.[2] The two figures combined suggest a matrix of processes that can be managed by automation: a clinical laboratory system that acts as a process control system. It is not, however, tightly coupled. It produces materials for people to work with, supports the quality assurance process, and requires human interactions to make adjustments.

There now are many turnkey systems available, and several custom systems also have been exported for use by other institutions. It will suffice to note that the systems are designed to support the internal processing needs of the clinical laboratory. Unlike the billing systems previously discussed, however, clinical laboratory systems can be designed with functions that support patient care.

TABLE 2.3. Characteristics of clinical laboratory data (hypothetical 500 bed hospital).

Laboratory section	Analytical techniques employed	No. of body sources for specimens	No. of different tests performed	Usual result type	Interim reports needed	No. of pt. specimens received per day	Time required in lab for processing	Specimens in processing at any time
Chemistry (incl. in vitro radio diagnostic procedures	Many automated spectrophotometric instruments; other chemical and physical methods	2–3	200 +	Numeric	No	500	Minutes to hours	500
Hematology (incl. coagulation)	Automated cell (particle) counters; microscopy for cell counting and morphology	2–3	10–20	Numeric and short literal	No	300	Minutes to hours	300
Serology	Mostly manual immunochemical methods	2–3	30	Numeric and short literal	No	50	Minutes to hours	50
Urinalysis (clinical microscopy)	Simple manual chemical methods; Microscopy	3–5	10	Short literal	No	100	Minutes to hours	100
Microbiology	Cultural and fermentation techniques for variety of organisms	100 +	20	Moderate length literal	Yes	200	Days to weeks	2000
Blood bank	Manual immunologic techniques. Blood inventory control. Donor recruitment.	1	20	Short literal	No	40	Minutes to hours	40
Surgical pathology	Histologic staining techniques. Microscopy.	100 +	2–3	Lengthy literal	Yes	50	Few days	200
Cytopathology	Cytologic staining techniques. Microscopy.	10	2–3	Short literal	No	50	Few days	100

Adopted from materials provided by R. E. Miller, personal communication.

The laboratory request sequence

Transition between steps			Check of steps	
Logical Controls	Logical Lists	Sequence of Operational Steps	Numerical Calcu-lations	Numerical Controls
		request	request/ M.D.	physician assessment
order controls	phlebotomy list	↓		
		specimen	spec./ patient	patient assessment
acquisition control	master list	↓		
		acquisition station	spec./lab/ day	measure of demand
distribution control	work list	↓		
		work station	workload	personnel control
work verification	work list check off	↓		
		measurement	quality control	quality control
exception control	error recognition	↓		
		data	delta check	consistency check
completeness control	master list check off	↓		
		report	significant results	measure of impact
urgency control	critical value list	↓		
		response	predictive variables	relevance check
delivery control	pending test list	↓		
		chart	data/ prognosis	utilitzation review

FIGURE 2.1. The laboratory request sequence. (From T. L. Lincoln, *Medical Instrumentation* 12: 233–234, 1978. Reprinted with the permission of the Association for the Advancement of Medical Instrumentation.)

Nevertheless, within the laboratory, they are primarily used as (a) a data capture device to record results and intermediate values and (b) a process control device to manage the flow by printing out work lists and data collection forms. The contribution of the clinical laboratory system is that it enables the clinical laboratory to operate at the desired level at a reasonable cost.

2.2.3. Patient Monitoring

Patient monitoring may be considered the *in vivo* analog of the *in vitro* clinical laboratory tests. This monitoring may be continuous, e.g., electrocardiogram (ECG) monitoring, or periodic, e.g., collection of vital signs. The data collection device may be noninvasive, e.g., a strain gauge to measure respiration, or evasive, e.g., a catheter used to inject dye to measure cardiac output. The data may be recorded for later processing, telemetered for remote processing, processed to identify events, or simply displayed without retention. The monitoring may be done for diagnostic purposes, e.g., in the emergency room, for therapeutic purposes, e.g., in the operating room, or for surveillance purposes, e.g., in the intensive care unit (ICU).

Patient monitoring does not imply the use of computers; indeed, most physiological monitoring units are completely analog. All monitoring units use a sensor to collect physiological activity and convert it to an electrical signal. All monitoring systems also have some form of signal conditioning for amplification and shaping the signal so that it may be further processed or displayed. Computer-supported monitoring systems, in addition, provide a logic module that processes the conditioned data. This processing may be limited to simple comparisons with a reference signal level, or it may involve sophisticated analysis to recognize events such as cardiac arrhythmias.

The early monitoring systems were entirely analog and were used to display continuous tracings of physiological signals on a cathode-ray tube (CRT) screen. The attending nurse was required to watch the screen to identify abnormal events. Such events were critical but relatively rare (perhaps one per patient day). Since there was a tendency to miss events, the use of automation to aid in signal processing and event detection was an obvious application.

Yet the automation of physiological monitoring represents a far more complex problem than the data processing and process control applications previously discussed. Which parameters should be collected, monitored, and displayed and how would they be useful in clinical care? Could the data be presented in ways that were meaningful to the users? How accurate were the data, and how did they correlate with other types of data? Could the health care team use the equipment, or would it be over-designed? How much data are enough?

Not all these questions have been answered to this day. For example, consider the last question. In one study, a group of physicians was asked to diagnose respiratory illness based on the data presented. The data ranged from 4 to 20 items. When only 4 or 5 items were presented, diagnostic success was low, but it increased as the number of items available increased. However, as the number of items began to approach 20, the diagnostic success fell off to the earlier levels. The conclusion: too much data are as difficult to deal with as too little data. Therefore, even if one could answer the question on how much data are enough, the next question becomes: What data?

One area in which computer-supported physiological monitoring is in widespread use is the coronary care unit (CCU). As a result of the improving emergency treatment modalities and the general knowledge of cardiopulmonary resuscitation (CPR) techniques, more patients with myocardial infarcts survive long enough to be treated by a hospital. Once in a CCU, monitoring ECG tracings for arrhythmia is considered a prudent approach to the early detection of life-threatening events. Computer-generated alerts are desirable, but the high incidence of false-negative alerts and the poor rate of artifact rejection limit their success. Clearly this is a case in which more needs to be learned about the problem. (One can anticipate that at the time of writing there are better systems than those I referenced in the literature; moreover, by the end of the decade even more problems will have been solved, and systems should exist that can consistently and accurately report the desired data.)

Once the monitoring system collects and processes the desired data, it can be sent to a central unit where it can be examined as information, e.g., average hourly heart rate, number of premature ventricular contractions (PVCs) counted by time, reconstruction of the ECG waveform, times of drug administration. Most systems that provide this capability have a very narrow scope and do not retain any data beyond a 24- or 48-hour period. Thus, although they are clearly information systems, they will not be further considered in this book.

Physiological monitoring—with and without the use of computers—is in widespread use. The initiative in this application came from electronics and not computers; the computer was introduced to improve the analysis. As suggested above, the computer processing of monitored data is not as robust as one would desire, but it is bound to improve. Still one must question the efficacy of the monitoring systems and the ICUs. It is a somewhat controversial subject, but the evidence suggests that the ICU has little impact on outcome (e.g., survival) but does improve patient comfort. Comparisons between units with and without monitoring show that more nursing time is freed for patient care activities when a monitoring system exists.

Although the ICU may have limited medical benefit, its cost impact is significant. Consider the following statement by Simborg regarding the relationships between medical technology and cost.

Louise B. Russell of the Brookings Institution conducted extensive studies during the 1970s of the factors involved in the adoption and dissemination of new medical technology. One technology examined was the intensive care unit (ICU). In the late 1960s and early 1970s ICUs proliferated at an astounding rate. By 1974, ICUs alone accounted for 10 percent of all hospital costs, whereas they were virtually non-existent in the early 1960s. When examining the factors leading to this dissemination Russell made some interesting observations. Medical efficacy was not the prime determinant. In fact, at the time of this dramatic proliferation there had not been any major controlled clinical trials that showed that intensive care units reduced mortality. Even today there is debate regarding this issue, especially regarding coronary care units. Perceived need in the community, likewise, was not a factor. As coronary care and other intensive care units proliferated they did not occur in areas lacking such facilities. Russell found that there was a greater probability of ICU adoption if there was a higher percentage of hospitals in the area having such facilities already than if there was a lower percentage. The attitude seemed to be that if someone else on the block had one I had to have one, too, to remain competitive. (From D. Simborg. Technology in hospitals—the effect of prospective reimbursement. In: *Pro-*

ceedings of the Seventh Annual Symposium on Computer Applications in Medical Care, 1983, p.20. Copyright 1983, Institute of Electrical and Electronics Engineers, reprinted by permission.)

As we examine these and other computer applications, we must always consider their cost/benefit ratio. The business and clinical laboratory systems previously presented are readily justified; one could not meet the demands for financial reporting and test processing without computers. Reduction in computer capabilities would result directly in a reduction in service; in these cases, cost is not the central issue. Computers are not a major factor in the debate about the cost-effectiveness of the ICU. Yet, computer applications are medical technology and, as such, should be evaluated with respect to benefit and cost. Clearly, they ought never be accepted only on the basis of local competition or folklore.

2.2.4. Diagnostic Systems—ECG Reporting

The computer has been linked to physiological monitoring sensors to process and interpret the signals for diagnostic purposes. This signal processing is one of the earliest applications of computers. In the field of medical computing, there has been considerable success in both research laboratories and commercial applications. The application with the most widespread use is the analysis of the ECG, and we limit our discussion to it.

The mechanical work of the heart is accompanied by electrical activity that slightly precedes the muscle contraction. The ECG is a recording of that electrical activity. The heart is a four chambered organ. Two chambers—the atria—are thin walled holding chambers whereas the other two chambers—the ventricles—use their thick-muscled walls to pump the blood through the lungs and body. Control of the heart muscle is regulated by special nerve fibers and self-excitable muscle fibers. The heart pacing in normal hearts is regulated by the sinus node in the right atrium which generates impulses at a rate of about 70 beats per second. Once activated, impulses proceed down nerve pathways in the heart (a) causing the atria to contract and thereby fill the ventricles, and (b)—after a delay—causing the ventricles to contract and pump the blood.

During the muscle contraction, there is depolarization in the heart muscle and a dipole field is created. About half a second later, there is a repolarization of the muscle that is accompanied by a dipole field with reversed polarity. These fields can be sensed with electrodes on the surface of the body to produce the characteristic curve shown in Fig. 2.2. The curve is divided into three waves:

P wave corresponding to the atrial depolarization and contraction
QRS complex corresponding to ventricular depolarization
T wave corresponding to ventricular repolarization.

The PR segment represents the time during which the ventricles are filling and the ST interval is the period of ventricular contraction. The atrial repolarization takes place during the ventricular depolarization and, therefore, cannot be detected. The shape of the curve depends on the placement of the electrode sensors.

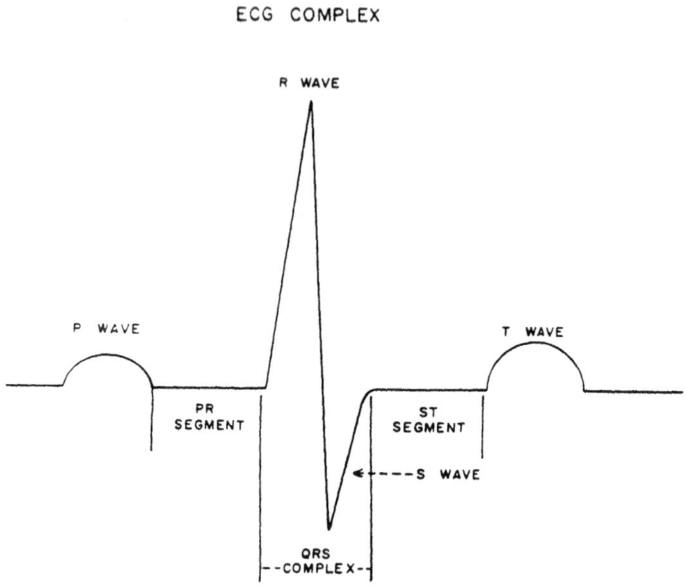

FIGURE 2.2. Schematic representation of the normal electrocardiogram. (Reprinted with permission from J. D. Bronzino, *Computer Applications for Patient Care,* Addison-Wesley, 1982, p. 65.

There are several different placements; fortunately there are standards for placement that allow comparability of data from different patients. Abnormal ECG patterns may suggest diseases or problems. Thus the ECG is an excellent diagnostic tool.

Two types of data may be derived from the ECG curve: quantified data such as rate (generally measured between R waves), the PR, QRS, and ST intervals, the P, R, S, T wave amplitude, etc., and subjective data such as the shape of the curve. Clearly, computers are very adept at matching data against a baseline configuration and computing descriptive values. Conversely, cardiologists are very effective in recognizing patterns in an ECG tracing. The physician's skill and the computer's calculations complement each other.

The processing of ECG data is considerably simpler than the monitoring of ECG data. Artifacts can be removed, the period of data collection is very brief and easily monitored, and the objective is to construct a typical curve rather than identify infrequent events. The first step in developing the technology was the representation of the ECG curve in a form that could be managed by the computer, e.g., recognition of the P, R, and T waves. From this one could measure amplitude and interval length. This type of pattern recognition is a general problem applicable to many nonmedical situations.

The next step was to translate the processed data into information that would be diagnostically useful. The computer could average several beats and print quantified results: a process the cardiologist finds cumbersome. It could also recognize abnormal patterns (such as an elevated T wave) and suggest possible causes. Since not all ECG curves are as clear as that shown in Figure 2.2, several different algorithms and systems have been developed to identify the curve features and interpret the results.

The technology is now sufficiently advanced to support both in-house and remote service center interpretive systems. Both employ an ECG acquisition cart with (a) data entry for patient identification and lead placement and (b) electrode connections for data recording. The in-house system uses a small dedicated computer; the remote system transmits the signals over telephone lines for interpretation at a service center. Each system offers the advantages of reduction in reading time, standardization of terminology, improved quality controls, and reduction in clerical duties. The service center—generally used by institutions requiring fewer than 50 ECG readings per day—also provides access to a cardiologist who reviews the data and prepares the final report.

2.2.5. Applications Using Graphics—Radiation Therapy Planning

The term computer graphics normally refers to line drawings generated by the computer. The line drawings can be the plot of a function, the tracing of a curve, a line drawing of a three-dimensional object, etc. Imaging, on the other hand, implies continuous tone displays. The graphic display is created from lines; its creation is a tracing operation. Conversely, an image display is created from primitive elements called pixels (picture elements). The creation of an image is a parallel process: the display of the gray or color scale value for each pixel in the output device. With some of the more modern systems, it is difficult to distinguish between graphics and images. This section shall illustrate how graphics are used in a specific application—radiation therapy planning.

There are three major therapy modalities used in the treatment of cancer and benign tumors: surgery, chemotherapy, and radiation therapy. Chemotherapy is the most appropriate for systemic disease, e.g., the migration of cells from the primary tumor to initiate secondary (metastatic) tumors. Surgery and radiation therapy, on the other hand, are most efficacious for local control. Frequently, the modalities are combined to produce an integrated therapy plan.

Radiation therapy uses radiation to kill tumor cells. It offers the potential to achieve local tumor control while preserving organ function. However, the radiation that kills tumor cells can also kill healthy tissue. Consequently, the objective of treatment planning is to determine how to eliminate all tumor cells while preserving as many healthy cells as possible. Fortunately, normal tissue is generally more resistant to radiation than tumor cells. Thus, the treatment strategy is one of (a) administering a dose just large enough to kill the tumor cells without destroying the surrounding tissue, and (b) shielding healthy cells from unnecessary exposure. Underdoses will have no beneficial result; overdoses may be life-threatening.

Without going into further detail, it is sufficient to note that the dose—total energy deposited per unit mass by the irradiating beam—is a function of the initial source and the attenuation resulting from the passage through air and tissue. Tumors on the surface will be treated with low-energy types of radiation that do not penetrate to deeper layers. Tumors within the body, on the other hand, must be treated with higher energies which might endanger the healthy tissues between the source and the tumor. This is further complicated by the fact that different tissues exhibit different sensitivities to radiation. Finally, functions such as the patient's general health and age also affect the planning process.

Clearly, the planning process is too complicated to be automated. Yet the computer can be used to assist in the preparation of a plan. It does this by managing data about the patient, merging it with known data about the therapy mechanisms, and then presenting it in a graphic form that allows the therapy planners to evaluate alternatives and select the most effective plan. One begins by plotting cross sections of the patient that show the patient's contour and location of the tumor and critical organs. For a selected machine and dose, internal isodose lines—lines of constant radiation exposure—are then superimposed on the patient contour. From this it can be determined what dose will be received by the tumor, critical organs, and healthy tissue.

The patient's contour is normally constructed from a plaster cast and the locations of the tumor and organs are determined from radiographs and—in some cases—computerized axial tomography (CAT). Different treatment prescriptions can be simulated by changes in the entry angle, field size, use of blocks to shield organs from radiation, etc. Fig. 2.3 illustrates a typical plan.

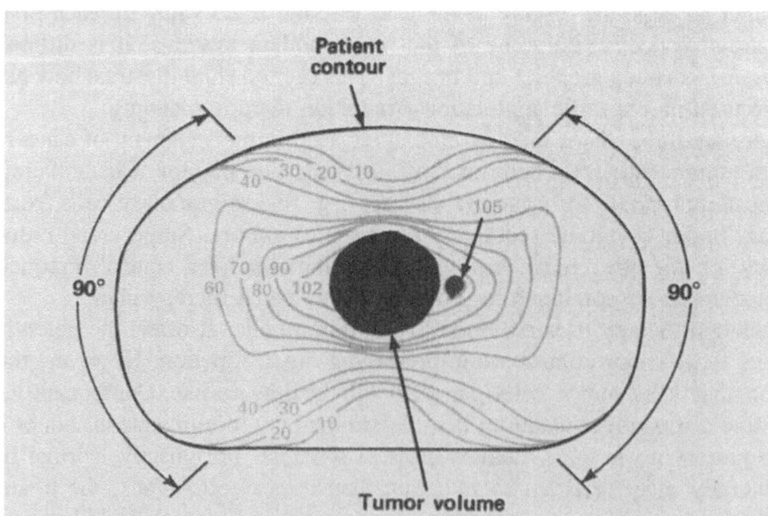

FIGURE 2.3. Sample treatment plan. Computer-aided treatment planning is used here as rotational arc therapy. An 8.5-cm^2 beam is rotated through two arcs (45°–135° and 225°–315°). Isodose lines are normalized to the center of the tumor volume (i.e., dose per 100 rads at isocenter). Much of the tumor is covered by the 102% isocontour. The distribution has a "hot spot" of 105%. (From DG Grant. Radiation Therapy Physics. *Johns Hopkins APL Technical Digest* 4(1): 27–41, 1983. Reprinted with permission.)

There are several commercial systems that support radiation therapy planning. Each comes with a digitizing device that allows the user to trace the patient data and produce an internal representation, mathematical models to compute the isodose lines, plotting hardware to print the therapy plans, and display terminals to assist in the planning process. In some cases, the computer is embedded in the system; in other cases the application is run from a general purpose computer. In either event, the computer is viewed as an integral (and dedicated) component of a clinical device.

2.2.6. Imaging Applications

At one time, virtually all medical images were in the form of radiograms recorded on film. Computers are altering this by providing (a) alternative views as in the case of CAT and (b) alternative storage media, i.e., digital databases rather than film. Images also are being derived from ultrasonography, thermography, and other sources of radiant energy.

The availability of images in digital form allows the use of techniques such as image enhancement, pattern detection, and displays using false color (i.e., the use of artificial color values within an image to improve contrast or establish relationships). In this section, we shall consider only a few applications.

We begin with a discussion of CAT. Introduced in 1972, the CAT scanner combined modern x-ray equipment with the computer to produce images of previously inaccessible structures of the body. This device so revolutionized diagnostic imaging, that Allan Cormack and Godfrey Hounsfield shared the 1979 Nobel Prize in physiology and medicine for their independent contributions: Cormack's 1963-64 papers which demonstrated the mathematical basis for image reconstruction and Hounsfield's work at EMI Limited in the production of the first commercial CAT instrument with high resolution images.

In reflecting on his early work, Cormack wrote

> In 1955 I was a Lecturer in Physics at the University of Cape Town when the Hospital Physicist at the Groote Schuur Hospital resigned. South African law required that a properly qualified physicist supervise the use of any radioactive isotopes and since I was the only nuclear physicist in Cape Town, I was asked to spend 1½ days a week at the hospital attending to the use of isotopes, and I did so for the first half of 1956. I was placed in the Radiology Department under Dr. J. Muir Grieve, and in the course of my work I observed the planning of radiotherapy treatments. A girl would superpose isodose charts and come up with isodose contours which the physician would then examine and adjust, and the process would be repeated until a satisfactory dose-distribution was found. The isodose charts were for homogeneous materials, and it occurred to me that since the human body is quite inhomogeneous these results would be quite distorted by the inhomogeneities—a fact that physicians were, of course, well aware of. It occurred to me that in order to improve treatment planning one had to know the distribution of the attenuation coefficient of tissues in the body, and that this distribution had to be found by measurements made external to the body. It soon occurred to me that this information

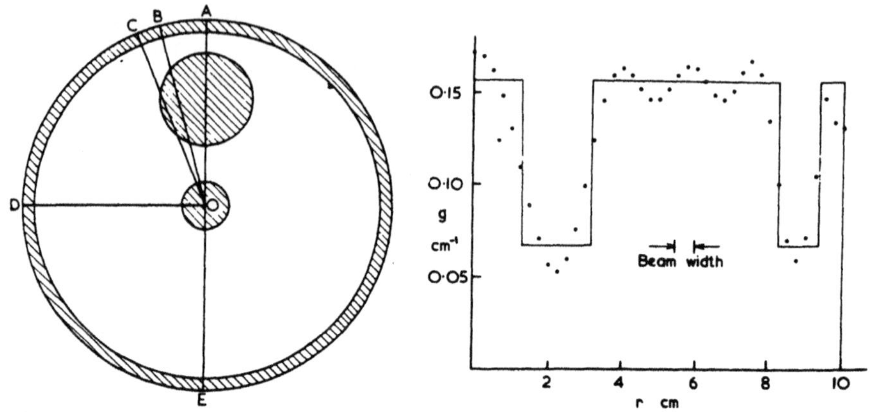

FIGURE 2.4. Figures from Cormack's papers. (From AM Cormack. Early CAT Scanning and Recent Developments, *MEDINFO* 80: xii, 1980. Reprinted with permission, North-Holland, Amsterdam.)

would be useful for diagnostic purposes and would constitute a tomogram or series of tomograms, though I did not learn the word tomogram for many years.[3]

Although the exponential attenuation of x- and gamma-rays was well understood for homogeneous slabs of material, Cormack could find nothing that generalized this for inhomogeneous materials. He translated the problem to a mathematical one and as early as 1957 did an experiment using a cylinder of aluminum surrounded by an annulus of wood. Intermittent work continued over the next 6 years, and by 1963 Cormack was ready to do an experiment using a circular phantom with an outer ring of aluminum (representing the skull), a Lucite interior (representing the soft tissue), and two aluminum discs (representing tumors). He was assisted by an undergraduate, David Hennage, "who wanted to know whether I had a numerical problem for him to work on so that he could learn FORTRAN and learn how to use a computer." The results of the experiment are illustrated in Fig. 2.4 taken from the 1963 and 1964 papers he published in the *Journal of Applied Physics*.

There was virtually no response to Cormack's papers. "The most interesting request for a reprint came from a Swiss Centre for Avalanche Research. The method would work for deposits of snow on mountains if one could get either the detector or the source into the mountain under the snow!" Less than a decade later, computer technology had advanced so far that Hounsfield could apply this knowledge to produce a CAT scanner.

In conventional x-ray imaging, a broad beam source is used to produce a perpendicular projection of the phantom or human body on film. In tomography, the source and film are mounted on opposite sides of a movable device each at a 45 degree angle. Both the source and film rotate 360° around a fixed point, thereby defining a plane of the body. The result is an image in which everything outside that plane is blurred and seen only as "noise" superimposed upon the image of the plane. Computerized tomogrpahy uses a point source with an x-ray detector rather than film. Rotation is used as in tomography, except that the plane of rotation is perpendicular to the body. Data collected in this plane are processed by a computer, using the mathematics of x-ray attenuation in inhomogeneous materials, to construct an image of the patient's cross-section, which shows all internal structures.

The CAT scanners were rapidly accepted by the medical community. During the first years of distribution, there was experimentation with their use and redundant tests were ordered so that CAT imaging could be compared with other procedures and tests. By now it is clear how CAT imaging can improve the diagnostic process. The availability of less expensive equipment, the avoidance of alternative invasive procedures, and the ability to clearly examine otherwise inaccessible structures all have contributed to an improvement in patient care.

CAT technology was designed to display spatial relationships, that is, anatomical details. Once the image reconstruction technology was developed, however, other sources could be used to provide even more powerful tools for medical diagnosis and biological investigation. Positron Emission Tomography (PET) goes beyond displaying structure; it can record changes in metabolism. In this case, the patient is injected with a short-lived radioactive material and the sensors record the source and intensity of the gamma radiation emitted by the isotope. Corrections are made for the effect of attenuation, and the result is an image that can represent blood flow distribution, metabolic activity, and receptor site concentration. Because short-lived isotopes are used, a colocated cyclotron to produce them is an essential—and expensive—component of the PET scanner.

Another imaging technique, nuclear magnetic resonance (NMR), also can provide information beyond the basic anatomical structure. This type of imaging is based on the fact that most elements have at least one abundant isotope whose nucleus is magnetic. These nuclei absorb and emit electromagnetic energy when a weak radio frequency magnetic field stimulates changes in their orientation relative to the direction of a strong static magnetic field. The frequency of this nuclear magnetic resonance phenomenon is a function of the magnetic field and the magnetic moment of the nucleus. NMR spectroscopy can be used to identify these frequencies to give information on molecular identity and structure.

Spatial distribution information for creating images can be gained by varying the magnetic field in a known manner. The strength of the signal at each frequency can be interpreted as the density of the hydrogen nuclei in the plane where the magnetic field corresponds to that frequency. Different planes may be used and an image may be reconstructed.

There are also two other parameters of biological importance: T_1, the spin-lattice relaxation time and T_2, the spin-spin relaxation time. They too can be measured to give information about local tissue conditions. As can be seen, there are many parameters containing much information. NMR imaging is still in its development stage. It provides a way to measure and display free water content, relative flow, and concentrations of some molecular species and contrast agents.

To date, we have only limited experience with diagnostic tools such as PET and NMR which show function as well as structure. Nevertheless, these new devices can be expected to produce as significant an impact as we have seen with the first of the computer aided imaging tools: the CAT scanner.

2.2.7. Implantable Microelectronics

This section on data oriented applications began with the mundane and will conclude with the exotic. With electronic miniaturization has come the possibility of creating implementable devices that contain either microprocessors or sensors designed to communicate with external processors. Table 2.4 presents a matrix of currently available implantable biomedical instruments.[4] This type of application represents a leading edge for the third generation of biomedical data processing systems.

2.3. Information Oriented Applications

Information-oriented applications combine data in ways that emphasize the meaning represented by a collection of data. Unlike the previous data-oriented examples, the emphasis is not on the transformation of data to new forms of data or data display (e.g., imaging), but rather on the collection and coordination of data for comprehension by the user. All information systems are assumed to retain a permanent database from which the desired elements can be retrieved; the technology is primarily one of data retrieval and not computation. Unlike a process control system in which the output is used as an input from the next system iteration, in an information system the output is directed to a human user who integrates the information to determine the subsequent actions. This distinction between data and information systems is artificial, but is useful in providing an organizational structure.

Information systems may be further subdivided according to where they are used. The most common clinical systems are:

- *Hospital information systems:* those systems located in acute care facilities to manage the communication of clinical data within the facility
- *Ancillary service systems:* those systems used by an ancillary service to manage their internal processing control, e.g., a clinical laboratory system. These are frequently integrated with a Hospital Information System.
- *Ambulatory care systems:* those systems used to treat ambulatory patients. They include emergency room systems, hospital outpatient systems, health maintenance organization systems, and private practice systems.
- Special applications for:
  Tertiary care
  Long term care
  Research

TABLE 2.4. Biomedical instrument matrix.

	Function				
Location	Research	Diagnostic	Monitoring	Therapeutic	Prosthetic
Subcutaneous	Microelectronics for totally implantable telemetry of flow, pressure, and dimension, for example	Totally implantable telemetry for coronary bypass graft monitoring	Cerebral pressure telemetry microtansducers and electronics	Microelectrodes for nueral stimulator for pain relief	Cardiac pacemaker microelectronics auditory prosthesis microelectronics
Supercutaneous	Microtransducers for animal backpack telemetry of flow and pressure, for example	Ingestible pH telemetry capsule	Ambulatory care ECG telemetry with active microelectronics	Microelectrodes and electronics for bladder stimulator	Hearing aid
Percutaneous	Implantable biopotential and temperature microtransducers with externalized leads	Catheter-tip blood gas sensor	Transvenous pacing lead for monitoring and stimulation; catheter-tip pressure sensor	Electrical stimulation of bone for enhanced healing	Microsensors for left ventricle assist device
Transcutaneous	Gamma ray microtransducer arrays for radioisotope imaging; blood pressure sensor array with piezoresistive microtransducers	Computerized x-ray tomography detector arrays	Piezoelectric transducer arrays for ultrasonic imaging; blood gas monitor microsensors	Microtemperature sensors for hyperthermia; microsensors for defilbrillators	Microoptical sensors and tactile stimulators for optical-to-tactile reading aid for the blind
Extracutaneous	Electron microscope	Mass spectrometer; cell sorter	Miniature silicon gas chromatograph for breath analysis	Microsensors for kidney dialysis machine	Voice-actuated wheelchair controller

From J.D. Meindl. Biomedical Implantable Microelectronics, *Science* 210: 263–267, 1980.

Patient interviewing
Automated multiphasic health testing (AMHT)

For the purposes of this book, the term clinical information system (CIS) will be defined as an information system that manages clinical data to support patient care and medical decision making.

We now have a decade of operational experience with such systems, and the CIS is entering its second generation of application. It has the potential for improving the delivery of health care. Unfortunately, few commercial systems offer the tools to do this, and few providers are aware of the potential benefit. One objective of this book, therefore, is to increase the awareness of their power and potential. Chapters 7 through 9 provide descriptions of systems and their features. The remainder of this section will be limited to an overview of the benefits of the CIS.

2.3.1. System Evaluation

Evaluation in a health care setting implies the confirmation of some previously defined hypothesis or objective. The clinical trial provides an excellent illustration. To evaluate a hypothesis, a homogeneous patient population is selected and a limited number of alternative therapies are administered according to preestablished criteria. At the end of the trial, the hypothesis is evaluated; that is, there is a statistical test to determine if the objectives of the new therapy have been realized. Except for the controlled changes in alternative therapies, it is assumed that there are no characteristics of the patient population or uncontrolled inputs that bias the conclusion.

Compare the clinical trial with the evaluation of a health care system. In the trial there are many patients; individual variability can be averaged out by increasing the sample size. In health care systems, there is generally only one sample. In a clinical trial, most variables are held constant; this is impossible to do in a dynamic health care system. Finally, in a clinical trial, the objectives are very specific and readily evaluated; in a health care system, on the other hand, the objectives are more generally stated.

Flagle presented a general cost/benefit model that is shown in Fig. 2.5. Inputs to the system are divided into those that are controllable (generally by the allocation of dollars) and those that are uncontrollable. The outputs are divided into benefits and cost. The evaluator may choose to modify some of the controllable inputs and look for predetermined changes in the outputs. Since only a limited number of the inputs can be controlled, the number of variables is large, and the sample size is usually limited to one, the evaluation of a CIS is subject to considerable uncertainty.

The story is told of a site visit during the early days of computers. The investigator demonstrated his clinical patient registration system and the program performed perfectly. "That's an interesting system, have you evaluated it?" asked one of the visitors. In shocked fury, the investigator responded, "What do you mean, evaluate—it's working, isn't it?" Although the definition of evaluation

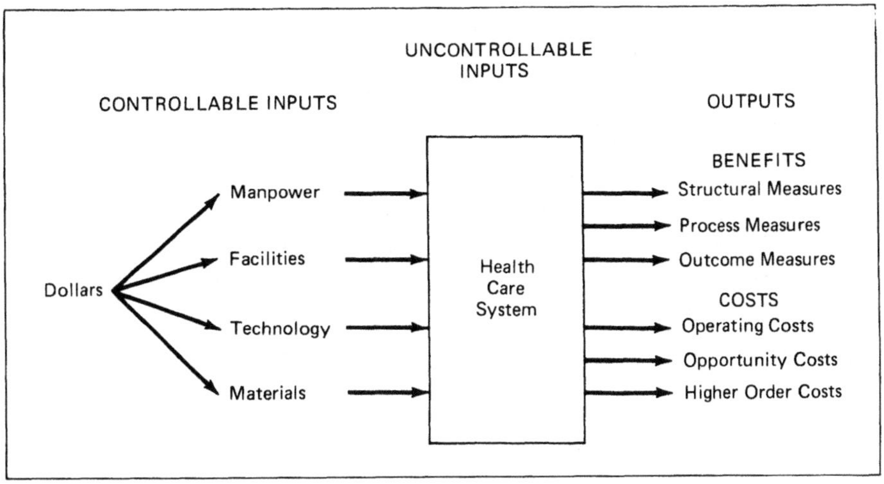

FIGURE 2.5. Cost–benefit model of a health care system. Adopted from C. D. Flagle, 1973.[5]

still may be subject to debate, we have at least come beyond the concept of acceptable being equivalent to the absence of failure. In the remainder of this subsection, we shall review the terminology of evaluation.

There are two stages in the evaluation of health care systems. In the *formative* stage, the evaluation is performed by the developer. The product typically undergoes changes, and a final revision is installed that best meets the developer's objectives. This is followed by a *summrative* evaluation in which the product is evaluated in the operational setting against the intended service objective.

Clearly, the formative evaluation is performed by the investigator. Where there is high risk, it is not certain that a satisfactory product will emerge, and the investigator constantly must make tradeoffs between performance or scope. As technology advances, the risk for a given application declines. (In this sense, formative evaluation is the equivalent of acceptance or system testing as described in Chapter 6.)

Once the product has demonstrated that it can meet its design requirements, there is the larger question of how well it meets its service objectives. That is, once it is agreed that it works, does it do what it was intended to? For example, if a hospital information system (HIS) was installed to reduce the time that nurses spend doing clerical tasks, does it indeed reallocate nursing activities?

As shown in Fig. 2.5, the benefits of a health care system are generally organized into three categories:

- *Structure*. This deals with the capacity of the facilities and the capacity and qualification of the personnel and organization. For example, a HIS may change the structure by allowing increased patient days with no change in staffing, altering the patient/nurse/support staff ratios, etc.
- *Process*. This relates to the volume, cost, and appropriateness of activities

of preventive, diagnostic, therapeutic, and supportive activities. In the HIS example, changes in the process may be seen in modified test ordering patterns that result from more rapid reporting of results, better retrieval of information resulting from better medical records, etc.

- *Outcome.* This is the change in health status attributed to the care or information system. In a clinical trial, outcome is easily defined: survival, reduction in tumor size, elimination of rash, improvement in limb mobility, etc. In the HIS example, it is more difficult to define outcome; examples are reduced length of stay, lower morbidity resulting from a reduction in evasive tests, reduced infection rates, etc.

In general, one is constrained to measuring changes in the structure and process. One begins with a hypothesis of how the information system will alter the structure or process and then collects data to test this hypothesis. It is not always clear that what is being measured addresses the key issues. It has been suggested, for example, that (a) outcome measures may not be valid resources, (b) process attributable measures may not reflect an impact on patient care, and (c) protocol adherence evaluation may be biased.

Further, it is not always possible to separate the impact of the CIS from changes in the health care system. In some cases, the CIS acts as an enabling tool: the process could not be performed without it even though the CIS is only a small part of the total system. We have seen how the computer enabled the clinical laboratory to improve throughput, reduce costs, and meet greater volume demands. In the same way, there are clinical activities that would be very difficult to implement without a CIS. However, the outcome benefits from these are derived from a synergistic combination of improved medical knowledge, trained health care teams, specialized facilities and equipment, plus the CIS. In such situations, it is impossible to identify the contribution of the information system technology—it is part of an integrated whole.

Too often, the final evaluation of a system is left to the pragmatics of the marketplace or the biases of the developers. Nevertheless, there is sufficient evidence to identify clearly some major CIS benefits. These are summarized in the next subsection.

2.3.2. Overview of the Demonstrated Benefits

Most clinical information systems have been evaluated only in larger institutions. The reasons for this are obvious: these institutions have the needs and resources that justify the relatively large outlays required to install and evaluate an information system. Thus we know the most about hospital information systems. We also know a good deal about ambulatory care systems in teaching and research environments. We know the least about the use of systems in smaller practices. In what follows, we group the benefits as follows:

- *Administrative support*: mostly changes in structure with some impact on process

- *Medical decision making assistance*: mostly changes in process Little has been established regarding outcome.
- *Cost Impact*: mostly measures relating to institutional operating costs

(More detailed evaluations are presented in Chapters 7, 8, and 9.)

2.3.2.1. Administrative Support

The process of patient care requires many administrative functions that range from those involving patient interaction (e.g., appointments and schedules) to those of a strictly clerical nature (e.g., charting). The CIS provides benefits to the practitioners and patients by performing the same functions either more efficiently or more effectively. Four areas are identified where changes have been measured.

- *Modify work flow*. The CIS can be used to support reorganization of the work flow in order to (a) reduce redundancy of information processing and (b) reassign clerical tasks that are normally performed by health care professionals. The greatest impact has been measured in hospitals with respect to the nursing activities.
- *Improve timeliness*. The CIS has the ability to transmit information once it has been recorded. This results in more rapid access to information such as laboratory and radiology reports. Again, the primary focus is the hospital. However, as communication costs fall, similar facilities may be used to link practitioner offices and ancillary support groups.
- *Reduce errors*. The CIS can be programmed to reject unreasonable inputs and query questionable entries. Further, systems can be designed with consistency tests and scheduling to provide lists of orders and other actions. These tools have been demonstrated to reduce errors. However, error identification can be employed effectively only in situations where a process is frequently repeated.
- *Provide access to new functions*. The availability of a database and computational tools provides access to many functions that could not be considered in a manual setting. Examples in resource utilization, quality of care, and facility management have been documented.

2.3.2.2. Medical Decision-Making Assistance

A computer has the ability to apply limited rules routinely to vast bodies of structured data without fatigue. The practitioner, on the other hand, has the ability to integrate a large number of analog sources. By combining these two capabilities, a CIS can improve patient care. It is the author's belief that this is the area in which the CIS will have its greatest impact. The existing capabilities are organized as follows:

- *Display clinical information*. The orderly display and organization of clinical data ensures reliable access to a complete and accurate database. The data may include medical text and laboratory results; the formats may be tabular or plotted. Some systems provide facilities for maintaining a completely automated medical record; other systems are less complete.

- *Automatic surveillance*. Since the CIS has access to all of a patient's clinical data, there is the potential for it to review all new inputs and evaluate them with respect to a set of predetermined criteria. This facility is most commonly implemented in hospital settings to produce alerts for drug-drug interactions and similar potential problems. The technique has also been used in an ambulatory setting to follow up on positive test results.
- *Automatic reminders*. These represent a special class of surveillance reports in which the provider routinely receives reminders for each patient encounter based on a preestablished set of rules. The rules vary in complexity from a reminder for inoculations to a suggested reevaluation of therapy. Where reminders or surveillance alerts are available, they have clearly altered provider behavior in a positive way.
- *Decision making support*. A growing number of tools are being developed to support medical decision making. These include the implementation of clinical algorithms, the use of Bayesian analysis to predict the outcome for one patient based on the outcome in a larger population of similar patients, and the use of expert systems. Most decision making support tools have a limited distribution, but this is an area of major research activity.

2.3.2.3. Cost Impact

The final factor in the evaluation of a system is the cost for the benefits provided. This is difficult to measure with large systems, and perhaps even more difficult with smaller systems. Drazen has analyzed the methods used in evaluating the costs of hospital information systems.[6] She concluded that (a) few rigorous studies have been conducted, (b) most of this work is prospective in nature, and (c) little work has been done in validating the predictive methodologies. She also suggested that improvements in information flow constituted the major motivation to implement an Automated Hospital Information System.

One study of automated billing systems for small practices found little—if any—cost benefit after 2 years of use. The major unmatched cost-saving was found in staff time. "Office administrators endeavoring to improve their billing effectiveness should not regard computerization as a panacea," warned the investigators.[7]

Thus, the cost benefit studies suggest that health care systems are not structured to benefit greatly from automated support. There are applications that require automation to enable their operation; the use of computers also allows the introduction of new functions at no change in cost. But the installation of information systems simply to replace current manual activities does not seem to have a significant cost benefit.

2.4. Knowledge Oriented Applications

We have organized this discussion of medical computing leaving what we call knowledge oriented applications for the last. Of course, all applications apply knowledge. In the case of data oriented systems, the knowledge is encoded in the form of an algorithm. For example, the ECG processing of input signals (i.e., data) uses our knowledge of what these signals represent in a physiological model. The results are repeatable and exact (within the limits of statistical error). The algorithm defines how the data shall be processed. All possible decisions have been encoded before the program can be used.

Information systems add another dimension to this encoding of knowledge. As before, there are algorithms. For example, the listing of a medical record organizes the patient's clinical data in a format that is helpful to the provider. The general structure of this medical record is fixed; it has been defined by an algorithm (in a program). However, the information system also allows the provider to extract additional information from the data base. It provides tools to submit queries, group data in new ways, and perform analysis. However, it can only supply information that is available in the database. The knowledge used by the application is limited to (a) what is encoded in the algorithms and (b) what the user explicitly applies in the query or analysis.

In knowledge-based applications, on the other hand, the knowledge is organized so that it can use inference to supply more information than has been given. Thus, the range of questions that a knowledge oriented system can answer will be greater than the number of explicit facts at its disposal; through inference, it will be able to provide solutions to problems that had not been anticipated. Moreover, because the knowledge is structured as a database, it may be added to and modified. Consequently, knowledge bases can be cumulative. Finally, since the knowledge is stored as text, it can be used to explain actions and recommendations.

To provide a slightly different view, consider human memory. Questions seem to be answered in three different ways:

- By searching memory for information, e.g., what is the capital of New York?
- By examining a mental image, e.g., does Lincoln's profile on the penny face to the left or right?
- By using inference, e.g., does an elephant eat more food in a day than a lion?

Both data and information systems are limited to the first type of problem solving; they only can search their databases using their algorithms. The second technique—the use of mental images—does not seem to have a computer analog. However, the third tool—inference—is precisely the added dimension that knowledge-based systems offer.

Currently there are two classes of medical systems that are considered to be knowledge-oriented. The first organizes knowledge so that it can be retrieved in ways that help the user identify and extract the knowledge. Once integrated by the user, it can be used to determine a course of action or arrive at a solution. An example is the structuring of the medical literature to provide direct access to the information desired as opposed to simply retrieving a document that might contain the information. The second category of system is the more common interpretation of a knowledge-based system; here artificial intelligence techniques are used to produce an expert system for diagnostic or therapeutic advice. The following subsections briefly consider these two types of systems. Chapter 9 contains a more complete discussion of expert systems as they are used in medical decision-making.

2.4.1. Bibliographic Knowledge Bases

One standard form for representing knowledge has been the printed document. Access to this knowledge is either by reading or secondary citation. The citation may be referenced in another document, verbally communicated within collegial circles, or embedded in "common knowledge." As the quantity and scope of this knowledge base has grown, tools to access its contents have become increasingly important.

The automated approach to managing bibliographic materials is referred to as information storage and retrieval. Each document is represented by a surrogate—for example, title, authors, publication, and keywords (indices). Information retrieval technology is used to select that subset of the database that satisfies the user's request. Recall measures the proportion of the appropriate material that has been retrieved; precision refers to the portion returned that is relevant to the user's needs. The use of interactive processing assists the user in modifying the search to improve precision.

The result of a search is either a collection of citations, author-prepared abstracts or indexer-prepared extracts. Because of the high cost of technical abstracting, there is an emphasis on automated text processing to determine the contents of a document and produce indices. As the storage media become less expensive, it is common to retain more of a document—such as the abstract— available on line. Nevertheless, the fundamental process remains one of storing segments of knowledge and using information retrieval techniques to access them.

In the field of medicine there are many online bibliographic tools available from the National Library of Medicine and other government and commercial sources. Most identify citations of journal articles and books. The largest and most frequently used of these systems is MEDLINE (MEDLARS online, where MEDLARS stands for MEDical Literature Analysis and Retrieval System). MEDLINE provides online access to biomedical journal articles from the current and preceding 2 years. It covers some 3,000 journals published in the U.S. and 70 foreign countries. Where an English abstract exists, it frequently also is available. Other online databases available from the National Library of Medicine include Health Planning and Administration, TOXLINE (Toxicology Information), TDB (Toxicology Data Bank), and CHEMLINE (Chemical Dictionary). Some databases from other sources include PRE-MED, a current index to 109 journals offered by Bibliographic Retrieval Services, CANCERLIT supported by the National Cancer Institute, and variations of the MEDLINE database available through different vendors and microcomputer networks.

The use of the online files normally requires special training and orientation which often limits the conduct of searches to librarians. This has led to the development of systems that provide an easy-to-use interface to access a database tailored to a specific environment. One such system is PaperChase[8] which supports searches to the journals maintained in one teaching hospital. It was found that—if the search tool was accessible and easy to learn—it would be used. In its first year of operation, over 1,000 individuals tried it and, of these, half conducted five or more searches and 14% conducted over 20 searches. About 40% of the searches were for patient care, 30% for research, and 20% for teaching. Thus, even though the search only provided a citation and the journal article still had to be located and read, it is clear that an effective index to the literature is useful.

Online access to the knowledge—as opposed to citations and abstracts—requires that the knowledge be extracted from the literature and structured for retrieval. Reggia has proposed an intelligent textbook "composed of synthesized knowledge bases that (a) could be read by physicians for its informational content just like a textbook, and (b) could be applied by computer to information about a specific patient to generate a differential diagnosis, estimate a prognosis, stage a disease process, recommend laboratory tests or potential therapy, and so forth."[9] But this concept is still in the research stage.

However, the National Library of Medicine has demonstrated how a knowledge base can be constructed and used as an online reference source. Its Hepatitis Knowledge Base (HKB)[10] was designed to contain substantive answers to questions posed by practitioners and, at the same time, provide answers that are both current and reflective of the consensus of a group of experts. The knowledge base was constructed by first performing a MEDLINE search which yielded more than 16,000 postings. From these, a hierarchical structure was defined, and the information was extracted and rewritten. Finally, the knowledge base was reviewed by a group of experts; new material was added and revisions of the text were made. The result was a dynamic knowledge base of some million characters (200 pages) with tables, references, and some graphics.

The HKB is organized as a hierarchy with each node containing a heading statement and a synthesis statement. At the bottom level are "twigs" that may contain data (i.e., highly specific text statements), references, or tables and figures. The perusal of the HKB is supported by either a table of contents type search or a natural language query. For example, Fig. 2.6 illustrates the paragraph which is the "best match" to the query, "Can an infected mother transmit the disease to her fetus?"

The use of bibliographic tools and extracts from references represents one method for accessing the large stores of knowledge that are accumulating. In this case, the use of the knowledge requires integration and synthesis by the reader (user of the system). As can be seen in the HKB example, there is considerable experience in the management and manipulation of text and bibliographic files. As more journals are published electronically (i.e., provided in a computer retrievable form), one can expect more emphasis on the development of tools to extract the knowledge from textual sources. The obvious difficulty in doing this is that the source materials were designed to be read and understood

Rank = 1 Similarity = 199.6% # roots matching unexpanded query = 2 Points = 159567

932 Transplacental infection occurs. In one case, the mother developed hepatitis at six months gestation and became antigen-negative before delivery; yet the cord blood was positive, and the baby has been HBsAg positive since birth. This represents in utero infection. The antigen in the cord blood was produced by the infected neonate rather than by the mother

. . .6/29

78 seconds have elapsed since receipt of your query.

FIGURE 2.6. Sample searches of Hepatitis Knowledge Base. From R. E. Williams, *ANNOD A Navigator of Natural-language Organized (Textual) Data,* Lister Hill National Center, National Library of Medicine, June, 1983.

by people. In the next section we shall examine some trends in which the emphasis is on the structuring of knowledge so that it can be processed by machines.

2.4.2. Artificial Intelligence and Expert Systems

The field of artificial intelligence (AI) is frequently traced back to a 1956 conference at Dartmouth College. The view at that time was that intelligent behavior was based on smart reasoning techniques; once ad hoc techniques were identified, intelligent programs would follow. The initial focus was on general problems such as natural language translation. Yet, as Lockheed was to learn about hospital information systems, the problem was deceptively complex. For example, it is said that when the statement, "The spirit is willing but the flesh is weak" was translated into Russian and back to English, the result came out, "The wine is good but the meat is spoiled."

True computer intelligence has proved to be allusive. In fact, even the term intelligence defies definition. (One researcher states: "Intelligence is what an intelligence test measures.") Nevertheless, after some 25 years of experience, there is a growing consensus of what constitutes AI. Figure 2.7 presents Nilsson's onion model of AI which displays the basic elements and applications.

As shown in the inner circle, AI systems have some representation of knowledge—generally called the knowledge base. This knowledge is specific to a domain; e.g., medical diagnosis, oil prospecting, linguistic analysis. The systems also have access to domain independent knowledge—generally called common sense reasoning. These two sets of knowledge are searched to produce useful results for a specific query. The search process is not formally defined as an algorithm; rather it uses general "rules of thumb" referred to as "heuristics." Finally, the AI system is written in a language and uses programming tools. The most common language in the United States is LISP; PROLOG was selected for the Japanese Fifth Generation Computer project.

Four classes of applications are shown in the outer ring. Interest here is limited to expert systems. We have already alluded to the fact that the early attempts

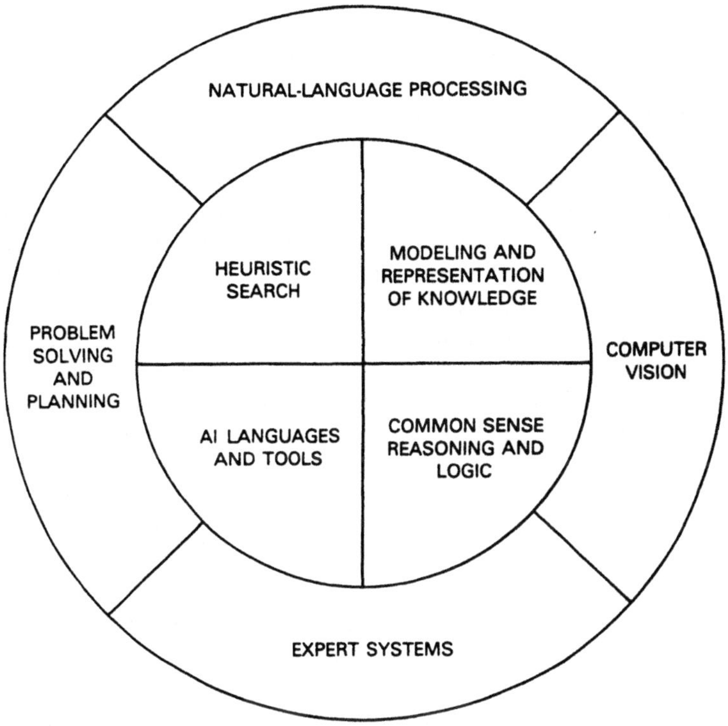

FIGURE 2.7. Elements of artificial intelligence. From W. B. Gevarter, NASA Technical Memorandum 85836, 1983.[11]

to find generalized smart reasoning techniques met with only limited success. It was also found out that the most elementary body of knowledge—common sense—was too difficult to codify. Thus, one potential area for success lay in the collection of knowledge in a narrow domain and the development of heuristic search tools tailored to that knowledge base. If this could be done, the knowledge base could grow and be cumulative. In time it could be expected to exceed the capabilities of the individual experts who built it. Moreover, the knowledge base could be used to infer new information that was not explicitly recorded in the knowledge base.

An illustration will help. One of the earliest expert systems was DENDRAL which was developed at Stanford University by Lederberg and Feigenbaum. The system was designed to analyze molecular structures using instrument data from a mass spectrometer and a nuclear magnetic resonance spectrometer. It was soon realized that if one first limited the molecular families to be studied and then applied a set of general rules for identifying plausible candidates, it then would be possible to use a computer to achieve expert levels of performance.

In the case of DENDRAL, the heuristics operate in three phases. First there is a plan that makes some rough guess as to what the solution should be. Next there is a generate phase that develops plausible solutions consistent with the plan constraints. Finally, in a test phase, each plausible solution is tested by having the computer generate expected instrument data and test it against the reported results. Close fits are ranked and saved. All phases use the knowledge about the type of compound under investigation.

In the DENDRAL example, the solution is constructed by using a heuristic search of its knowledge base. By way of contrast, a data oriented solution would require that an algorithm be used to construct each possible solution and then test it for validity. Although this approach may be feasible for small problems, the combinaterial explosion (i.e., the increasing number of possible cases) makes it impossible for most real applications. An information processing approach, on the other hand, might query a database such as the National Library of Medicine's CHEMLINE chemical dictionary. This provides online access to molecular formulas, names and synonyms, links to other Library files, information about ring systems, etc. Of course, if the data have not been entered and indexed, the information system will not be helpful. Thus, each of these two approaches has obvious limitations. The limitation of DENDRAL, however, proved to be the small subset of organic molecules for which it could generate plausible solutions. By introducing a more powerful structure generator (CONGEN), the original system has been extended beyond the restrictions originally imposed by the use of NMR and mass spectral data.

Clearly, expert systems have major advantages over other implementation approaches. Their current shortcomings include the need for a specialized knowledge base with the tools to build and maintain it, the lack of generalized domain-independent heuristics, and the relative inefficiency of the fourth generation computers for symbolic inference processing. Still, there already are commercial successes. For example, Digital Equipment Corporation uses an expert system (XCON) to configure their VAX computer systems: they estimate it saves them tens of millions of dollars a year.

The use of expert systems in medical applications is discussed in more detail in Chapter 9. Most systems are experimental; few are in operational use. Nevertheless, it is obvious that AI and expert systems represent a major area of investigation, and one can reliably predict the existence of effective knowledge-oriented applications in the coming decade.

2.5. Concluding Remarks

This chapter began with a historical introduction and followed with a survey of three decades' accomplishments. The results were organized into three categories:

- Data-oriented applications which emphasize the scientific and engineering aspects of computers and medicine
- Information-oriented applications which are the central topic of this book
- Knowledge-oriented applications which represent the new frontier

This final section asks if there are any unifying principles that link these applications, or are they simply a collection of diverse products used by a single industry? In other words, is Medical Informatics a discipline or simply a categorization of users.

The term Medical Informatics is European in origin; the term used more frequently in the United States is Medical Information Science. The advantage of the former is that it makes no statements about the scientific nature of the field. It may be a science—the discovery and demonstration of underlying principles—or a method—the application of techniques to produce a predicted result. Van Bemmel offers the following definition.

Medical Informatics comprises the theoretical and practical aspects of information processing and communication, based on knowledge and experience derived from processes in medicine and health care.[12] (From J. van Bemmel. The structure of Medical Informatics. *Medical Informatics* 9(3), 1984. Reprinted with permission of Taylor & Francis, London.)

Van Bemmel feels it is too early to say if Medical Informatics is a science or not; his definition considers both the theoretical and practical. Shortliffe, on the other hand, addresses the issue of scientific content as follows.

It can be argued that medical informatics is still in a "prescientific era.". We build artifacts, our papers describe them, but an underlying theory has thus far failed to emerge. In the field of pure computer science, courses in the mathematical theory of computation exist, but even so, much of that field is characterized by individual experiments and reports of their success or failure. The field of medical informatics has underlying fundamental principles, but we tend to identify and articulate them poorly, and those basic science issues that exist are not generally recognized or accepted. Rarely are scientific activities in the field viewed on an equal level with traditional "pure science medical research."[13] (From E. H. Shortliffe. In: *Information Science and Medical Education*. North-Holland, Amsterdam. Reprinted in *Medical Informatics* 9(3), 1984. With permission.)

The reluctant conclusion, therefore, is that most of the near term advances in medical computing will result from the pragmatic application of other disciplines to a health care setting. It is too early to identify the underlying rules of a medical information science, and emphasis will remain on the utilization of the computer as a tool. Does it matter? In a way, yes. With no clearly defined discipline, there is no focus for research, education, or career advancement. This distributes the already limited expertise, delays the establishment of professional standards, and encourages persons with only a marginal training to become active in the field.

Perhaps as knowledge applications develop, the AI community will be able to use medical knowledge engineering as a focus for a true discipline of medical informatics. In the near term, however, we must recognize that the data oriented applications are in the domain of specialists in bioengineering and medicine, whereas the knowledge-oriented applications are research projects for physicians and computer scientists. The clinical information systems, on the other hand, represent the application of existing knowledge and technology. Their implementation is a branch of engineering and not a science. A great deal is already known about the CIS, and advances will be made only by building on this knowledge.

We are now developing the second generation of medical information systems. Experience with these applications is broad; the knowledge of the technology is vast. The VLSI revolution has allowed us to produce practical solutions that leap beyond the obsolescence of older systems. Yet, advancements are constrained by the facts that the field requires expertise in both computers and health care delivery, that the literature is diverse and difficult to evaluate, and that the technology is changing so rapidly that it is not always clear how past experience relates to new applications.

The basic thesis of this book is that CIS represents a mature technology that can (and will) have a major impact in the way in which health care is developed. To understand how to apply this technology one requires a basic understanding of computer science (Part II) and a knowledge of the medical systems that already exist (Part III). Since the technology is changing, the goal is to present an understanding of the framework upon which future CISs will be built. Although there is no guarantee that the insights presented in this book are correct, they will at least orient the reader to avoid old errors and to build upon our decades of experience.

For Further Reading

There is a growing number of books that deal with what we have chosen to call Medical Informatics. B. Jacobson and J. G. Webster have assembled a useful text in *Medical and Clinical Engineering*, Prentice Hall, 1977. As the title suggests, it is more concerned with the application of engineering than the use of computers. J. D. Brenzino has produced a thorough survey in *Computer Applications for Patient Care*, Addison-Wesley, 1982. This contains chapters on materials not included in this text such as the clinical laboratory, automated multiphasic health testing, diagnostic support systems, patient monitoring, and medical imaging. Several of the classic books are now out of print and somewhat dated. An excellent modern introduction to the field is D. A. B. Lindberg, *The Growth of Medical Information Systems in the United States*, Lexington Books, 1979. A text with a European viewpoint is F. Wingert, *Medical Informatics*, Springer-Verlag, 1979.

Artech House has prepared two good collections of reprints: V. Sondak, H. Schwartz and N. Sondak (eds), *Computers and Medicine* (1979) and N. Sondak and F. Kavaler, *Computers in Medical Administration* (1980) (which includes more than its title suggests). Springer-Verlag has a Computers in Medicine series which also includes reprints. The first volumes are B. I. Blum (ed), *Information Systems for Patient Care* (1984) and J. A. Reggia and S. Tuhrim (eds) *Computer-Assisted Medical Decision Making* (2 volumes, 1985). P. Szolovits has edited a volume called *Artificial Intelligence in Medicine*, Westview Press, 1982. W. Clancey and E. Shortliffe have also edited a collection called *Readings in Medical Artificial Intelligence: the First Decade*, Addison-Wesley, 1984. The September 1979 issue of the *Proceedings of the IEEE* was devoted to Technology and Health

Care; it contains a fine collection of papers on that topic. For office practice systems there is B. B. Oberst and R. A. Reid (eds), *Computer Applications to Private Office Practice*, Springer-Verlag, 1984. Among the texts in process which I have not seen are *An Introduction to Medical Information Science*, edited by E. Shortliffe, G. Weiderhold, and L. Fagan on medical informatics and an introductory outline of the field by D. Levenson, *Computers in Clinical Medicine: An Overview*, MacMillan, 1985.

For persons interested in clinical information systems, there are two annual U.S. meetings of interest. One key source is the Symposium on Computer Applications in Medical Care (SCAMC) which holds an East coast meeting in October or November. The proceedings are a rich source of current work. The American Assocation for Medical Systems and Informatics (AAMSI) is a membership organization with a principal interest in this field. They hold an annual West coast Congress each May; there also are proceedings. The major international meeting is MEDINFO. It is triennial and last met in 1983.

Few journals are devoted to clinical information systems. Indeed, much of the literature is diffused throughout the medical journals. This makes the identification of works somewhat difficult and also leads to articles of varying technical quality. The bibliography for Chapters 7, 8 and 9 includes many of the most common sources.

References

1. Adopted from materials provided by R. E. Miller, personal communication.
2. Lincoln, T. L., Computers in the Clinical Laboratory: What We Have Learned, *Med. Instr.* 12:233-236, 1978.
3. Cormack, A. M., Early CAT Scanning and Recent Developments, *MEDINFO 80*, North-Holland, 1980 ix-xii.
4. Meindl, J. D., Biomedical Implantable Microelectronics, *Science* 210 (17 October 1980) 263-267.
5. Adopted from C. D. Flagle, Evaluation of Health Care Systems in M. F. Driggs (ed), *Problem-Directed and Medical Information Systems*, Year Book Med. Pub., 1973, pp. 187-194.
6. Drazen, E. L., Methods for Evaluating Costs of Automated Hospital Information Systems, in B. I. Blum (ed) *Information Systems for Patient Care*, Springer-Verlag 1984 427-437.
7. Nelson, E. C. and B. Bise, Evaluation of a Computerized Billing System for Small Primary Care Practices, *Proc. Sixth Annual Symposium on Computer Applications in Medical Care*, 1982 p 467.
8. Horowitz, G. L. and H. L. Bleich, PaperChase: A Computer Program to Search the Medical Literature, *N.E. J.Med.* 1981 305:924-930.
9. Reggia, J. A., T. P. Pula, T. R. Price, and B. J. Perricone, Towards an Intelligent Textbook of Neurology, *Proc. Fourth Annual Symposium on Computer Applications in Medical Care* 1980 190-198, reprinted in J. A. Reggia and S. Tuhrim (eds), *Computer-Assisted Medical Decision Making* Vol. II, Springer-Verlag, 1985.

10. Bernstein, L. M., E. R. Siegel, and C. M. Goldstein, The Hepatitis Knowledge Base—A Prototype Information Transfer System, *Ann Internal Med,* 1980 93: (Part 2) 169-181.
11. From Gevarter, W. B., *An Overview of Artificial Intelligence and Robotics, Vol. 1—Artificial Intelligence*, NASA Technical Memorandum 85836, 1983 p4.
12. Van Bemmel, J., The Structure of Medical Informatics, *Medical Informatics* 1984 9(3). This special issue of *Medical Informatics* is devoted to the proceedings of a workshop on a Framework for Medical Information Science.
13. Shortliffe, E. H., The Science of Biomedical Computing, J. Anderson, F. Gremy, A. Levy and J. C. Pages (eds), *Information Science and Medical Education*, North Holland, 1984. Reprinted in *Medical Informatics* 1984 9(3).

Part II. Computer Systems

3
Overview of Hardware and Software

3.1. Introduction

In the early 1940s "computer" was a job title. A person was given a calculator and a set of formulae and then called a computer. The meaning of computer today is quite different. The computer now is something seen as an external, controlling force (as in "the computer is down"), or extension of one's persona (as in "*my* personal computer"), or simply as a useful tool. It is in this last role that we should consider the computer: that is, as a tool that performs some useful work. In this chapter we shall describe the computer system: the equipment and materials required to support computation and user applications.

It is common to divide the computer system into two basic units:

- *Hardware*. This includes all equipment used in computation for and interaction with the users of the computer system.
- *Software*. This includes all instructions used by the computer to carry out the users' requests. Software also includes documentation; in fact, all software is simply a form of written text.

Both hardware and software can be further subdivided as follows:

- *Computing unit*. This is frequently the least expensive hardware component. It contains (a) a central processing unit (CPU) that performs and controls the computation, (b) a memory to store the programs and data required for the processing, and (c) electronic paths (each called a bus) to other hardware units (called the peripherals).
- *Peripheral units*. These hardware units manage the transfer of information to and from the computer. Called input/output (or I/O) they also retain data and programs for longer term storage. Examples of I/O units are the terminal, which uses a cathode ray tube (CRT), a printer, and a bar code reader.
- *Systems software*. This is the collection of computer programs used by the hardware to manage its operations and also to transform and run application programs.
- *Application software*. These are the computer programs that provide services to the user.

There are no clear cut dividing lines separating these four categories. However, the separation does facilitate discussion. The hardware and systems software are typically purchased or leased. Frequently, one vendor will provide all components. It is also common for users to purchase components from multiple vendors or from a single integrating vendor. Many users also purchase or lease application software. A system as complex as a hospital information system is seldom developed locally. Where applications are developed locally, this is done through the process of system design and programming.

With this brief introduction, we shall now review how a computer works. As we have seen in Chapter 1, there have been four generations of computers: the vacuum tube, the transistorized integrated circuits (IC), and the two generations using chips with large scale integration (LSI) and very large scale integration (VLSI). The second-generation computers are the easiest to understand; they are a direct implementation of the von Neumann model. The fourth generation computers are essentially the same model; however, their larger size and scope make them a little more difficult to explain. We shall, therefore, begin with a description of the modern analog to the second generation computer system: the single user personal computer. Next we shall consider how the architecture has been modified to meet the needs of the current generation of large scale computers. Finally, we shall consider how computers can be networked to provide a unified resource.

3.2. The Personal Computer

A typical personal computer system consists of a processing unit, a keyboard for input, a display device for output, a printer, and a disk unit for permanent retention of programs and data. The processing unit, in turn, contains the central processing unit (CPU) and memory. This may be packaged as one or more physical units. A schematic diagram is shown in Fig. 3.1. Note that each of the units interfaces with the central processing unit, which manages all communication and coordination in this model.

3.2.1. Computer Memory

The memory contains the information immediately required for processing. It is organized in units called words. When processing is over, the contents of the memory are usually written over or erased. Thus, it is referred to as working memory. In Fig. 3.1, the working memory is divided into four sections. The top two contain system programs (fixed memory and variable memory), which are used by the computer to manage the processing of applications. Fixed or read only memory (ROM) can be read but not written into (changed) or erased. Variable or random-access memory (RAM) can be both read and written into. Both types of memory are read by supplying the address (location) of the word desired.

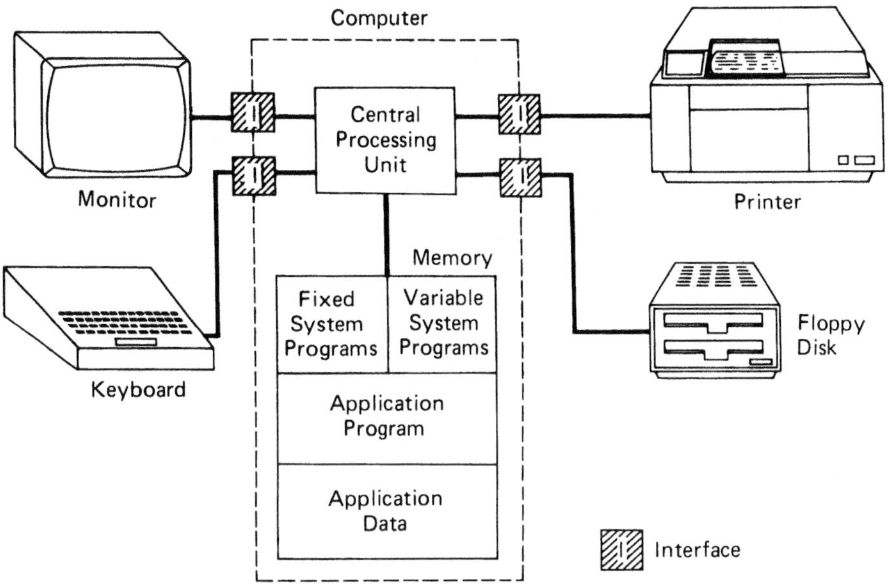

FIGURE 3.1. A typical small computer system.

Originally, all computer memory was RAM. An early technique was to use tiny doughnuts of magnetic material through which wires were passed. The direction of the magnetism was determined by the electricity flowing through the wires. These doughnut-shaped elements were called cores and acted as permanent (nonvolatile) memory for temporal changes in the current. Even today, RAM is often referred to as core memory even though the technology has changed.

Since core memory required mechanical assembly, it was relatively expensive. That has changed with the advent of the silicon chip, which can hold thousands of circuits. These memories represent data as a series of gates, which are either open (conducting) or closed (nonconducting). Today, most memories are comprised of metallic oxide semiconductors (MOS), and are called MOS memories. Unlike core memories, MOS memories lose all their information when the power is turned off; they are therefore said to be volatile. Larger computers normally use backup batteries to prevent loss of the contents of the MOS memory in the event of a power failure. An alternative to MOS is complementary metallic oxide semiconductors (CMOS), which are memories with very low power requirements. They can be powered by flashlight batteries, making them ideal for portable computers.

The advantage of ROM is its permanence; it stores programs that must be available and unchanged. There are several varieties of ROM. The standard ROM is designed for mass production. Programmable read only memory (PROM) is slightly more expensive than the standard ROM, but it allows the user to insert his own code. It is best in situations where ROM capabilities are desired, but mass production is inappropriate. Erasable programmable read only memory (EPROM) and electrically alterable programmable read only memory (EAPROM) have all of the permanence of ROM, but also allow writing into the memory under certain circumstances.

Memory is organized in units called words and bytes. (The byte has a fixed size; word size is a function of the computer design.) The working storage contains all of the instructions and data used by the CPU. Recall that Babbage used separate cards for the Analytical Engine's instructions (program) and variables (data). In the modern computer, both are stored in the same device, usually in separate areas. Each word (or byte) of program instruction or data is directly accessible by its address. The address is a number from zero to the number of bytes (or words) in memory (minus 1). For example, in a 64K memory, the addresses go from 0 to 65,535. (The symbol K represents 2^{10} or 1,024.)

3.2.2. The Central Processing Unit

The CPU performs all the processing by manipulating some special words called registers. It can transfer the contents of a word in memory to a register or from a register to memory. It can use the contents of a register to find the address of a word, and it can manipulate the contents of a register. Fig. 3.2 contains a more detailed view of the CPU. Note that it shows four types of registers:

- *Accumulators*: to perform arithmetic and logical functions (two accumulators—register 1 and register 2—are shown in Fig. 3.2; the number and types of registers varies with the computer)
- *Program counter*: to tell the address (location) of the next instruction to be executed
- *Data counter*: to hold the address of the data to be processed
- *Instruction register*: to hold the next CPU instruction to be processed.

In general, the application programs primarily use the accumulators. The other registers are used by the CPU to keep track of what it is to do (the program counter and instruction register) and where it is to get or store data (the data counter). Besides these registers, the CPU also contains a unit to perform addition, called the arithmetic and logic unit (ALU). Despite its name, the ALU does more than just arithmetic; it also must do shifting, complementing, Boolean logic, and other simple tasks.

To manage all this processing, there must be a control unit (CU). It transfers words to and from memory, loads the registers, and interprets the instruction register. It also processes the sequence of basic instructions used to produce more complex operations such as division and multiplication. In fact, the CU is a computer within a computer. Its instructions may be hardwired or written as microcode programs and stored in ROM.

The CPU connects the memory and peripheral interfaces through electrical pathways called buses. There is more than one type of bus. A data bus carries data from the ALU to and from the registers. An external bus communicates

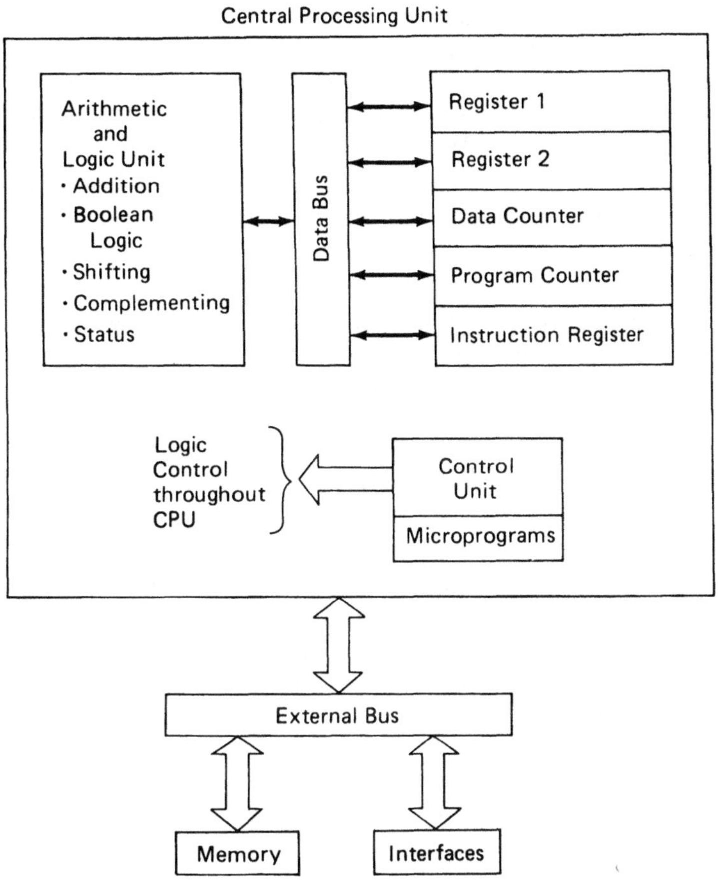

FIGURE 3.2. A central processing unit.

between the computer and the peripheral interfaces. This bus must carry all signals to and from the I/O devices.

Another integral part of the CPU is the clock. It produces regular, periodic voltage pulses that initiate and synchronize all the actions of the CPU. Clock frequency (or machine time) is measured in millions of cycles per second or megahertz (MHz). The clock also synchronizes activities throughout the entire computer; therefore, it must be located on the bus that links the memory and interfaces with the CPU.

The CPU contains some of the initial instructions of the computer, but not all of them. We start the computer by using some fixed code stored in ROM called the bootstrap. It does some processing and then sets the program counter so that another set of instructions can continue the processing. The program branches from one set of instructions to another by changing the program counter. Transfer of control goes from the bootstrap to the operating system which then manages the operation of the application programs.

A simple illustration will help to explain how the CPU coordinates processing. Consider, for example, the problem of adding A to B and storing the result in C. Three instructions would be given to the CPU as follows:

1. Take the number stored in location A and bring it to accumulator register 1.
2. Take the number stored in location B and add it to the contents of accumulator register 1.
3. Store the number in accumulator register 1 in location C.

This three-line sequence could be written as three instructions in an assembly language. To see what the CPU must do to carry out this sequence, consider the internal processing of the first instruction.

Assume that the program counter is pointing to the first instruction to be executed; i.e., load the contents of the word at memory address A into register 1. The CPU does the following:

1. Gets the word identified by the program counter and loads it into the instruction register.
2. Looks at the instruction, which indicates that the address of a word follows.
3. Adjusts the program counter to point to the next word of the program.
4. Loads this word (the address of A) into the data counter.
5. Starts processing the contents of the instruction register.
6. Reads the word whose address is indicated by the data counter and places it in the accumulator register.

While this may seem like a great deal of processing, the computer can perform millions of these steps in a second.

Note that we have used three levels of abstraction in this example:

- The problem statement:
  Let C = A + B
- The assembly language sequence (in simplified form):
  LOAD A into Register 1
  ADD B to Register 1
  STORE C from Register 1
- The microcode sequence.

The microcode is always delivered with the computer; it is designed by the development engineers. The assembly language programs are normally used only for some of the systems software. Thus, the general user is able to interact with the computer using some higher level language or application package. To understand how the higher level languages operate, it is necessary to learn how the contents of the words are formatted.

3.2.3. Word Contents and Formats

We know that all information in the computer is stored in the form of 1s and 0s, voltage on and off, gate open and closed. In this section we shall examine how these binary digits (bits) can be organized to represent data and support computation. We begin with a discussion of binary arithmetic.

3.2.3.1. The Binary Number System

When speaking of number systems, we say that the number of distinct digits is the base. In the decimal system, for example, there are 10 digits (0, 1, 2, . . . 9) and so the base is 10. Every number in this system is expressed as the sum of products of a digit and power of 10. For example, 3,409 is a short notation for

$$3 \times 10^3 + 4 \times 10^2 + 0 \times 10^1 + 9 \times 10^0$$

When we add two numbers, we line them up by their powers of 10, add the digits, and carry any amount over 9 to the next highest power of 10.

This concept is easily generalized for bases other than 10. In the case of the binary system, i.e., to the base 2, there are only two digits (0,1). As is true for any number system, every number is written as a sum of products of digits and powers of the base. Since there are only two binary digits, all binary numbers are strings of ones and zeros. For example, 10101 is the binary equivalent of the decimal number 21. To see why, consider

$$\begin{array}{llllll} 1\times 2^4 & + 0\times 2^3 & + 1\times 2^2 & + 0\times 2^1 & + 1\times 2^0 & = 10101 \text{ binary which is} \\ 16 & + 0 & + 4 & + 0 & + 1 & = 21 \text{ decimal} \end{array}$$

To avoid confusion, we sometimes write the base as a subscript after the number, e.g., $10101_2 = 21_{10}$.

With this introduction, there should be no trouble in counting to 10 in binary.

Decimal	Binary	Sum of Powers of 2
1	1	1
2	10	2+0
3	11	2+1
4	100	4+0+0
5	101	4+0+1
6	110	4+2+0
7	111	4+2+1
8	1000	8+0+0+0
9	1001	8+0+0+1
10	1010	8+0+2+0

3.2.3.2. Binary Arithmetic

Arithmetic for binary numbers (or numbers to any base, for that matter) is essentially the same as for decimal numbers. To add two numbers, we line up the digits according to the base power and add them up from the right. If the sum for any column is greater than that which can be expressed with the digits (0,1,2,. . . . 9 for the base ten, 0,1 for the base two), then we carry a 1 to the next highest base power. We call this an overflow if the next higher power has not been implemented, and thus a carry is not possible.

Without even concerning ourselves with the decimal representations of the following numbers, it is easy to see how they are added.

$$\begin{array}{r} 100101110 \\ +\ 110011011 \\ \hline 1011001001 \end{array}$$

Long binary numbers are hard to read. For this reason, there is a convention of grouping the bits by threes or fours starting from the right. We will follow the latter convention. It is also customary to write each set of 4 bits as a digit in a hexadecimal system (to the base 16). These digits are 0,1,2,. . .,A,B,C,D,E and F. Thus 0011 is 3 and 1111 is F. In the remainder of this section we shall use the binary notation for the sake of clarity.

To best explain subtraction, it is useful to present a concept of modern algebra called the additive inverse. Whenever we add a number to its additive inverse we get 0. For example:

$$3 + (-3) = 0$$

Mathematically, subtraction is possible because every number has an additive inverse. In fact, subtraction is really just the addition of an additive inverse. The following two problems are the same.

Subtraction	Addition
minuend	addend
subtrahend	inverse of subtrahend
difference	sum

This is important because the CPU has logic for addition. If we can convert subtraction to addition, then we can use this logic. We can compute the additive inverse in two steps. First we form a number which is called the ones complement. Wherever the original number has a 1 bit, this has a 0 bit, and vice versa. Then we add one and call this the twos complement. For example, consider the following 8 bit numbers

```
0010 0101 Number
1101 1010 Ones complement
1101 1011 Twos complement
```

Note that if you add a number to its twos complement, then the sum is a power of 2. Hence its name. In the above example

```
   0010 0101 Number
+  1101 1011 Twos complement
------------------------------
 1 0000 0000 Sum as a power of two
```

If we disregard all but the rightmost 8 bits in this example, then the answer is indeed 0.

Multiplication follows the same process used in decimal arithmetic except that the multiplication table is much smaller. Consider the following multiplication example without being concerned with the decimal values.

```
   101
 x 101
 -----
   101
  000
 101
 -----
 11001
```

Since we multiply by only 1s and 0s, we can convert the multiplication problem into a series of additions and shifts by looking at the bits in the multiplier. If the bit is a 1, we add the multiplicand to the partial product and shift the multiplicand 1 bit position to the left; if the bit is a 0, we simply shift. Since the CPU has logic for shifting as well as adding, we now understand how the computer does multiplication.

In this case we see that what to us is a single operation becomes to the computer a sequence of primitive operations. The result is that multiplication is more complicated to perform, and it takes longer. In fact, the length of time it takes to do a multiplication will depend on the number of 0s in the multiplier. The fewer the 0s, the more additions and the longer the processing time. The lesson from this: not all instructions have the same processing speed, and some processing speeds will vary with the data.

Division is carried out in much the same way as long division is performed with decimal digits. Subtraction is used instead of addition. The answer to a division operation contains two values: the quotient and the remainder.

3.2.3.3. Representing Numbers

In the normal use of decimal numbers, we write the numbers with varying lengths, for example 7, 3,461, and 83. In the case of a computer, the numbers of a given type are stored in words of a fixed length. This implies that the numbers must be stored in units of a fixed size with leading zeros. One standard unit for organizing bits is the byte: a sequence of 8 bits. As will be seen below, the byte has become the standard unit for all character codes. For this reason most machines use a word size that is a multiple of 8 bits.

The largest number that can be stored in a byte is 1111 1111 or $2^8 - 1$ or 255. If we set aside the first (leftmost) bit to serve as a sign bit, then the numbers that can be stored in a byte range from -127 to 127. One solution to storing larger numbers is to combine two consecutive bytes. In 16 bits one can fit a positive number as large as $2^{16} - 1$ or 65,535. If we use one bit to be the sign bit, then the range becomes -32,767 to 32,767. This size number is large enough for many applications; it is generally called an integer and the 16 bits are called the integer format.

Still, some problems require larger numbers or fractional values. We might deal with still larger numbers by employing 4 bytes (32 bits) as a unit. That leaves the problem of representing fractions, e.g., ⅔, 3.14, or 1.98. There are two ways of managing this: scaling the integers or using a form of scientific notation.

Scaling is simply the use of the binary equivalent of a decimal point. For example, in decimal arithmetic we normally add a decimal point and convert the fraction to an acceptable approximation. Thus, ⅔ rounded to four decimal places becomes 0.6667. When we add, we first line up the decimal points and then add in the normal manner. To do this in a computer, one uses a binary point. Since there is no way to record the binary point within the binary number, the user program must keep track of where the binary point is. In other words, the user program must know how the number is scaled. The use of scaling is common in applications where processing speed is critical. Yet, the use of this technique involves careful analysis to avoid inadvertent changes in scale. Fortunately, there is a more general and effective approach called floating point.

In scientific notation we normalize our numbers by representing them as a product of a value and a power of 10. For example,

$$.32 \times 10^{-4}$$
$$.765332 \times 10^{2}$$

We can modify this concept by storing a number as 4 bytes. The first byte will represent the signed exponent (as a power of 2) and the remaining 3 bytes will contain the signed value. The former is called the exponent or characteristic, the latter is called the mantissa. If we number the bits from right to left starting at 0 (i.e., the powers of 2), then the number might be stored in a format that looks like this:

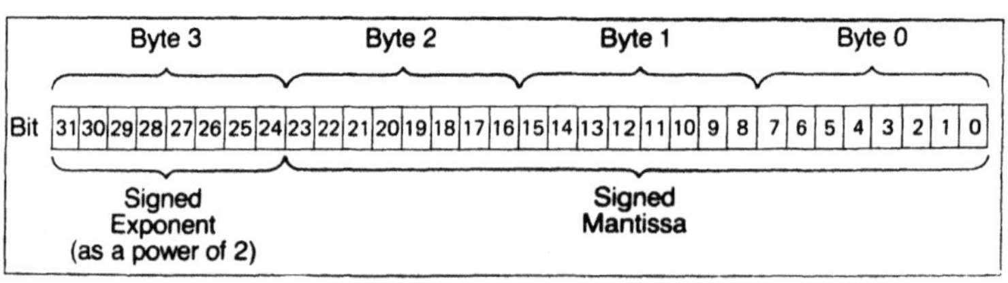

This is called floating point. Multiplication (division) involves adding (subtracting) the exponents, multiplying (dividing) the mantissas, and adjusting the exponents by removing leading zeros in the mantissas. Addition and subtraction are done by shifting the mantissa to get identical exponents and then adding or subtracting.

With floating point numbers, the absolute values range from 0.29×10^{-38} to 0.17×10^{39}. This is the most flexible representation for numbers, and it is essential for scientific computation. But one pays a price for this generality. Remember that the CPU operates using a sequence of primitive operations. In some machines, the use of floating point may result in 50:1 reduction in processing time. Fortunately, there are floating point hardware units designed to speed this operation; such hardware is standard for all larger computers.

In many cases, the floating point format does not provide sufficient accuracy. There are only 23 bits for the mantissa value which can store a number of about 4 million. This means that the result will be accurate to only 6 decimal places (i.e., there are decimal numbers of 7 or more digits that are too large to be represented in 23 bits). To store these numbers, double precision floating point is required. In this case, 8 bytes are combined to form a number with 1 or 2 bytes serving as the exponent and the remaining 7 or 6 acting as the mantissa. For some applications, triple precision is used.

3.2.3.4. Representing Characters

Virtually everything that passes to or from the computer begins or ends up as characters in some alphabet. The computer's alphabet contains 26 uppercase and 26 lowercase letters, 10 digits, some dozen punctuation marks, and several dozen special control characters that the hardware recognizes. Each of these characters has a unique code that can be expressed in one byte. For example, when the user types in "57" at a terminal, he actually enters an 8 bit code for "5" followed by an 8 bit code for "7." The computer's system software may then convert these codes to the binary number 0011 1001 which can be used for computation. In the same way, every time something is to be printed, the system software must convert the data to a string of codes that can be listed or displayed.

To eliminate errors in transmission, computer systems add a parity bit to detect invalid codes. If the parity is odd, the parity bit is set to either a 1 or 0 to guarantee that the code has an odd number of 1 bits. (There is also an even parity.) It is easy to design hardware to test the parity of each character processed and detect invalid codes. This is particularly useful when reading data stored on a magnetic media, such as a disk, in which specs of dust could cause a temporary error. When a parity error is detected, the system software will normally try to reread (rewrite) the character a fixed number of times. If the error persists, the job then aborts.

The use of 1 bit for parity checking will make the character longer. However, this is not really a problem since there are fewer than 128 codes in the computer's alphabet, and 128 codes can be expressed in 7 bits. The eighth bit, therefore, is available for use as the parity bit.

The American Standard Code for Information Interchange (ASCII) is the code used by all microcomputer applications. Each character is written as 7 bits. For example,

```
100 0001 stands for A
110 0001 stands for a
100 0010 stands for B
```

There is also a second code called the Extended Binary Coded Decimal Interchange Code (EBCDIC). This is an 8 bit code developed by IBM for larger computers. It does not require a parity bit because the hardware that processes it adds a parity bit. That is why we refer to 9-track tape—8 bits for the EBCDIC or ASCII code and 1 bit for parity. Many memories also use a ninth parity bit to verify their contents. Such parity bits are processed by the hardware and cannot be used by programs.

3.2.3.5. Logical and Physical Representations

It is a common practice when dealing with computers to differentiate between logical and physical entities. Logical entities are those that convey meaning. For example, an 8-bit character code, a 16-bit integer, a 32-bit floating point number, a 64-bit double precision number are all logical units. The word, on the other hand, is a physical unit. The word size is the number of bits that can be accessed as a unit. In an 8-bit microcomputer, the word size is 8 bits. To read a logical floating point number requires the reading of four physical words. In a 32-bit computer, the logical floating point number is stored in a single physical word. Four characters also fit in one physical word. Thus, the instruction set for the 32-bit computer normally provides facilities for accessing only part of a word, e.g., a specific byte.

3.2.4. The Peripheral Units

Although the CPU and memory are the essential components of a computer, peripheral units are required to make the computer an effective tool. These units include those that support human interaction and those that provide long-term or permanent storage. Both operate as I/O devices interfaced to the CPU.

3.2.4.1. User I/O Peripherals

A keyboard is still the standard means of communicating with the personal computer, although other modalities such as the mouse, touch screen, and voice are increasingly available. Each time a key is depressed an 8-bit code is sent to the computer. The computer then echoes that code back to a video display; the computer controls what is on the screen. The keyboard sends these 8-bit codes to the computer as fast as one can type.

The number of bits sent to the computer from a peripheral, such as a keyboard, in a fixed period of time is called the data rate. It is usually measured as bits of information per second (sometimes incorrectly called baud). You can estimate the number of characters sent per second by dividing the bit rate by 8.

Video output devices can display full pages (or screens) of output. Since this is done electronically, it can be done very quickly. The computer can write any character in any position on the screen. All that is necessary are the commands and circuitry to indicate where and how the character is to be printed, for example, upper- or lowercase, reverse video, half-tone, or blinking. Standards for these character placement modes are emerging; nevertheless, different terminals use different codes. From the viewpoint of data transmission, however, all character placement commands are just character strings to be sent to the output device.

Many computer systems are implemented so that the user can send output to alternative output devices. In this case, sending characters to a video display screen is the same as sending them to a printer. The only difference is that the printer is a mechanical device and cannot process the data as rapidly. Slower printers can operate at 30-45 characters per second. Higher speed printers on small computers can operate at 120-600 lines per minute. Larger computer systems, of course, use faster printing devices. Some nonmechanical laser printers, for example, print thousands of lines per minute.

When data are sent to a printer at a high baud rate, control signals are essential so that the printer can signal when it is ready to accept more characters. Where the system needs to transmit characters as fast as the device can print them, a buffer (temporary storage unit) is necessary. The buffer may be located in the computer memory, in the peripheral, or in special interfacing electronics. Characters are sent to the buffer, and the printing mechanism reads from it. This eliminates the need to synchronize the sending and printing as is necessary in some personal computers.

In some cases, the computer can store more than one line in a buffer; this way, the entire line is listed from the buffer. Some printers list every other line starting from the "back" of the buffer. This allows the printing mechanism to type left to right on one line and right to left on the next. All of this bidirectional logic is in the printer.

3.2.4.2. Permanent Storage

It is convenient to think of the personal computer's memory as working storage. It is relatively small—generally large enough for only one program at a time—and volatile—i.e., its contents vanish when the power is removed. What is desired, therefore, is a storage medium that is relatively large, comparatively inexpensive, and nonvolatile. We call this permanent storage.

The cheapest medium for permanent storage is some type of magnetic material. It is permanent, erasable, and reusable. Magnetic materials are available in several forms; the oldest and least expensive are rolls of tape. Many of the early, low-cost microcomputer systems used inexpensive tape recorders and tape cassettes as input/output devices. Input/output (I/O) was very slow and somewhat unreliable. Duplicating everything compensated for the unreliability, but it made the entire process even slower. The main disadvantage of magnetic tape, however, is that it is a serial device, meaning that one must read through all of the earlier contents of the tape to get at material at the end. One cannot quickly jump around. Nevertheless, magnetic tape exchange for larger computers has been standardized, and it remains the most reliable and inexpensive exchange media for data and programs.

The disk (or disc) is a flat storage medium covered with a thin film of magnetic material. It is read and written onto by a unit that spins the disk and places a magnetic read/write head over any portion of the disk. Unlike the tape, the disk is a random access device; you can quickly access any part of it. Disks are available in several forms. The floppy disk is a small (usually 3½, 5¼ or 8 inches in diameter), flexible disk of magnetic material encased in a protective envelope. The Winchester disk, one type of hard disk, has one or more rigid disks coated with a magnetic surface and mounted in a hermetically sealed container. Still another form of disk allows you to load and unload the disk packs (the recording media) into the disk unit (the read/write device).

The data on the disk are recorded in a series of concentric circles called tracks. Within these tracks, data are broken down into blocks (or sectors). Each block can contain from a fraction of a K to several K bytes depending on the size of the computer. The block is the physical unit for the disk just as the word is the physical unit for internal memory.

To read data from a disk, you must first indicate which track you want. There is usually only one read/write head per surface that moves radially from the outer to the inner margin of the disk, track to track. If the disk has more than one surface, these surfaces are mounted on top of one another, like the records in a jukebox. Each surface has its own read/write head, and all the heads move together over the same track. The set of tracks for all surfaces is called a cylinder.

Much of the outer portion of the surface is left blank. You can tell where a block begins by formating the disk; codes are written out that indicate the location and contents of each block. Disks also have a physical mechanism to provide them with a fixed reference point. In the case of a floppy disk, it is the small hole in the cover near the center. This allows the disk to synchronize as it senses a physical mark.

The speed at which a disk can be read or written depends on how fast the disk spins and how densely recorded the data are. Floppy disks run slowly. The read/write head rests directly on the disk and could damage it if the disk spins too quickly. The capacity of a floppy disk can be increased by using both sides of the disk (double-sided) or adjusting the number of tracks recorded. Depending on the format, double-sided, floppy disks currently store between 380,000 and 1,200,000 characters.

Since hard disks do not let the read/write head touch the surface, they can spin much faster. But hard disks have their problems, too: dust or dirt can scratch the magnetic surface, and the read/write head must be aligned and maintained. As the disk spins faster, the storage density increases, and the tolerance to dust, dirt, and misalignment decreases. Winchester disks have overcome these problems by sealing the unit in a clean chamber and using servos (to control the head position). The accuracy required for these units has been compared to the flight of a 747 jet at an altitude of 0.1 inch off the ground covering a distance of several miles without bumping its wheels. When the head touches the disk surface, it is called a head crash and the unit is physically destroyed. The data stored on the disk are lost.

To protect against loss of permanent data due to hardware failure or human error, devices are normally copied using a process called backup. For removable disks, a spare disk is mounted and the latest version of permanent storage is copied onto it. Generally three generations of permanent storage are retained (the grandfather system). Since Winchester disks are not removable, they need something to back them up. For smaller units, this means copying to a floppy disk. For larger units a high-speed, dedicated tape unit may be provided.

3.2.4.3. Interfacing the I/O Devices

There are two types of I/O interfaces: one for the relatively slow devices, such as keyboards and video displays, and one for faster devices, such as disks. The interfaces receive their signals from the computer's external bus. At the other end, the I/O devices also communicate through interfaces. When these interfaces share the same connections and logic, the computer can communicate with the I/O device.

Interfaces can be serial or parallel. Serial transmission sends 1 bit at a time (together with control signals); parallel transmission sends one or more bytes at a time. For slower data rates, a serial interface is used; for high data rates, a parallel interface is used. For most personal computers, the interface between the CPU and the CRT/keyboard terminal is designed to send one ASCII character at a time. This is called asynchronous ASCII transmission; it allows the easy interchange of data. In some larger systems, data are sent in a continuous stream of characters at one time. This block mode is called synchronous transmission. It is faster, but requires more specialized terminals and I/O ports. In general, all smaller computers use serial transmission for these slower character-by-character transfers. The exception is the printer that can be configured with either a serial or a parallel interface.

Every computer has a fixed number of interfaces for I/O, and each interface is called an I/O port. It consists of a buffer and a connection. The transferring of data to or from this device is done by loading or unloading the contents of the buffer. For example, when one depresses a key on the keyboard, an 8-bit code is selected, sent across the communication lines one bit at a time, and stored in the I/O port's buffer. When transmission is complete, the computer reads the contents of the buffer to a register, then stores it in RAM, echoes it to the video display, or does whatever the operating system has programmed the computer to do with it. The peripheral may also have a device of its own for communications and error checking. This is called a controller and normally comes on a printed circuit that can be plugged into the computer's bus.

Control signals govern the communication between the I/O device and the computer. In the data transfer just described, the buffer is used to hold and pass the data. However, if the CPU does not read the contents of the I/O port's buffer quickly enough, the next input to the buffer will write over the previous input and the data will be lost. There are two ways to avoid this. In smaller computers the system may be placed in a mode of constantly examining control (status) bits to see if the transmission is complete. But the processing of I/O transfers is considerably slower than the processing of data in the CPU (e.g., 1,200 baud compared to 10 MHz). Thus the constant examination of status words is an inefficient use of the computers' resources. As a result, many smaller and all larger systems initiate an I/O operation and resume with the processing of other functions. When the I/O process is completed, an interrupt is issued that stops the CPU processing and passes a message (i.e., status word). Interrupts are a common method for managing error detection (e.g., a hardware fault), I/O processing, and program control.

To avoid having to send each transmitted character through the CPU, a technique called direct memory access (DMA) is used to link the I/O device directly to a block (or buffer) in memory. The use of I/O interrupts and DMA allows the computer to process programs asynchronously and I/O concurrently. Of course, if the computer is organized to perform only one task at a time, there may be nothing for the CPU to do during the I/O process. The management of the CPU resources is one of the responsibilities of the operating system: the topic of the next subsection.

3.2.5. The Operating System

The operating system is the system software that directs the hardware processes in performing the tasks specified by the application programs. In general, the operating system does even more. It also provides an environment for the easy development and execution of applications. To gain an understanding of what functions the operating system must perform, we consider a very simple single user computer system.

As shown in Fig. 3.3, a computer memory can be subdivided into four logical components:

- *The fixed system programs*. These are stored in ROM. The bootstrap program is an example of such a program. When the computer is turned on it causes other programs to be loaded and executed.
- *The variable system programs*. These are normally retained in permanent storage and are loaded into working storage as they are needed. The bootstrap program generally causes one or more of these programs to be loaded. Because RAM is volatile, these programs are lost when the power is turned off. Thus, they must be loaded each time they are used; alternatively they may be provided as part of the fixed system (ROM).
- *The application programs*. These are always retained in permanent storage. The operating system must load the desired program into memory and then transfer control to it, i.e., allow the CPU to process the application program instructions.
- *The application data*. As we have seen, all memory is organized as words. It is impossible to determine from the contents of a word if it is an instruction, an integer, or part of a double-precision floating point number. Consequently, most operating systems separate the programs (which should not be altered) and the data (which normally are altered). Each is stored in a separate block and only certain privileged programs (i.e., programs operating in a privileged mode) are allowed to modify the contents of an application program.

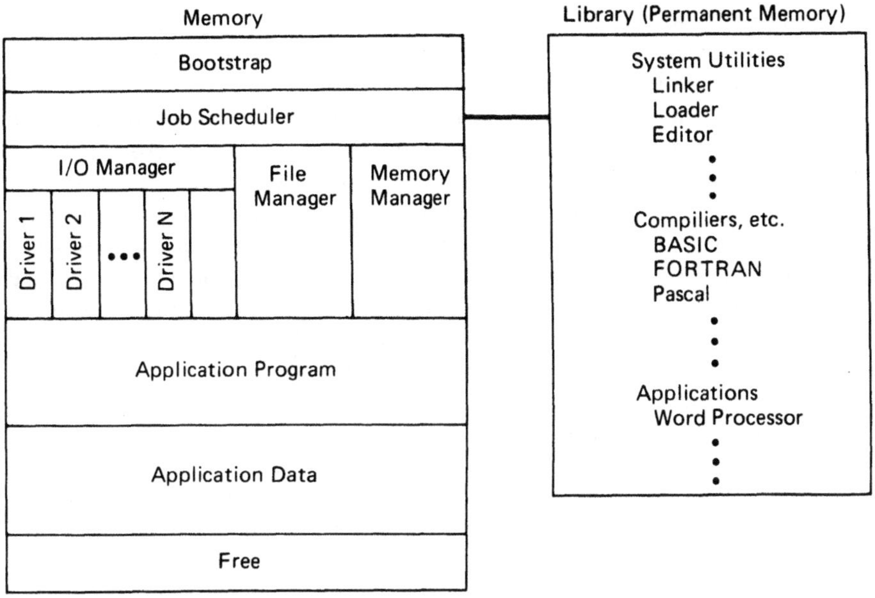

FIGURE 3.3. The operating system and memory.

Given this allocation of memory, consider the sequence of operations that must go on from the time the computer is turned on until an application is run. In this case, the application NAME will ask for a patient's name and print it on a form. The sequence begins with turning on the machine.

- The bootstrap program is initiated. It loads a control program from permanent storage into working storage and transfers control to this program.
- The control program requests commands from the user to establish what the computer is to do. The command is to run the application NAME.
- The control program now loads the NAME program and initial data from permanent storage to working storage. It then sends control to the first instruction in NAME.
- NAME writes a message to enter the patient's name and waits until a "return" has been entered. It stores the data entered before the "return" in its application data memory area and then starts to print out the required form.

In this brief scenario there are several I/O activities. The loading of the bootstrap and control programs each brings data from a device (normally a disk) into memory. Data on the disk are stored in blocks of about 1K bytes. These must be stored in specific locations in working memory (or, hereafter, simply memory). A second type of I/O activity were the queries to the user. The first query was by the control program to find what should be done, and the second was by the application program to find the patient's name. Each of these requests resulted in a wait until the user enters in the request or name or the "return" to signal that the entry was complete. Finally, there is an I/O to the printer to list the forms with the patient's name.

Four I/O operations were identified: to the disk, to the terminal screen, from the keyboard, and to the printer. For each kind of device, a separate device driver (or handler) is required. The device driver prepares data to be sent or received, waits if the device is not ready to receive additional data, manages faults, indicators, and sends interrupts to the CPU. An I/O Manager coordinates the requests from the system and application programs and directs them to and from the device drivers. Among these functions are the opening and closing of a device to establish and relinquish ownership. (This eliminates the possibility of two tasks listing on one printer at the same time.)

The process of loading a program from the disk (i.e., permanent memory) involves two issues. First, the program to be loaded must be found on the disk; that is, its logical name (e.g., NAME) must be associated with the blocks on the disk that contain the program. All data in permanent storage are organized in logical units called files. The application programs, in this case, are simply data to be processed by the operating system load program. To find the desired data, a file manager program is used. It accepts the logical name and—by using a series of directories—identifies the physical device and physical location. This information is then passed to the I/O manager to access and load the program.

Once the program is loaded in memory, it is stored in words and must contain all the information necessary for processing. For example, in the previous C = A + B example, we suggested that this could be implemented with the assembly language sequence

```
LOAD     A into Register 1
ADD      B to Register 1
STORE    C from Register 1
```

In this case, the address of the words containing A, B, and C must be known. These addresses can be expressed in one of two ways:

- *Absolute address*. For example, the address of A is set to the word with hexadecimal address 1A00. This disadvantage of absolute addresses is that the program must be designed to be loaded in a specific section of memory and no other program can use that memory at the same time.
- *Relative address*. In this case, the memory is divided into pages of from 256 bytes to several K words. Each page has a starting address and each storage location is given as a value relative to that starting address. For example, the address of A might be hexadecimal A2 plus the starting address of the page containing the application data. Using this technique, the application data can be loaded into any available page of memory; the addressing of an individual word takes advantage of the CPU register's ability to add the page address to the relative address.

Clearly, all modern computers use some form of relative addressing with the identification of free pages. The computing of the page address is part of loader program's responsibility.

Closely associated with the loader is a linker or linking program. Its responsibility is to allow communications among programs in an application. In general, programs are divided into smaller logical units called subroutines that are combined to form the application. Examples of subroutines are programs to list a file, compute a square root, or read an input from the keyboard. Most subroutines are used with many applications. It is the responsibility of the link-loader combination to identify the required subroutines and load them into memory so that they may communicate with each other.

Finally, the operating system provides utilities to support program development. For example, there is normally an editor used to enter and modify programs. There are normally one or more languages supported by a system. These may include an assembly language (which, as in the above example, is very similar to the actual machine instructions), or some high order languages (HOL) such as BASIC, FORTRAN, or Pascal. Each program is written as source code in the programming language. This source code is converted into object code by a compiler (for HOLs) or an assembler. The loader program uses only the object code.

The contents of memory for a single user system is shown in Fig. 3.3. Most of the memory in this example has been allocated. The free space is generally used as buffers for I/O. Because the speed of I/O devices is slow relative to the CPU speed, it is sometimes effective to store blocks of data in buffers in the free space. If these blocks are requested again, they may be retrieved from the free space more rapidly than they could be from the permanent memory device. In some cases, however, there may not be enough room in memory for the entire application. When this occurs, one may design the application as separate parts that can be loaded into the memory as units. This is called overlaying the program. Alternatively, the operating system may be designed to treat each page of memory independently. Pages will be entered into memory as space is available. During execution, if a page is required that is not in memory, then processing stops while the page is loaded on top of a page that the system believes to be no longer necessary. Processing then can resume. This is called a virtual memory system. It allows the execution of programs that are logically far larger than the physical memory. In the case of overlays, the designer must manage how the limited memory is to be used; with virtual memory this is all controlled by the operating system.

3.2.6. Summary of the Personal Computer

We have described how a computer works by using the single user personal computer as an example. These systems have been designed to support just one user. This simplifies memory management and limits the number of processes that must go on at one time. In some computers, no processing is done while waiting for a user to enter data from a keyboard; in other cases the computer can print output or process a disk in parallel with the input process. Nevertheless, the personal computer provides a good model for understanding how the second generation computers worked and how they were supported by their operating systems.

In the next section we shall discuss how the size and speed of the third- and fourth-generation computers added complexity and how the architectures and operating systems were modified to meet these new needs.

3.3. The Multiuser Environment

The availability of inexpensive, large-scale integration (LSI) transformed the second-generation computers from batch-oriented, one-job-at-a-time devices into computers that were too large and too fast to justify dedication to a single job. The result was multiprogramming in which more than one application program resides in memory and the CPU shares its time among the programs. Since the computer still uses the von Neumann architecture, there is a single path between the CPU and memory. The apparent parallelism is managed by distinguishing between the periods that an application program can use the CPU and the periods when the program is waiting for some other activity to complete. During the latter times, the CPU can be assigned to a different program.

3.3.1. Multiuser Hardware Configurations

To understand this process better, consider the functions a computer can perform and the length of time it takes for each function to be completed. As we have seen, the CPU can read from and write to memory and manipulate data in its registers. With larger computers this process is measured in units of millions of instructions per second (MIPS). Input and output to users is considerably slower. The typical CRT terminal operates at 9,600 baud, which is about a screenful in 1 or 2 seconds; far slower than the CPU. Printing devices have comparable speeds. Few mechanical printers can produce a full page in less than a second or two; nonmechanical printers may be an order of magnitude faster.

The computer also reads and writes blocks of data for the purpose of permanent storage—generally on an electromechanical device, a disk. Three steps are required to perform this function. First the write head must be positioned over the track that contains the desired block. Next the mechanism must remain in a wait state until the desired block is positioned under the read head. Finally, the block must be read or written. The slowest of these processes is the first: seeking the proper track. It is primarily a physical activity. Because the time to access a block will depend on the relative positions of the read head and the desired track, the time to read a block will vary. In mid-sized systems, the total transmission time will vary from 25 to 100 milliseconds for a 1,000-character block.

Thus we see that computer operations include processes in the CPU that are measured in nanoseconds and I/O processes that are measured in miliseconds. For efficiency, the CPU must manage the I/O processes as separate tasks rather than remain idle while waiting for an I/O process to complete. Task management is supported by both hardware and the operating system. The method is straightforward. Say, for example, that a computer is to write out some data. First the data are moved to a block of words in memory called a buffer. Once the data have been moved to that buffer they have been logically written out; that is, the application program has completed the process of writing and can no longer access or modify what it has written out. After the buffer has been filled, a request to write the buffer to the desired device (disk, printer, CRT, etc.) is entered into a queue. Depending on the operating system, this queue may be periodically examined or be processed by using interrupts.

The actual transfer of data from the buffer to the output device generally relies on a separate device—the device controller—with its own microcomputer system. This is given a sequence of commands that define where the buffer is to be found and where the data are to be stored. Once started, the controller can operate independently. By using DMA (direct memory access) it can read (or write) directly from (to) the buffer. In the case of a disk, the controller is responsible for moving (some or all of) the data to its local buffer, positioning the read head over the proper track and block sector, and then transferring the data.

While this is being done, the CPU is free to perform other functions. When the transfer is complete, the controller sends an interrupt to the CPU to indicate that it has completed successfully (or with a failure). When interrupted, the CPU saves the key registers so that it can resume its current processing after the interrupt has been examined. Interrupts have priority levels associated with them, and the operating system may elect to act immediately or simply save some key information for later processing. After an interrupt has been processed, the saved registers are restored and the machine is restored to its state before the interrupt. Processing resumes with no perceptible change to the application that had been interrupted.

Thus, as we have seen, the disparity in speeds between the CPU and the I/O devices requires parallel processing (or concurrency) for efficiency. However, if only one program were available to be processed, there would be little for the CPU to do once an I/O operation was initiated. Fortunately, the large memory size allows the storage of more than one program at a time. Thus, when one program initiates an I/O activity, the I/O is begun and the program is placed in a wait state (i.e., the contents of the key registers are saved for later resumption of processing.) The operating system then selects the next program in memory that is not in a wait state, loads its registers into the CPU, and resumes operations of that application. Processing of the application terminates when either it requests an I/O activity, or it exceeds a predetermined period of processing time. It is then placed in a wait state, and the process continues.

In this way the CPU can be allocated to many different programs in turn.

Generally, interrupts require little computation and are processed at once. The overlap between I/O and computing allows several processes to continue concurrently. When there is little I/O activity, the CPU spends most of its time processing applications. In this case, we say that the system is compute bound. That is, the throughput (i.e., work performed) is limited by the processing speed of the CPU. Conversely, when there is a great deal of I/O activity, the CPU may be idle because all the active programs are waiting for an I/O activity to terminate. In this case, the system is said to be I/O bound.

Most systems have a balanced workload that is neither compute- nor I/O-bound. Some applications, however, involve a great deal of computational processing. Fortunately, in many of these cases, the data to be processed can be organized as vectors, e.g., a triple such as wind speed, temperature, direction for a weather-modeling application or shades of red, green, blue for a picture element (pixel) used in an image processing application. For these applications, vector processors (sometimes called array processors) have more than one CPU so that they can perform the identical processing on each element of the vector in a single processing cycle. That is how the large "number crunching" computers such as the Cray-1, ILLIAC-IV, and Star-100 are configured. Smaller scale versions of this architecture are also used in image processing.

When a system is I/O bound one can add more devices and controllers to manage them. However, if all the controllers must access memory using a common bus, the bus may become a bottleneck. Thus, most large data processing configurations use a more complex architecture than that described for the personal computer. In this case the bus is called a channel and more than one channel can be used for I/O at one time.

Finally, we note that the computer architectures described are based on the von Neumann model. There is a single processor and path to memory. For I/O applications, the processor can initiate an I/O process and allow it to be completed asynchronously. For vector processors, a group of CPUs can be operated in tandem with a single path. Thus, in each case there is a serial path to the CPU(s) that controls all operations. Concurrency exists only to the extent that it is initiated and controlled by the CPU.

This form of the multiuser system became popular as soon as the CPU became so fast and the memory so large that one could not justify dedicating so powerful a system to a single application. We now see VLSI technology advancing to the point where it will be economically feasible to replace the single CPU with multiple processors. Indeed, to achieve the next step in performance improvement, it will be necessary to have multiple processors and multiple paths between processors and memory. This will no longer reflect the von Neumann model, and it will have a major impact on operating systems and programming languages. When there is true parallel operation, how does one break a serial process into many independent processes that can be performed concurrently? This, and similar questions, are being addressed today. It is not clear what the outcome will be, but it is reasonably certain that the computer technology of the fifth generation will provide some answers.

3.3.2. Multiuser Operating Systems

The purpose of an operating system is to facilitate the use of the computer system. In the case of general purpose, multiuser systems this involves (a) providing an environment that is easy to use and (b) managing the application functions so that they can be processed by the computer system. That is, from a user's point of view, the operating system is the interface between the application and the hardware.

Within the computer system, the operating system performs the following:

- Manages the processor by interleaving periods of CPU activities for programs. These programs are both application and system programs. (To the operating system, the system is the application.) It also handles interrupts and must synchronize access to shared resources. A shared resource is a facility that may be used by more than one application, for example a disk unit or a file on a disk.
- Manages the memory by allocating memory to programs as they require it. The basic memory unit is the page. Virtual systems read pages into memory as they are required and release pages as space is required. Some machines also have a very fast memory, called cache memory, that can be more rapidly accessed by the CPU. In this case, the operating system must also manage cache contents for the most efficient processing.
- Manages the peripheral devices by initiating I/O requests, maintaining queues, and reporting completion. The completion may be normal or abnormal. In the latter case a decision to alarm, retry, abort or take another action is required.
- Manages program initiation and interprogram communication. Program initiation generally requires access to data residing on a disk (i.e., use of the device management function) and the loading of the data into memory (i.e., use of the memory management function). Thus, the programs in an operating system sometimes are processed as application programs by the operating system, and the programs on disk are treated as data by the operating system.
- Manages data by supporting the creation, opening, closing, reading, and writing of files. Files are the logical sets of data stored in permanent memory. Files may contain programs or application data. Opening a file indicates that that file is assigned to a given application. To avoid conflicts, many systems will allow a file to be opened by only one program at a time. The close releases the file.

The external structure of an operating system may be very simple or very complex. The MUMPS operating system was designed to support only the MUMPS language (see Chapter 4) and applications written in that language. Since its goals are limited, it can be activated with half a dozen keystrokes. Once active, one can either create programs or run programs without any further operating system interactions. With a general purpose system, however, there are many more options to choose from and the process of selection can involve a great deal of user/operating system interaction. In what follows, two common operating systems are examined.

3.3.2.1. IBM MVS Operating System

The IBM 360 computer was the first of the third generation computers. Therefore, the first third generation operating system was developed for it. Called OS/360, this system has undergone continuous evolution. The 360 computer has been succeeded by the 370 and then the 30XX and 43XX computers, and OS/360 has evolved into the Multiple Virtual Storage (MVS) operating system. It is clear from the previous discussion that MVS must support multiprogramming, virtual storage, workload management, etc. In what follows, we shall identify a few of the additional functions a general purpose operating system such as MVS must manage.

In the MVS terminology, a task is the execution of a program. (Other systems call this a process.) A task may be an application program, a compiler, or a portion of the application program. A sequence of tasks may be scheduled with files used to communicate between independent tasks. For example, suppose a source program (i.e., in the programming language) exists in a file and it is desired to compile that program, save the resulting object (i.e., compiled) program, and then execute the program if it was compiled successfully. By using a job control language (JCL), one would indicate to MVS what file contained the source code, what file should contain the resultant object program, what compiler should be used, and on what condition the compilation should be followed by an execution of the compiled program.

In this sequence, the compiler uses a logical name for the input (source) and output (object) files, for example, INFILE and OUTFILE. Through the JCL, one can associate specific source and object files with the compiler's input and output. These source and object file names are logical names that are linked, using the JCL, to physical devices and locations. Thus the compiler can accept an input file from a disk, or magnetic tape, or floppy disk. This property is called device independence, and one function of the JCL (and the operating system) is to link the logical name of a file with the specific file (and associated device) that is to be used, i.e., its physical location.

Because a system such as MVS supports many applications at the same time, it must manage the output to avoid conflicts. For example, if 10 programs are running at one time, each producing printed output, it is necessary to control the printing of the output so that no job can access the printer until the current job is completed. This is done through a process called spooling. A task writes to an output file. The output file "looks like" the printer to the task program, but it is really a device independent file. When the task is completed, the output file is closed and placed in a queue for the printing program. When the printer is free, the file is opened as an input to the print program and the printing device is opened as the output device. In this way, only one task will print at a time. Further, since the original task is now complete, the printer can operate at full speed; there will be no delays for task computations.

Table 3.1 summarizes the features of MVS and also suggests the evolution of IBM operating systems from the 701 to the systems of the 1980s. Many of the advanced features of the IBM operating systems are transparent to the user. The very power of the system, however, frequently forces a user to communicate with the operating system using JCL. For frequently executed processes, such as compile and execute, there are catalogued JCL procedures that allow the user to simply specify file names or other selected parameters. For many other tasks, however, the JCL is clumsy and time-consuming. This awkwardness of the JCL is not limited to the IBM operating systems. Since the JCL was developed as a solution to problems in batch-oriented environments, JCL remains an integral part of most operating systems with batch origins.

3.3.2.2. The UNIX Operating System

The UNIX* Operating System provides an interesting contrast to MVS. MVS is part of an evolutionary development designed for a broad range of applications to be run on a large number of different computer configurations. The diversity of the target computers requires generality in the design. UNIX, on the other hand, was initially designed for internal use only. Its success can be attributed to three basic factors. First, it provides an effective user interface that is very natural for program development. Second, because UNIX operates on minicomputers and the UNIX license was almost free for educationl purposes, UNIX has become a standard programming environment in many computer science departments. Finally, because UNIX and look-alike systems become available for many manufacturer's equipment, it provides an alternative standard for hardware independent government procurements.

UNIX was designed for interactive use, i.e., time sharing. Rather than apply the JCL concept, UNIX uses a command interpreter called the shell. All user interactions are with the shell; the shell creates tasks to be executed by the kernel of the operating system; pipes can be used to transfer data between programs (tasks). The result is a very flexible environment that is well suited to a modular, "tool set" orientation. To understand how UNIX differs from systems such as MVS, one must first understand how tasks are normally managed.

In the single user environment described earlier in this chapter, an application program is loaded into memory as two parts: the program (in a write protected area) and the data (in an area that can be both read and written). The application must be complete; this means that all the subroutines it will use (e.g., the square root subroutine) must be loaded with it. As we have seen, it is the responsibility of the link-load function to combine the complete application before control is passed to it. Once loaded in memory, the application has access to every function it may need to use.

To illustrate this, assume that one of the functions of an application is to compute a standard deviation. The application may have to load a subroutine to

---

*UNIX is a trademark of AT&T.

TABLE 3.1. Capabilities of MVS and its IBM predecessors.

		Extensions of function	
Generation	Operations	Hardware functions	Applications functions
Preoperating system (early 1950s) with, e.g., the 701	Manual (e.g., each job step required manual intervention) No multiple-application environment support	Symbolic assembler Linking loader	Subroutine libraries in card tubs, manual retrival
First generation (late 1950s and early 1960s) with, e.g., FMS, IBSYS on the IBM 704, 709, and 7094	Automatic job batching Manual device allocation, setup, work load scheduling No multiple-application environment support Off-line peripheral operations	Higher level languages—FORTRAN, COBOL Primitive data access services with error recovery	Subroutine libraries on tape, automatic retrieval Primitive program overlay support
Second generation (late 1960s) with e.g. OS/360 on System/360	Multiprogramming Primitive work load management Primitive tuning (device, core allocation) Spooling, remote job entry Operator begins to be driven by the system Primitive application protection Initial multiprocessing (loosely and tightly coupled)	More higher level languages—PL/1, ALGOL, APL, BASIC Device independence in data access First random access data organizations Primitive software error recovery, full hardware ERPs Array of hardware function extensions Supervisor call routines	DASD subroutine libraries Full facilities for programmed overlays Interactive program development support Primitive automatic debugging aids First application subsystems Checkpoint/restart
Third generation with e.g., MVS OS/VS on System/370	Integrated multiprocessing (loosely and tightly coupled) Work load management extensions More self-tuning, integrated measurement facilities Less operator decision-making, fewer manual operations Full interapplication protection, data and program authorization Primitive storage hierarchies for data	Virtual storage Device independence extended Hardware error recovery extended to CPU, channels Operating system functions begin to migrate to hardware	Growing libraries Overlay techniques obsoleted by virtual storage Symbolic debugging aids Primitive data independence Integration of application subsystems Software error recovery for system and applications

From M.A. Auslander, D.C. Larkin, and A.L. Sherr, The Evolution of the MVS Operating System, IBM *Journal of Research and Development* 25:471–482, 1981.

compute the standard deviation. This subroutine, in turn, uses the square root subroutine which, in turn, must be loaded. In short, every program or function that may be required must be available *before* the execution of the application begins. In a virtual memory system, the programs may not be physically stored in internal memory. Nevertheless, all application and system programs are logically combined before any can be used. Thus, although the application program may be very general, it will not be able to perform any functions that have not already been linked and loaded. For example, when a personal computer user is working with a spread sheet program and wishes to integrate the output with some text, he must write the spread sheet text to a file, load the word processing application, and then read the file just created to edit it. (This assumes that the file formats are compatible.)

The same basic structure is also used in a typical multiuser environment. We will use the analogy of how the spooler accepts output from one program and then uses this file as input to a printing program. We spoke of device independence as being a factor that made the printer and the output file "look" the same to the application program. The application that produces the output is, of course, a complete package; once loaded it cannot perform any functions beyond those it was programmed to perform. The spooler is also a complete package that performs a different, but limited, number of functions. For the application (and the spooler) the machine state is defined by the program and data contents of memory; the application program processes its data and sends output to be printed. It sends the output to a file; this output can be thought of as a "message" to the spooler. In general, the message is not sent until the last line of output has been sent. The message then is, "Processing complete, please enter this file into the queue for printing by the spooler." Conceptually, one could think of each output line as being the message, "Put this line in the output queue for printing by the spooler as part of this program's output."

Notice that there are two distinct processes going on. In one process, the application program uses its data and all the subroutines already loaded to perform its desired functions. In the second process, it sends "messages" to another independent program to perform some function that the application program was not programmed to do. (In the case of the spooler, the function is the management of the printer and the interleaving of multiple outputs.) One can make the application program more powerful by adding to its functions and making it longer. Alternatively, one can use the operating system to facilitate communications (message passing) between independent applications. In this way, each application still must be complete, but a job may be constructed by sequencing a series of smaller applications and having them communicate by the passing of messages. The MVS operating system previously discussed treats each application as a complete program; message passing is limited to selected system functions such as spooling. UNIX, on the other hand, is designed to support communication between independent applications.

The primary mode of communication is the file. In UNIX, all files "look" alike to the applications, and therefore it is simple to transfer them between programs. The files are considered long strings of characters. That is, even though they may be physically broken into blocks that are stored in tracks on a specific disk, the logical view of the file is one of a continuous string of bytes. Thus one can request the first 10 bytes of the file, the 120 characters following the last byte read, etc. The files are named in a directory; the directory is itself a file. The fact that the physical structure of the file is transparent to the user program makes it very easy to interface independent tasks.

For example, consider a program to copy data from one file to another. There is a UNIX program, COPY, that does this. The shell command interpreter (which takes the place of JCL) requests an input and an output. One can enter

```
COPY FILE1 FILE2
```

to copy the contents of FILE1 into FILE2.† Since the format of the file is already known and the directory (and hence location) of the files is established during the process of logging on, no further information is required. To copy the file to the printer, one could write

```
COPY FILE1 /DEVICE/PRINTER
```

(That is, copy FILE1 to the device called PRINTER.) To list a tape one could write

```
COPY /DEVICE/TAPE /DEVICE/PRINTER
```

In each case COPY is a program (task) that copies the contents of the first named file to the second named file. COPY has been compiled, linked, and loaded and is a complete program. It derives its generality from the fact that it is not bound to a specific input or output file. (MVS provides programs that perform the same function using JCL.)

In this simple example, the user communicates with the shell which then sets up the programs to be executed. In some cases, the shell will execute a series of programs when one command is entered. The shell is, itself, a program that can be modified. Thus, the user can even tailor the command language to his needs.

Another example will clarify further how UNIX operates. Files contain data; the list of files for a given user is contained in a directory that is defined when he logs in. The program LS will list on the terminal the names of the files in the current directory. The program PR will print a file in multiple columns with headings, and the program LPR will send a file to the spooler for printing. Table 3.2 illustrates two ways of sequencing the commands to print every file in the current directory in a four column format. The first technique uses intermediate files; that is, the output of one step is used as the input to the next step. The second technique uses a pipeline (or pipe) to connect the processes. This causes

†UNIX normally uses lowercase in commands. Uppercase is used here to improve legibility.

TABLE 3.2. UNIX command sequence examples.

<table>
<tr><th>UNIX command</th><th>Comment</th></tr>
<tr><td>(a) Use of temporary files</td><td></td></tr>
<tr><td>LS > FILELIST</td><td>LS normally copies the list of files to the terminal. The character > indicates that the output is to be redirected to the file FILELIST.</td></tr>
<tr><td>PR -4 < FILELIST > TEMP</td><td>PR uses the parameter -4 to define how many columns are to be used in the output. The < FILELIST specifies the input file and > TEMP the output file.</td></tr>
<tr><td>LPR < TEMP</td><td>LPR sends a file to the spooler for printing. < TEMP indicates the input file.</td></tr>
<tr><td>(b) Use of pipelines</td><td></td></tr>
<tr><td>LS | PR -4 | LPR</td><td>The symbol | is a pipe that connects the output from the program on its left to the program at its right. There are no temporary files.</td></tr>
</table>

From B.W. Kernighan and J.R. Maskey. The UNIX programming environment. *Computer* 14(4), 12–24, 1981, copyright 1981, Institute of Electrical and Electronics Engineers; reprinted with permission.

each output of the first program to be sent as input to the second as it becomes available; the need for temporary files is eliminated. In effect, each output of the first program is sent as a message to be used as input to the next program.

Notice how UNIX allows the user to create small building blocks that can be combined. The interactive support, the common file interfaces, the flexible shell, and the use of pipes have made UNIX an effective environment for program development and document preparation. Because of the large number of users and the modularity of the programs, many tools are available. Of course, UNIX also has its limitations; nevertheless, it does represent an operating system philosophy with a large and growing following.

3.4. Networking Computers

We have seen how computers have grown in size and capability. As they become more powerful, their architectures are redesigned so that the fastest components need not be delayed by the slower ones. The I/O processes have one or more channels through which they send their requests. The channels operate asynchronously with the CPU; they have their own, smaller processors to manage the I/O operations. Communication with the CPU is in short, fast bursts. The use of expensive resources is maximized; the processes of monitoring and waiting is relegated to slower, less expensive devices.

Thus, what seems to be a single computer is in reality a network of processors designed to act as an integrated unit. The discussion of vector processors briefly alluded to how many CPUs can be integrated to produce a single supercomputer. In each case, the end product is a single, independent unit. But technology is also moving in another direction: the unification of many independent units to produce an integrated resource. Called networking, this philosophy blurs the distinction between the application and the machine that runs the application. That is, the user accesses resources without any knowledge of which computer or computers are being used.

3.4.1. The History of Networking

The concept of computers as a resource can be traced back to the 1960s when multiprogramming first became practical for large scale commercial applications. Timesharing was introduced as a means for an organization to have partial access to a computer. Through the use of telephone lines, terminals, and remote job entry stations (RJE, usually a card reader and printer combination), customers were able to purchase only as much computer time as they required. Most applications were batch jobs; the terminals would be used to write programs, submit jobs, and review results. Because the communication costs were relatively high, charges were made for both CPU and connect time. Thus, there was an incentive to log on, use the system, and then log off.

As computer costs fell, many users purchased their own facilities. The time sharing vendors also began to link their computers so that there would be automatic backup in the event of a failure. Next they began to link computers within their network so that resource users could access several machines. With a nation wide enough to span four time zones, major vendors could level computer loads on the network for all but the peak 5 hours.

In 1968, what is now called the Defense Advanced Research Projects Agency began a project to develop a resource-sharing network. Named the ARPA network, or ARPANET, it provided a laboratory for the engineering of efficient communications among diverse hardware, software, and data resources. In 1975, the operational system was turned over to the Defense Communication Agency; by the end of 1981 the network contained almost 100 nodes at some 90 separate sites. The geographic distribution of these sites is shown in Fig. 3.4.

The microcomputer revolution of the late 1970s and early 1980s produced a large number of small computers and computer based systems. Some were packaged as independent personal computers, and some were packaged as specialized work stations, e.g., the word processor. The proliferation of these many small computers led to decentralization; frequently it was more cost effective simply to purchase a small system with the desired application than to implement it using the central facilities. In parallel with this trend, however, was the growing awareness that data are an important resource that must be shared. Consequently, there was a need to unify as well as diversify.

Improved communication technologies have shown how text, images, and voice can be communicated. New tools for the office environment—called Office Automation—have created new and lucrative markets. The sheer number of small devices has made old methods of communication obsolete. The result has been creation of local networks designed to allow a single group of users to pool their resources (LAN or local area network). There are also long haul networks

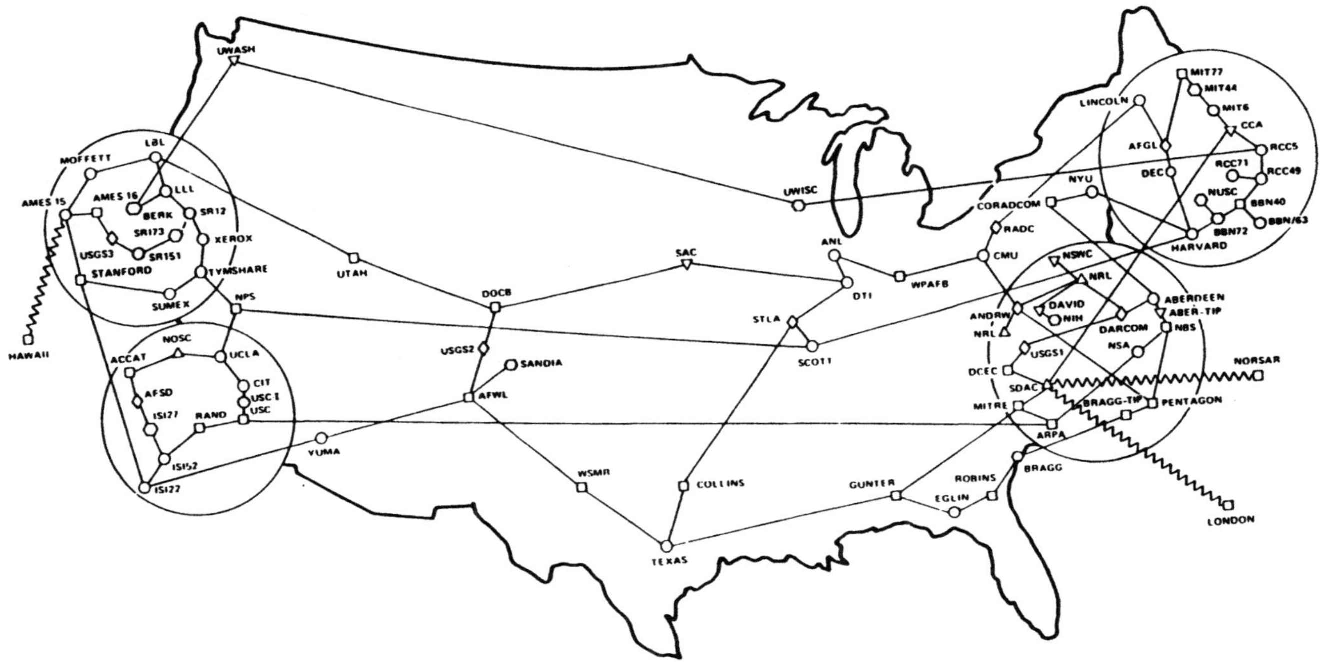

FIGURE 3.4 Advanced Research Projects Agency (ARPA) Network in 1981. From J.S. Sobolowski, The ARPA Network, in A. Ralston and E. Reilly (eds) Encyclopedia of Computer Science and Engineering, Second Edition, Van Nostrand Reinhold Co., 1983, p. 108. This figure is originally from the ARPA Network Information Center, 1981. All rights reserved.

designed to link users and LANs within much larger networks. Someday computer networks will provide plug-in access to computational resources just as today's generator networks provide access to electricity. When that day comes, the personal computer will be like the telephone instrument; an interface to a networked resource. And it will be difficult to distinguish between the function of an individual computer and its role as a component in a larger system.

3.4.2. Some Communications Fundamentals

The basic concepts used in computer networks can be described in terms of the telephone communications model. In the case of the telephone, each user has an instrument and a device to link into the network (the dial or touchtone). Older systems used a crank to get the operator's attention; the operator then used a plugboard or a manual switch. There is a single line from the instrument to an external drop where the line is joined to a pair of wires in a large cable, e.g., the lines on the telephone pole. One pair of wires is dedicated for each telephone number.

Once the wires reach the switching station, the signals from the calling instrument are routed to the called number. Although each number uses dedicated lines up to the switching station, the costs for dedicated lines between switches would be prohibitive. Thus, a single line is used to share many telephone calls (or signals). It does this by modulating the input signal on some base frequency, sending the signal at that frequency, and then demodulating the signal at the other end of the circuit.

The sharing of one line to carry many different signals at once is called multiplexing. When the "line" is made up of many smaller physical channels, it is called space division multiplexing. The cable on the telephone poles is an example. When the medium is divided into many smaller channels, each with a unique frequency assignment, it is called frequency division multiplexing. This is how we receive radio and television signals. Each station is assigned a frequency, its signals are modulated for transmission at that frequency, and the receiver (e.g., radio or television set) demodulates the signal for the speaker or video monitor.

The same principle is used with telephone signals. The major difference is that the air is essentially an unbounded medium. It can carry all frequencies at once. Wire, however, is a bounded medium and can carry only a limited number of frequencies at one time. The range of frequencies a wire can carry is called its bandwidth. The bandwidth is a function of the wire size and length and its resistance to noise, i.e., static or snow in the radio-television analogy. Normal household wire can easily carry the frequency required for voice signals. That is what is used to connect the telephone instrument to the drop. When many of the wire pairs are in close proximity, they can interfere with each other. By simply twisting the wire pairs we can randomize this noise and thereby eliminate its effect. Thus, the so-called twisted pair is the standard medium for narrow band signals; it is used to transfer voice signals to the switching station.

Once the signal is to be routed, economics of scale can be applied. First there are many fewer circuits for connecting telephone instruments than there are instruments. It is assumed that most instruments will be inactive most of the time. The charges provide incentives for short calls and the use of low activity times. The paths between stations are not fixed, and the long-distance switching between two stations may use different paths for different calls. Finally, wideband media are used rather than twisted pair. These media may be satellite communications or wire cables. The common form of wire used for wideband transmission is coaxial cable. It is composed of a single-wire conductor surrounded by some insulating material, then some conducting material shield, and finally an outer protective material. One standard is the ½ inch coaxial cable used for Community Antenna TV (CATV or "cable TV").

3.4.3. Comparing Voice and Computer Data

The requirements for transmitting computer data differ from those for sending voice. Consider first the telephone system. An acceptable frequency range for human speech is from 300 to 3,400 Hz (Hertz or cycles per second). The telephone system uses a frequency range of 4,000 Hz when multiplexing signals: 3,100 Hz for the voice and the rest to guard against interference with other frequencies. Given a cable with a 48,000-Hz bandwidth between the frequencies of 60,000—108,000 Hz, 12 voice channels could be sent over the cable simultaneously: the first at the frequency range 60,000—64,000 Hz, the second at 64,000 to 68,000 Hz, and so on. Because the cable is used to carry many different frequencies at one time, this is an example of frequency division multiplexing.

With a computer, the frequencies (data rates) are generally much higher. The lowest speed of computer communications is 300—1,200 baud (bits per second, but see the glossary definition). This is a transmission rate slow enough to transmit through normal telephone lines. Higher speed transmissions tend to become noisy. This noise is generally not noticed with voice transmission; it becomes critical with digital data transfer. Data transmission at 1,200 baud is too slow to be convenient. Most video terminals can accept data from the computer at rates of 9,600 Hz or 50 KHz. The CPU operates at a rate measured in MHz (i.e., millions of cycles per second).

Another difference between the voice and computer use of communications media is the manner in which they are used. Telephone conversations transmit information at about 150 words per minute. The initiation of a connection takes approximately 17 seconds and the duration of a call is measured in minutes. Computers, on the other hand, send data in short, intense bursts. A long connect time would be unacceptable; continuous connection when no data were available would be wasteful of the resources. Fortunately, there is an alternative method for multiplexing that better suits the requirements of computer transmission.

Time dimension multiplexing (TDM) uses a clock to separate the transmitted data into a group of time-sequential wideband bursts of data. In the above example of frequency dimension multiplexing (FDM), many channels transmit data con-

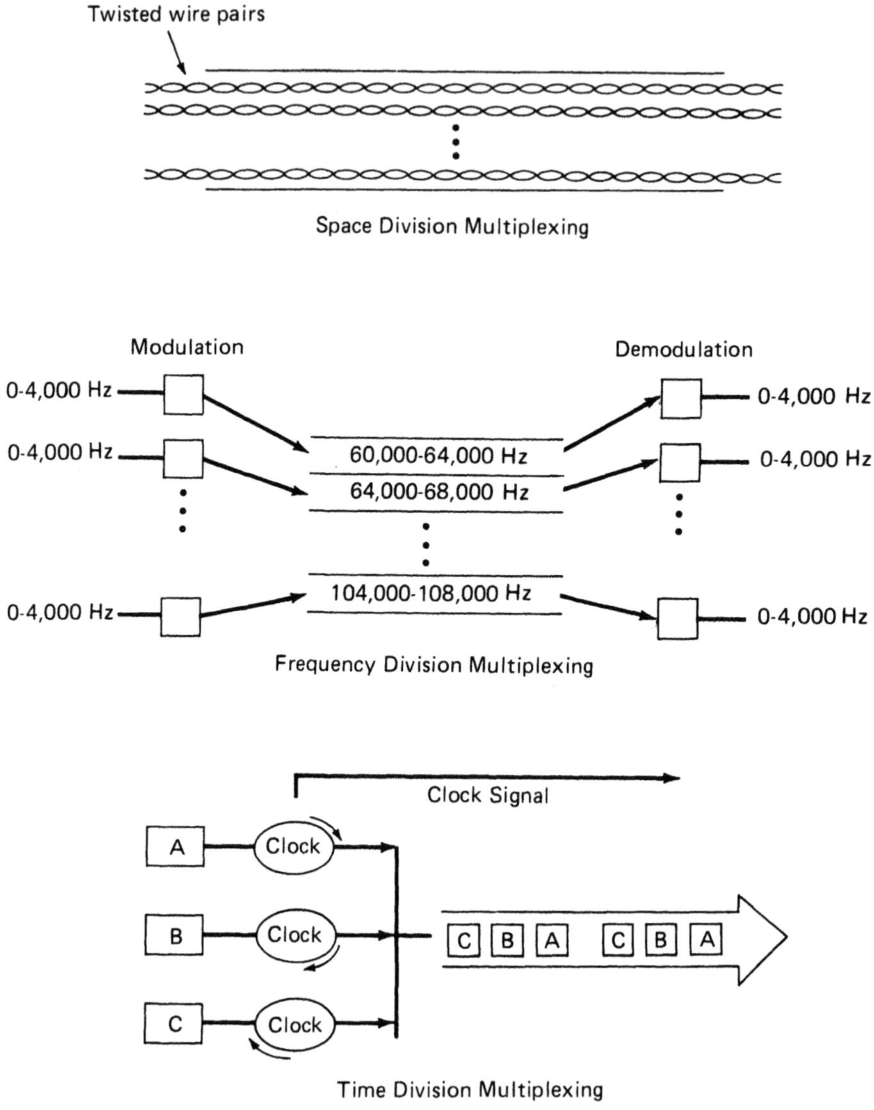

FIGURE 3.5. Three types of multiplexing.

currently; the different channels are identified by their frequency. In TDM, on the other hand, only one channel is transmitting at any point in time. It sends a burst of data called a packet. One must reference the clock and packet header to establish the identification of the current channel. The FDM allocates channels by frequency; therefore it normally uses an analog signal. TDM, however, can transmit digital data without conversion to and from analog. This reduces the error rate. The three types of multiplexing are shown in Fig. 3.5.

3.4.4. A Local Area Network

A Local Area Network (LAN) links the resources in limited geographic areas such as an office complex or building. These resources may include voice and video conversations as well as computer data. A long-haul network links computers over great distances. The ARPANET is an example of a long-haul network. Like the long-haul network, the LAN is designed to communicate with all computers in its network. The LAN also can communicate with other LANs or other computers that are part of a long-haul network. When the LAN communicates with a LAN of the same architectural type, it does this through a device called a bridge or repeater. When the LAN communicates with a device of some other design, it must communicate through a gateway. In what follows we shall limit the discussion to the communication within a LAN. First we shall explain how LANs are organized; then we shall examine how they can be used to provide a general purpose data utility resource.

The network topology describes how the links and nodes are arranged geometrically. The node may be a computer, terminal, printer, etc. and the link is the communication path between nodes. Physical links refer to the actual connections among links; logical links refer to the paths that can be used for communications between nodes. There are two basic types of links. Point-to-point links are circuits that connect two and only two nodes without passing through any other nodes. The connections between a computer and its terminals are generally structured in this way. Every other type of link is called a multipoint link.

Nodes in a network may be organized with one node responsible for the network. In this case, there is a master node with tributary nodes. Alternatively, a more democratic organization may be used with each node having responsibility for its actions. This is called distributed control. In either case, control implies providing access to network resources in an equitable manner.

The individual nodes are normally structured in one of three ways. In a star network there is a single control processor with all other processors communicating to it. The central node of the star is the master node; all communications between tributary nodes must pass through the master. A variation of the star is the tree. In this case, tributaries can coordinate communications among nodes subsidiary to them.

Ring networks link all the nodes in a closed circle. The nodes may be equal with respect to network management (i.e., distributed), or there may be a control node (i.e., master). The third basic topology is the bus network. This is similar to a ring network that has been opened. In both cases, each node in the network must examine each message to determine if the packet is addressed to it. In the ring network, the node actively participates in passing a message to the next node; in a bus network no such action is necessary. Physically, the bus network has an advantage over the ring in that it is easier to install in a building; all that is required is the bus (usually a coaxial cable). Ring networks, on the other

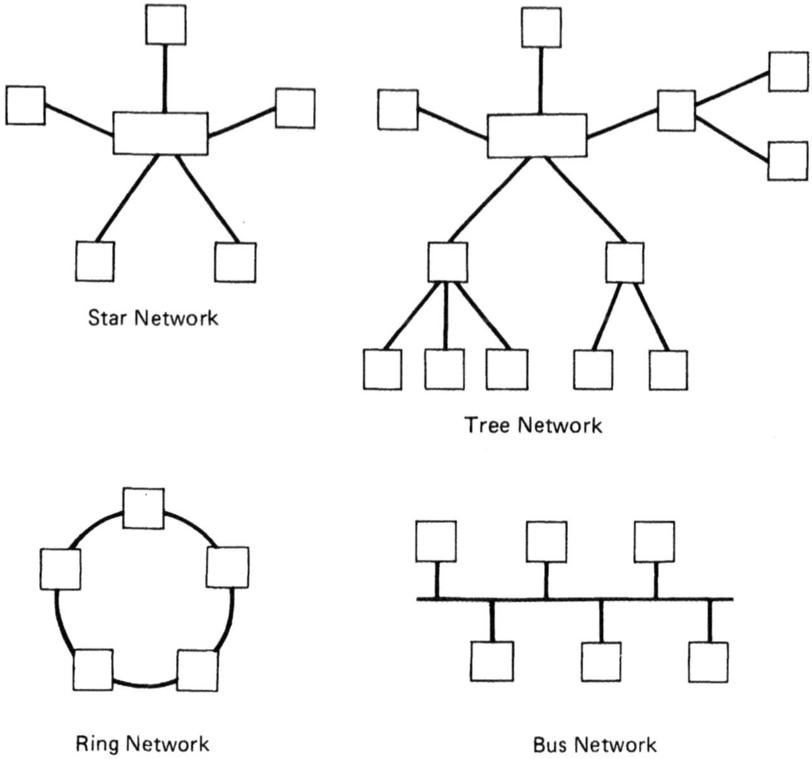

FIGURE 3.6. Typical network typologies.

hand, require point-to-point wiring to preserve the ring's connectivity. The topologies are illustrated in Fig. 3.6.

Communication within the network is accomplished by passing packets of data. Each packet contains the address of the destination node, the address of the sending node, and the data to be sent. In a star network, this is all managed by the control node. In a ring or a bus, some control must be established to avoid several nodes sending a message at the same time. One way contention is avoided is by use of token passing. A special message, called the token, is passed from node to node in the ring. When a node wishes to write out a packet to the node, it waits until it receives the token. It does not pass the token on; rather it writes its packet and then passes the token. With only one token, only one node can write out at any time. Another controlling mechanism used in rings is called the slotted ring. In this case, several fixed messages circulate through the ring. Each has positions (called slots) for messages. To transmit a packet, the node waits for a free slot and then inserts its message in the slot for forwarding. Because of the high transmission speeds, the slots tend to be relatively small.

In the case of a bus network, all nodes are connected to a single communication path. When there is a signal in the path, all nodes can read the signal. Each node can also send a message as soon as it senses that the channel is free of traffic. (It does not have to wait for a token.) However, if two nodes send messages at the same time, their signals will interfere; this is called a collision. To avoid this, bus networks use Carrier Sense Multiple Access with Collision Detect (CSMA/CD). Carrier sense is the ability of a node to detect traffic on the channel. It does this by "listen-before-talking." Multiple access refers to the fact that any node can write when the channel is free. However, even with "listen-before-talking," collisions will occur. For example, two nodes may start to send a message at exactly the same time. When this occurs, the collision is detected. At this point each of the transmitting nodes will delay a different period of time and retransmit.

Communications between units in a LAN is controlled by a protocol. A protocol is a formalized set of rules. In clinical research, the protocol describes the necessary steps to evaluate a hypothesis. In diplomacy, the protocol defines the rules for interaction among representatives of different nations. In communication, protocols are the rules for exchange of data between links and nodes. We have already talked of packets of information. In most cases, these packets contain from 128 to 1,024 bytes. Thus, a logical message may be decomposed into more than one packet. The packets are the physical units transmitted. They contain housekeeping information as well as the application message. When routing is used—as in the case of most long-haul networks—individual messages are sent to intermediate nodes in the network. At each intermediate node, a next node is determined based on network destination and workload. Thus a single logical message may be decomposed into many packets. Each packet may be routed by a different path and the packets from a given logical message may arrive at their destination out of order. This method of routing is called store and forward.

Compare this with the broadcasting approach used with the bus network, where each node has access to each message. The store and forward routing method can be used only for computer data; it would not be suitable for voice conversations. However, it makes the best use of a limited number of circuits. The broadcast method is suitable for both voice and data communications. Thus it is possible to combine both voice (e.g., telephone) and computer data networks using common cabling. Before we can understand how that is done, we must first examine how the packets are exchanged.

The transmission of data from one node to another in the network involves a variety of processes from the preparation of the logical message to be sent to the transmission of the electrical signals. The International Standards Organization (ISO) has organized these different processes into a 7-layered model. Level 1 of the model defines the electrical and mechanical connections. Level 2 is the data link; it defines bit formats and error checks. Level 3 is the network control that addresses and routes messages. Fig. 3.7 shows all 7 layers.

Each level communicates with other levels in the same node through interfaces. The rules for understanding what has been transmitted across the network are

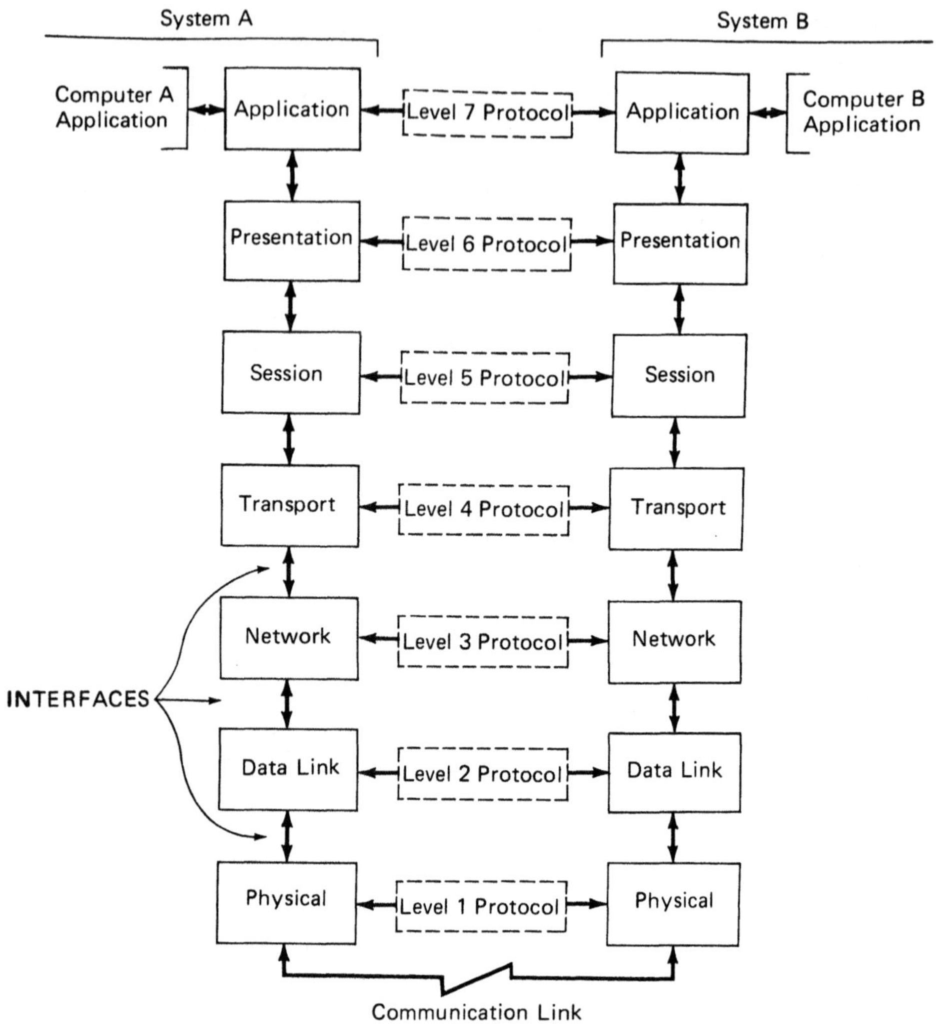

FIGURE 3.7. The International Standards Organization (ISO) Layered Protocol. The protocol layers allow logical communication between similar levels on different machines. The *solid line* traces the data path in actual transmission.

called protocols. There is a protocol that allows a level 1 module to communicate with another level 1 module in the network. Each level 1 module transforms its data to (or from) data it receives from a level 2 module. In this way, two level 2 modules in different nodes can logically communicate with each other. The level 2 node determines if a valid transmission has arrived. When it has, the data are sent to the network control level where the packet is processed. If all nodes in the network use the same rules for defining a packet, then the level 3 module in any node will be able to send packets to or receive packets from any other node in the network. In short, the protocol provides the ability to transmit data using a preestablished standard. There are several standards.

IBM's System Network Architecture (SNA) supports all 7 levels of the ISO model. Ethernet, on the other hand, supports only the first 3 levels, i.e., to the level of the packet. Some protocols are implemented in separate hardware; others are implemented within the computer. When using a protocol such as SNA, one operates at the level of the logical messages. When using a protocol such as Ethernet, it is necessary to have modules that can perform the functions of the top four levels of converting to and from packets and logical messages. Generally, this is supplied as systems software by the computer vendor. When communicating between networks with different protocols, protocol conversion is necessary. This is one of the functions of a gateway.

3.4.5. Some Local Area Network Implementations

We conclude this section on networking computers by illustrating several different ways the concepts just presented are being combined to produce networks. The three technologies currently in use are:

- *Private Branch Exchange (PBX).* This is an extension of the telephone systems that switch telephone calls within an organization and between the local and outside telephone network.
- *Broadband technology.* This is an adaptation of the video transmission technology. It provides a single environment for data, voice, and images.
- *Baseband technology.* This approach was developed to meet the unique needs of digital communications; it is well suited for implementation using VLSI technology.

Each technology has its advantages. Through gateways, all can be combined. We briefly discuss them in turn.

The PBX is designed to take advantage of the telephone wires currently in place. The wires can be used for either voice or data transfer. The cables carry only an analog signal, thus the computer signals must be *mod*ulated and *de*-*mo*dulated using a *modem*. Existing twisted pair wires are used. Because the lines are short and the switching limited, computer communications can operate at rates much higher than the 1,200 baud common for long-distance telephone communications. Nevertheless, PBX systems are optimized for voice use.

Newer versions of PBX technology use digital switching rather than electromechanical devices for connecting units within an organization to the outside lines. Called Computerized Branch Exchange (CBX), the switch processes digital signals using time division multiplexing (TDM). Since all input and output signals are analog, they must be converted by a COder/DECoder (CODEC) unit which is normally implemented as a VLSI chip. A variation of this approach is the

Digital Branch Exchange (DBX) in which the CODEC can be located in a microprocessor to which the telephone is connected. This provides the ability to record details about each outside call, compute the least-cost routing of a call, and use store and forward techniques for integrating voice with text electronic mail systems.

Broadband local area networks tap into a cable system and use frequency division multiplexing (FDM) to transmit data within the network. Recall that FDM assigns a frequency range to each channel and allows all channels to operate simultaneously. This means that some channels can be used for voice or video while others are used for computer data. All transmissions use analog signals and therefore a modem is required as an interface between the computer and the network. The bandwidth of the coaxial cable used with broadband networks is between 300 and 400 MHz. This is enough to carry over 50 standard 6 MHz color TV channels or thousands of voice grade and low speed data channels. Fiber optics offer even greater transmission capability: over 3 GHz, i.e., gigahertz or billion Hz.

The third technology is baseband. Here the initial signal is not modulated; it can be transmitted as digital signals that are optimized for data. TDM is used; most systems use a bus topology. Data are transmitted in packets and each node in the network examines each packet address to extract its packets. Transmission usually uses the CSMA/CD technique described earlier. Access to the bus is usually configured as a wall jack. Thus, a terminal, printer, or other device may easily plug into the LAN to send or receive.

3.5. Concluding Remarks

In this chapter we have described how the computer works. We started with the single user personal computer, then discussed multicomputer systems, and closed with a discussion of networks. Current LAN technology is blurring the distinction between voice, image, and data communications. A goal of the fifth generation computer is to integrate voice I/O with language analysis.

One can anticipate that future generations of computers will be quite different from those we currently use. The human interfaces will be different. It will be difficult to draw clear boundaries between where one computer ends and another begins; key components will be shared. Finally, one can expect computer resources to be available in two ways. First, as embedded devices, we will consider them parts of the tools we use. Second, as a networked resource, they will be as modular and accessible as our telephone systems. Much of this is available today.

Despite this progress in hardware development, we will continue to develop customized programs to meet our specialized needs. In that context, the computer is a tool that (a) supports the development and (b) operates the product. In the following chapters we shall examine the languages we can use to describe those products, the techniques used to organize the information in the database, and the methods for managing the development process.

For Further Reading

There is a vast body of literature in the field of computer hardware and system software. The key professional societies are the Association for Computing Machinery (ACM) and the Institute of Electrical and Electronics Engineers (IEEE) Computer Society. The ACM publishes a monthly *Communications* and *Computing Reviews*, a quarterly *Surveys*, and an annual *Guide to Computing Literature*. They also produce lists of recommended texts. The IEEE produces two magazines, *Computer* and *Software*. They also publish a large number of very useful tutorials that deal with many topics in computer science and software development. Both organizations also produce more specialized journals.

There are several major periodicals that deal with computer applications. *Datamation* is the most frequently referenced controlled circulation magazine; *Computerworld* is one of many paid subscription periodicals. For personal computers, *Byte* has a position of prominence among hobbyists; there are also many magazines for less well informed readers. *Scientific American* has periodic papers of interest. The December 1982 issue contained an excellent review of personal computers by H. D. Toong and A. Gupta.

Because the field is so vast and moving so rapidly, it is difficult to recommend books. For personal computers, I have found those of A. Osborne (McGraw-Hill) both readable and technically satisfying. A recent text on operating systems is available from H. Lorin and H. M. Deitel, *Operating Systems* (Addison-Wesley, 1981). For introductory discussions of networking, I have found some vendor documentations to be very clear and relatively unbiased. In particular, Digital's *Introduction to Local Area Networking* (EB-22714-18, 1982) is short and readable.

4
Programming Languages

4.1. Introduction

Languages are normally divided into natural languages, such as English and French, and artificial languages such as those used for programming, chemical formulas, and mathematical notation. A programming language provides communication between a developer and a computer through use of a stored program. All languages have a syntax, or set of rules, that defines the correct forms for the language. For example

The cow ate the hay.

is syntactically correct, whereas

The cow eated the hay.

is not. The latter is a common mistake of children who learn a general rule for changing tense (add "ed" to the verb) but have not yet learned the other rules that take precedence.

Languages also have semantics: the meaning applied to a sentence. The following

The hay ate the cow.

is syntactically correct, but (except for the most bizarre circumstances) semantically invalid. In languages for human exchange, there is also a property, pragmatics, which refers to the origins, uses, and effects of the language, i.e., the meaning received by a listener or reader. Since the target of a programming language is a machine, the design of programming languages is concerned only with syntax and semantics.

In the Old Testament, the Tower of Babel was used to explain how—since the time of Adam and Eve—so many languages had come into being. Within 15 years after the implementation of the first vacuum tube computer, Sammet's book on programming languages portrayed a new Tower of Babel on its cover. She was able to catalogue some 120 programming languages. Many still are in use; new languages also have been added. This raises two obvious questions.

What is a programming language, and why are there so many different languages? The answer to these questions is the topic of this chapter.

4.2. Survey of Programming Languages

We are so accustomed to the ubiquitous presence of computers that it is hard to realize that the concept of a stored program barely existed before the early 1940s. For example, consider the first vacuum tube computer: the ENIAC. In a 1943 report proposing its development, Mauchly and Eckert defined one of its components in the following way:

Program Control Unit: A unit which contains the necessary control circuits for initiating the various steps of the calculation in their proper order. The program control unit can be equipped, if desired, with a punch-card program selector to facilitate rapid set up of different problems. Usually only one punched card would be needed for any one problem. (Cited in Brian Randell, *The Origin of Digital Computers*, third Edition. Reprinted with permission, Springer-Verlag, Berlin, 1982, p.298).

The primary goal was to produce ballistics tables, and the sequence of instructions was limited. The first ENIAC "programs" were encoded by use of cables in a plug board. Within a year of its dedication, the programming method was revised so that programs could be rerun by using manually set function tables without changing any interconnecting wires. While this method exacted a penalty in performance, it did allow the programmer to think of the operation as a sequential series of steps.

In the next few years the use of the new computing devices was restricted to mathematical computations. Von Neumann developed a machine language for these computers and even wrote a sort program in 1944, 1 year before the ENIAC was complete. Yet the programs were implemented as ones and zeros or as holes in a Hollerith punch card. It was soon recognized that the computer could perform functions other than numerical computations; it could transform instructions suitable for programmers into instructions for computers.

4.2.1. Assembly Languages

The first major book on software appeared in 1951. Written by Wilkes, Wheeler, and Gill, *The Preparation of Programs for a Digital Computer* described how programs could be divided and joined within working memory. They also introduced the term "assembler" which has come to mean a program that translates a symbolic assembly language into a machine executable language.

To understand what a symbolic assembler does, consider the simple problem introduced in Chapter 3. We wish to add A to B and store the result in C. Let the computer that will run this program have machine instructions that perform the following actions:

"LOAD:" take the current contents of a word and store it in the accumulator.

"ADD:" take the current contents of a word and add it to the contents of the accumulator.

"STORE:" take the current contents of the accumulator and store it as the contents of a word.

We also assume the format for all instructions on this computer to be:

```
OPERATOR    WORD ADDRESS
```

where the operator is stored as 8 bits and the address as 16 bits. Logically, we would like the machine to take the following action:

```
LOAD    A
ADD     B
STORE   C
```

Since the machine instructions are written only as 1s and 0s, the assembler must transform "LOAD" to an 8 bit number that causes the computer to load the contents of a number to the accumulator. The next 16 bits of the instruction must contain the address of the word to be loaded. A is a symbol (in this case also a variable) that represents that address. The assembler must reserve a word in working memory at location A and then, for every occurrence of A, substitute the address of the word assigned for A. In this way, the user can communicate in a language that is more meaningful for his application, and the computer operates on a translation of that language that is efficient in its domain.

In the early 1950s the creation of an assembler was a challenging task; it had not been done before. Today, the process is well understood. Development of a symbolic assembler is frequently assigned as an undergraduate student project. It involves the following processes:

- Scanning of the input program. This includes testing for errors.
- Building a table of symbolic addresses. This table includes both the symbol (e.g., A, B) and the address of the word that will contain the contents.
- Translation of the instructions and word addresses into a form that can be interpreted by the computer.
- Generating the code and storing it in memory, on punch cards, or on a disk. In the early machines, absolute word locations were used; in modern systems, a relative address is generated by the assembler and converted to an absolute address during loading. (see Chapter 3).

Assembly languages were too inconvenient, and they were soon expanded to include macro-instructions. This allowed the user to introduce specialized user oriented instructions. For example, the macro-definition facility provided a tool that allowed the user to define

```
ADDM A,B,C
```

as a substitute for the previous three-line assembly language sequence. System-supplied macros were particularly useful in organizing sequences of input/output (I/O) commands to read from or write to a peripheral device.

Nevertheless, even macro assemblers had major deficiencies. Each was targeted to a specific type of machine; thus each program had to be written for that machine. Moreover, assembly languages were difficult to use. Although they had great power and potential for efficiency, there was an even greater potential for error. To use an assembly language, the user must think in terms of how the computer will implement his solution. Thus, he thinks less about the problem to be solved and more about how the computer operates. The next step in the development of programming languages improved this balance. It provided a more natural way to describe the problem to be solved and hid from view much of what the computer was to do. Assembly languages continue to be used for some systems software and in applications where there are extreme constraints on size and performance.

4.2.2. High-Order Language

A high-order language (HOL) is an application oriented language that defines the functions the computer is to perform. Since there are several different classes of application, many different languages have been developed. When cataloging the HOLs, one may organize them according to different characteristics, or one may view them in a historical context. The first of the HOLs were developed in the 1950s. The products of this period were concerned with performing useful work, and—as a byproduct—with the discovery of programming language concepts and implementation techniques. Up to this time there were few formal theories to link languages and automation. Methods for input analysis and statement parsing had to be developed. Even the flow of a symbolic assembler had to be established and refined.

By way of example, consider how to compute an algebraic expression. We have seen that the computation of

```
A+B
```

is quite direct, but how should

```
A*(B+C)
```

be evaluated? (Note, the symbol * is generally used in computer programming languages as the multiplication operator.) We intend that B be added to C and that sum be multiplied by A. How can these operations be sequenced to get the correct result? One answer was supplied by the Polish logician Lukasiewicz in 1951. He showed how an expression could be written without parentheses. Because of the difficulty in spelling his name, this representation has become known as Polish notation.

In its prefix form, Polish notation places the operator before the two operands. Thus, for the last expression, it becomes

$$*A+BC$$

One reads this as: "Multiply A and the sum of B and C." While this may seem unnatural, consider how easy this is for a computer to process if one reads from right to left. The sequence is:

- The first operand is C.
- The second operand is B.
- Add the first operand to the second operand and save the result as the first operand.
- The now-second operand is A.
- Multiply the first operand by the second operand and save as the first operand.

It should not be difficult for the reader to see how that sequence can easily be transformed to the sequence:

```
LOAD  C
ADD   B
MULT  A
```

Yet in 1950 this was a very difficult problem.

The next decade of HOL development built upon the experience of the previous period. There now was a technology base that could be analyzed and extended. There was also an understanding of formal languages that is used in today's compilers and parsers. (A compiler is a computer program that translates a HOL program into machine language. A parser, used in a compiler, is a computer program, or module in a program, that decomposes a statement into the components defined by the syntax.)

In addition to a theoretical foundation, there was a decade of experience with HOLs. It is interesting to note that three of the most popular languages of today were among the first of the HOLs. FORTRAN began as a language to support mathematical computations, and it remains the standard language for mathematics and engineering. COBOL was developed to provide an environment for business applications; today it is the most widely used of all mainframe languages. Finally, LISP was produced to manage symbolic data, and it remains a standard language in this country for artificial intelligence. A fourth early language, ALGOL, was never widely used in America; however, it did introduce many concepts that became integral parts of later languages.

In the following section, each of these languages will be described in some detail. From the historical point of view, it is important to note that each surviving language has gone through many changes and several official versions. The earliest language definitions had ambiguities and inconsistencies. Moreover, their compilers frequently were built using an imperfect understanding of the language.

The result was illogical special rules and compilers that were difficult to build and certify correct. Wirth described one of his earlier efforts as follows.

> Looking at it from the distance, that compiler was a horror; the excitement came precisely from having insight into a machinery that nobody understood fully. There was the distinct air of sorcery.[1]

The time was right for the building of a new generation of languages based on earlier research and experience.

This process took two directions. First, there was the creation of more powerful languages. PL/1 was designed to combine the best features of FORTRAN, COBOL, and ALGOL. ALGOL 68 was designed as a successor to the earlier ALGOL 60; it, too, added new functions. Each of these languages became quite complex and difficult to describe formally. In reaction to this trend toward complexity, Wirth developed Pascal. Although designed as a language to be used by students, Pascal had the advantage of a completely formal definition. It sacrificed functionality for clarity and simplicity.

The second major activity took advantage of time sharing to produce a new class of languages designed for a broad audience and intended to be used interactively. BASIC was designed as a variation of FORTRAN that could be used for introductory programming courses. APL provided interactive facilities for computational applications. MUMPS was developed to meet the text and database requirements associated with the processing of medical data. In each case, the language translator was implemented in a different way. Rather than compiling the program and loading it into working memory for execution, one interpreted the program one line at a time. That is, an interpreter would read each line of code, parse it, and execute it during an interactive session.

The advantage of this approach was obvious. If an error was encountered, an error message could be printed for the user immediately. The user had the ability to change the line of code or examine any of the data used by the program. This facilitated testing (called debugging) and learning. However, interpreters also produced programs that operated less efficiently than programs that are compiled. Fortunately, many languages now are supported by both compilers and interpreters and various intermediate processing.

The 1970s were characterized by a consolidation of the existing languages for the practical management of the computer environment. Because computers had become more powerful, the applications had become more complex. The languages of the 1950s were designed to allow computers to be used by persons who did not really understand how computers worked. During the 1960s the languages were refined to apply the results of earlier research. By the 1970s, however, it became clear that many of the available languages were too limited for the production of larger systems. A language called SIMULA had been developed for simulation applications. Because simulations have to manage the operation of several independent activities at one time, the features used by SIMULA provided new insight into the management of concurrency. (Recall

TABLE 4.1. Different forms for assigning the value of A+B to the variable C.

Language	Statement
FORTRAN	C = A + B
BASIC	100 LET C = A + B
COBOL	ADD A,B GIVING C.
Pascal	c := a + b;
PL/1	C = A + B;
MUMPS	SET C = A + B
Ada	C := A + B;

that the multiuser operating system must manage the I/O processing and user tasks concurrently.) Many of these ideas were incorporated by Wirth in MODULA-2, a successor to Pascal. The same concepts also were incorporated into Ada,* a new standard language for Department of Defense embedded computer applications.

Although there are dramatic differences in style, each language so far mentioned (other than LISP) is concerned with the management of words in the computer working memory. We began by describing an assembly language program that added A to B and stored it in C. One of the assembler's tasks was to assign the addresses for A, B and C and to allocate words to hold the values of A, B, and C. Table 4.1 contains some statements illustrating how several languages would write this statement. The process is called assignment, and each assignment statement alters one (or more) words in working storage.

In each of these examples there is the implication that the statements will be applied sequentially (one after the other). Given the architecture of the von Neumann computer, this is a very natural approach. But what if computers are to have many processors and use parallel processing? What type of programming language should be used for these new machines?

The alternative approach to the use of "imperative" languages (which concentrate on altering the contents of fixed storage locations) is called "applicative" or "functional" programming. Derived from LISP, the functional programming languages apply functions to the program and data to arrive at the desired result. There are no assignment statements. To illustrate the difference between imperative and functional programming, consider the mathematical function "n factorial" (written n!). This is defined for all positive integers; it is the product of the integer n and each smaller integer. For example:

$$3! = 3 \cdot 2 \cdot 1$$
$$7! = 7 \cdot 6 \cdot 5 \cdot 4 \cdot 3 \cdot 2 \cdot 1$$

In an imperative language, one might compute N! using the following procedure:

*Ada is a trademark of the U. S. Government.

1. Set a variable ANSWER equal to N.
2. Subtract 1 from N and store it in TEMP.
3. If TEMP ≤ 1 the program is finished
4. Multiply TEMP times ANSWER and store the result in ANSWER.
5. Subtract 1 from TEMP and store in TEMP.
6. Go to statement 3 and continue processing.

When the processing is finished, ANSWER will contain N!

A functional language would begin with the definition of N! which is:

$$N! = N\cdot(N-1)! \text{ for } N > 0$$
$$N! = 1 \text{ for } N = 0$$

Notice that two lines are used: one for N greater than zero, the other for N = 0. Also notice that N! is defined in terms of itself. For example:

$$7! = 7\cdot6!$$

One can compute 7! only if one can compute 6! This is called a recursive definition. Note that in this recursive definition we end up with

$$7! = 7\cdot6\cdot4\cdot3\cdot2\cdot1!$$

where

$$1! = 1\cdot0!$$

and that is why 0! must be defined to be 1. (What happens in the imperative example if N is 0? Obviously the procedure definition is not complete.)

Once the function has been defined, it may be used without any concern for the order of processing or where any of the data are stored. To illustrate how the imperative and functional languages differ in concept, we define three programming functions:

INPUT (N)	reads a value of N from the user
FACTORIA L (N)	computes N!
PRINT (N)	prints the value of N for the user.

In an imperative language, we could write a program to read a number, compute its factorial, and then print the result as:

INPUT(N)
Do FACTORIAL(N,ANSWER), i.e., the procedure described to compute ANSWER as N!
PRINT(ANSWER)

Notice that this program requires three sequential steps: first storing a value in N, then computing ANSWER from N, and finally printing the contents of the word with the address labeled ANSWER.

The functional language sets the input with

INPUT

which reads a number from the user. It uses the FACTORIAL for the computations. Since the input is processed by the function INPUT, the factorial function for this input is:

```
FACTORIAL (INPUT)
```

Once the factorial is computed, the above line represents the answer. Thus, to print the factorial of the value that was input, we use

```
PRINT (FACTORIAL(INPUT))
```

Notice that this approach does not indicate how the processing is to be done or even the internal sequence of processes. Moreover, since there is no need to save either the input (N) or the result (ANSWER), no variables are assigned to hold these values. Everything is implicit in the definitions of the functions.

The use of functional programming may seem awkward. As will be shown in the following sections, this approach is especially useful for the processing of symbolic information such as language. Thus many of the tools used by researchers in artificial intelligence are written in LISP or one of its dialects. (The Japanese Fifth Generation computers are an exception; they are designed to use the PROgramming LOGic language PROLOG). Functional programming is also used to support user friendly environments such as the children's learning tool LOGO and the development tool SMALLTALK.

4.2.3. Current Trends

As we enter the 1980s the major thrusts in language development are twofold. First, there is consolidation of the techniques used with imperative languages. Examples are the new languages Ada and MODULA-2. Second, there is the broader use of the functional programming just discussed. Each approach addresses the question of how to develop complex systems in a different way.

In addition to these new developments in languages, there are also changes to languages designed for interactive use with a personal computer. The BASIC language is continuously being enhanced. Specific environments have made new languages popular. For example, the fact that the UNIX† operating system was implemented in C has made C a language of general interest. The ability of FORTH to support complex applications in very small processors has produced a very enthusiastic following for that language. The use of data base management system (DBMS) tools has led to a class of data processing languages called Nonprocedural Languages (NPL) or Fourth-Generation Languages (4GL). These languages are designed for database applications and report generation. They are called fourth generation languages because they are an order of magnitude (10 times) "better" than the third generation language of COBOL. These 4GLs are sometimes implemented as languages, sometimes as interpretive application gen-

†UNIX is a trademark of AT&T.

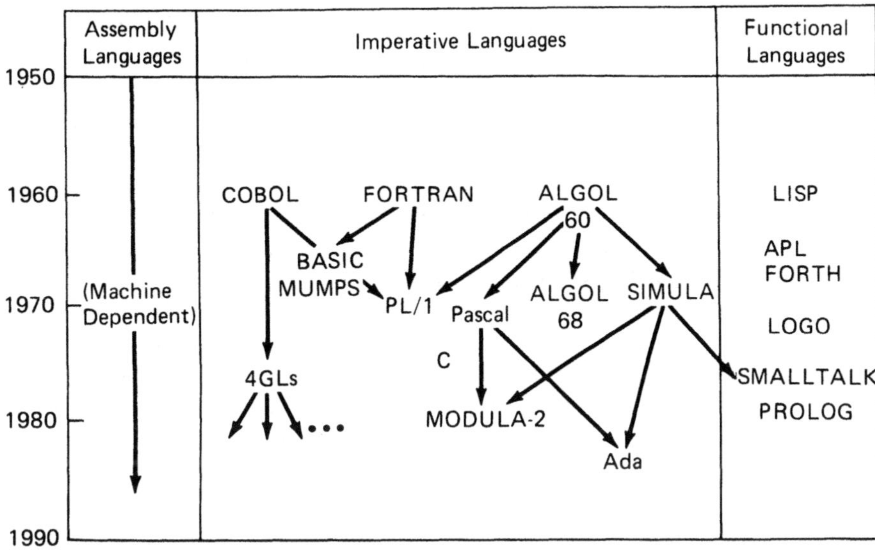

FIGURE 4.1. Overview of programming languages.

erators, and sometimes as program generators that transform user-friendly statements of what is to be done into programs written in a traditional language (e.g., COBOL). The key phrase here is "user-friendly." With more and more users, there is a major incentive to make the computer a natural tool for solving new problems. That demand has resulted in the development of the propriery products, called 4GLs, designed for data processing applications.

The programming languages of the 1990s probably will not resemble those we use today. Just as computer networks now obscure the physical distinctions among communicating machines, the new graphic, audio, and language interfaces will obscure the difference between using a computer and building new "programs" for subsequent use. That is, the computer will become a general resource and the process of "programming" will be seen as simply "using the computer."

4.3. Some Programming Languages

In the previous section, programming languages were surveyed. As shown in Fig. 4.1, they can be divided into categories:

- *Assembly languages*, which operate at the level of the machine instructions. These are machine-dependent. Although there is some activity regarding standard instruction sets, new instructions (and hence new assembly languages) will always be required. We shall not discuss these languages any further.

- *Imperative languages*, which are designed to manage the data in working storage. The three key original languages are COBOL, FORTRAN, and ALGOL. The functions of these three were combined in PL/1; BASIC was developed as a simpler version of FORTRAN. Most computer science activity has been based on the ALGOL model and its derivative languages, Pascal, SIMULA, Ada, etc. Some languages, such as MUMPS and C, have no clear derivation in this figure. The Fourth Generation Languages (4GL) are many and diverse. In what follows we shall discuss only FORTRAN, BASIC, COBOL, MUMPS, ALGOL, and Pascal.
- *Functional Languages*, which apply functions (recursively or by composition) to achieve its effect. There are many functional languages not shown in the figure. LISP is the root for most of these. Examples using APL and FORTH will be used to illustrate some concepts, and descriptions of LISP and PROLOG will follow. (PROLOG does not fit the definition for functional languages which we have given. This is a point that we choose to ignore.)

In the remainder of this section we shall describe each of the above programming languages. The descriptions, by necessity, will be brief and superficial. The primary goal is to introduce concepts associated with programming languages. It must be kept in mind that there is no "best" language. Moreover, almost any modern language can be made to solve almost any solvable problem. Frequently, the choice of languages is dictated by machine or operating system selection, and an implementer may have few choices. Nevertheless, some understanding of how programming languages are designed should provide useful insights into the workings of a computer system.

4.3.1. Imperative Programming Languages

In the following section we describe six different imperative languages. The common characteristics are that each relies on a sequence of instructions with assignment of data to variables. In general, the variable is associated with fixed locations in computer memory; however, interpretive languages such as BASIC and MUMPS use the assignment operator in a different way.

4.3.1.1. FORTRAN

The origins of FORTRAN can be traced back to a 1954 IBM document describing a Mathematical FORmula TRANslating System. The system was first issued in 1957. FORTRAN has been viewed as the "single most important milestone in the development of programming languages. It was developed at a time of considerable skepticism concerning the compile-time and run-time efficiency of high level languages, and its successful implementation provided an existence proof for both the feasibility and the reliability of high level languages."[2]

Because of skepticism regarding the efficiency of a high order language,

FORTRAN did not receive immediate acceptance. There were competing "English-language-like" and proven assembly language alternatives. A 1958 revision, FORTRAN II, achieved wider acceptance, and the 1962 enhancement, FORTRAN IV, became the standard language for scientific and engineering applications. Because each vendor produced his own variation of the language, a standardization effort was initiated that finally resulted in FORTRAN 77. For the purposes of this description, all versions are essentially the same; we shall use the syntax of FORTRAN 77.

The primary objective was to perform computations. Thus, FORTRAN required a facility to translate mathematical formulas in a natural way. The algebraic expression

$$(4x + y^5) / (xy)^3$$

had to be written using only the character set available to the computer. To facilitate parsing, multiplication had to be stated explicitly. The term $4x$ becomes 4 * X and xy is written as X * Y. Exponentiation is indicated by the operator **. (Note that even though two characters were used, it is considered a single operator.) Thus, the previous expression is written:

```
(4 * X + Y ** 5) / (X * Y)**3
```

The operators are ranked with the exponentiation (**) taking precedence over multiplication (*) or division (/); the latter, in turn, are executed before addition (+) or subtraction (−).

Once the language can compute an expression, it can store the value of that expression as the value of a variable. For example

```
Z = (4 * X + Y**5) / (X*Y)**3
```

assigns the computed value on the right side of the equal sign to the variable named on the left. In this case, the equal sign character is the assignment operator. The statement

```
X = X + 1
```

is a FORTRAN statement to increment X by 1; it is meaningless as an algebra statement, for no finite value of X can satisfy that condition.

As you may remember, there are many formats for storing a number. These are called data types. Examples of different data types are:

INTEGER:	A number with no decimal point
REAL:	A floating point number
DOUBLE PRECISION:	A double precision floating point number

Initially, FORTRAN used a naming convention that any variable beginning with I, J, K, L, M, or N was an integer; everything else was real. Later, type statements were added to specify the data type. For example

```
INTEGER   X,X1
REAL      I,J,JUNK
```

These are nonexecutable statements. They are used by the compiler and do not cause any processing at execution time. In general, every program will have both non-executable and executable statements.

We can now use what we know of FORTRAN to write a function that will compute N factorial (N!). The procedure we shall implement was described on page —. The FORTRAN program is

```
          INTEGER ANSWER,N, TEMP
          ANSWER = N
          TEMP = N - 1
   10     IF (TEMP .LE. 1) GO TO 100
          ANSWER = ANSWER * TEMP
          TEMP = TEMP - 1
          GO TO 10
  100     CONTINUE
```

There are six executable statements in this program plus a CONTINUE statement that serves only to hold the statement label. In the case of FORTRAN, the label is a number; 10 and 100 are statement labels that are used by GO TO commands to transfer the sequence of control.

In statement 10, the IF tests whether the logical statement in parentheses is true; if it is true, then the remainder of the statement is executed. (FORTRAN 77 allows more complex IF statements, which we shall describe in Section 4.3.1.4.) Notice that this program repeats the sequence of instructions from statement 10 through the next three statements. Such a repeatable sequence is called a loop; its repetitive execution is called iteration. Since iteration is common in mathematical applications, FORTRAN also provided an instruction for looping: the DO command. The factorial program can be rewritten using the DO as follows:

```
        ANSWER = N
        DO 10 I = N-1,2,-1
   10   ANSWER = ANSWER*I
```

In this program the DO will execute every statement from itself through the numbered statement (10) starting with a value of I set to N-1. For each iteration the value of I will be altered by the value in the third position (-1). The looping will end after the processing of I set to 2 (i.e., the value of the second parameter). Thus, the form of the FORTRAN DO is:

DO statement variable = start, stop, increment

For an input of N=7, there will be five iterations of line 10 with values of I equal to 6,5,4,3 and 2. Compare these two implementations of the N factorial problem. The second is more compact and much easier to understand. However, there is a question of what happens if that sequence is started with N = 1? In this case, N-1 is 0 which is smaller than the "stop" value of 2. If we were to execute statement 10, then the answer would be 0; otherwise it will be 1. Here is an example of where knowing the form of a statement (the syntax) doesn't tell how it is to work (the semantics). In the case of FORTRAN 77, the DO loop (through statement 10) will be ignored if the start value is less than the stop value. Hence, the algorithm works for N of 1 or greater. It does not work for N=0, for in this case it returns the value of ANSWER=0.

FORTRAN introduced the basic elements used in all subsequent imperative programming languages:

- The sequence of statements
- The IF statement (selection)
- The DO statement (iteration).

Other languages would develop better ways to express these structures, but FORTRAN provided all the features necessary to implement complicated programs. In general, these programs were divided into less complicated parts called routines or subroutines. Each subroutine performed a well-defined task; most were written to be reused in many different programs. For example, if the computation of a factorial were to be performed often from many places, it would be useful to have the ability to write

```
CALL FACT(N,ANSWER)
```

where FACT is a subroutine that accepts N as an input and returns ANSWER containing N!. The CALL operator transfers control from the current program (or subroutine) to the subroutine FACT.

FORTRAN allows each subroutine to be compiled separately. To do this, one uses SUBROUTINE and END statements that indicate to the compiler the beginning and end of a subroutine. A subroutine to compute the factorial might be:

```
      SUBROUTINE FACT(N, ANSWER)
      INTEGER ANSWER, N
      ANSWER=N
      DO 10 I = N-1,2,-1
10    ANSWER = ANSWER * I
      END
```

The variables in the parentheses are called the subroutine's arguments. The variables N and ANSWER are known only to the subroutine. The CALL to the subroutine may use any valid variable or expression, for example:

```
CALL FACT(I,J)
CALL FACT(4*K-J,A)
```

Of course, it is the responsibility of the calling program to use the subroutine in the proper way; in this case the first parameter is an integer greater than zero and the second will be altered to contain the result of computation. It is also good programming practice for the subroutine to test the inputs for validity. In this case there should be some initial code that tests to see if N < 1. If so, this is outside the range of the subroutine's algorithm, and an "error" return should be made (e.g., return with ANSWER = -1). Where this is done, it becomes the responsibility of the calling routine to test for the error condition and take an appropriate action when it is found.

Even disregarding the problem of the range of N, it still is very easy to make mistakes using even this simple example. For instance:

```
REAL X
CALL FACT(7,X)
```
(Second parameter is not an integer)

or

```
CALL FACT(1.5,I)
```
(First parameter is not an integer)

or

```
I = 3
CALL FACT(7,I).
```
(Second parameter (I) value is changed from 3 to 7!)

The use of FORTRAN subroutines had a major impact on the success of the language. Each subroutine abstracted a problem into a more general form that might be used with many different applications. If one understands how to use a particular subroutine properly, then one can reuse that subroutine without understanding its internal structure or design. In practice, we have built large libraries of FORTRAN programs that are available for most computational applications. The availability of these libraries has resulted in the acceptance of FORTRAN as a *de facto* standard for scientific programming. The investment in training and libraries is so large that one computer scientist has stated: We don't know what the language of the 1990s will be, but we do know it will be called FORTRAN.

4.3.1.2. BASIC

The Beginner's All-Purpose Symbolic Instruction Code, BASIC, was developed in the mid-1960s at Dartmouth College under the direction of Kemeny and Kurtz. Time sharing systems were becoming relatively inexpensive, and it was now practical to use an interactive environment for development and training. While several of the interactive languages produced during this time were designed to implement systems and solve problems, the primary objective of BASIC was education. It was seen as a tool to teach programming; the assumption was that the students would then be better prepared to learn and use more complete languages such as FORTRAN.

The style of BASIC was modeled after FORTRAN. The earliest implementations were quite limited. For example, all variable names were single letters. In time, features were added and BASIC became a complete language suitable for application development. Although the language has been used to implement sophisticated systems (for example, The Regenstrief Medical Record System, see page 258.), the general perception through the mid 1970s was that it had "great success in high schools, two-year colleges, and other environments concerned with teaching elementary programming."[3] That is, BASIC was a good teaching tool for users outside the computer science community. Moreover, the language was simple enough to be implemented in very small computers. And, of course, it was precisely these characteristics that led to its great popularity in the microcomputer revolution.

BASIC, like FORTRAN, was designed to implement computational applications with limited control logic. It provided a natural, easy to understand syntax for smaller applications. It differs from FORTRAN in that it was designed to be executed by an interpreter. This means that it ran one line at a time, and that each line had to be interpreted before it could be executed. Consequently, at the time of execution, the run time environment had access to the programs and data as they were currently defined. To illustrate this, consider the statement:

```
100  LET C = A+B
```

Note that each statement has a number. This serves as an index for the statement and establishes the order of statements in the program. The statement begins with a verb that is the command. That is, the parsing of the statement first identifies the command, thereby identifying what function the interpreter is to perform. (Some BASIC implementations omit the LET verb; it is implied by the statement syntax.)

Once the interpreter recognizes an assignment statement, it transfers the line to a section of the interpreter that computes the expression on the right side of the assignment operator (=) and assigns that value to the variable on the left. We have seen how an assembler performs this simple statement. In the case of the assembler the statement was known in advance and the code was designed for only the sequence C = A + B. In the case of an interpreter, on the other hand, it is not known that addition is required until the expression is parsed. Moreover, the interpreter does not know where A and B are stored. To find the value for A, it must look up the variable name "A" in a symbol table to find the address of the word in which the value for A is stored. As shown in Fig. 4.2, the variable A has an entry in the symbol table that points to word 132 in the program's data; this word contains the value of 200. By tracing the address of B we find the value of 100. The interpreter's assignment function adds the two values and then checks to see if C is already in the symbol table. If it is, the interpreter finds the address and stores the value of 300; if C is not in the symbol table, then the interpreter adds it to the symbol table and stores 300 in the address allocated for C. If either A or B is not in the symbol table when statement 100 is being interpreted, it is added and its value is set to zero.

The use of an interpreter has both advantages and disadvantages. Every statement must be parsed each time it is executed. All addressing of variables must go through a table look-up. Therefore, an interpreter will run slower than a compiled program. The advantages of an interpreted language include access to

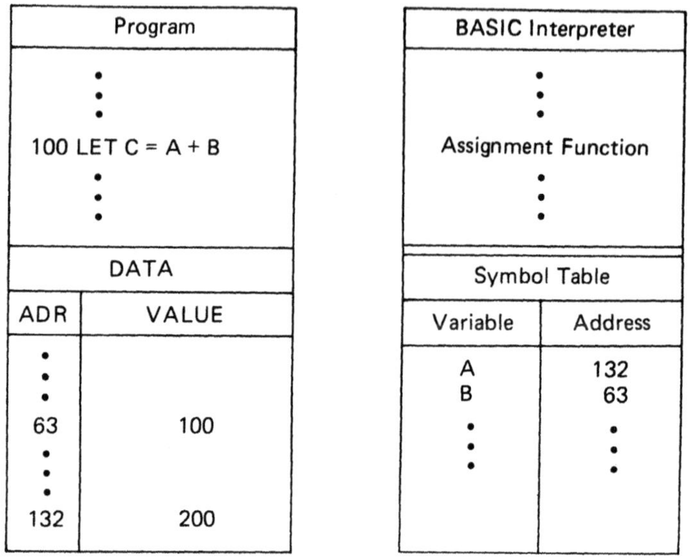

FIGURE 4.2. The BASIC interpreter.

data variables at run time plus the ability to modify and test the program dynamically. For example, if the program stopped after statement 100, one could PRINT C to find its current value. If, on reflection, it was decided that the statement should have been

```
100  LET C = 2 * A + B
```

then it could be edited and immediately rerun. Many implementations of BASIC offer both the interpreted and compiled modes of use. The former is used for development, the latter is used for production operation.

By way of summary, both FORTRAN and BASIC are similar in syntax. The major difference is that FORTRAN was designed to be compiled. The FORTRAN compiler builds a symbol table and then allocates all the space required by a routine during the compilation process. For efficiency, all compiled instructions directly access the words that contain variable values; the variable names (e.g., A, B, C) have no meaning to the compiled (object) program. (There may be a separate symbol table to be used in debugging or testing.) FORTRAN also was designed to link independent subroutines. Transfer to the subroutines is done using the CALL statement.§ In the case of BASIC, the initial goal was teaching and the programs are assumed to be small with the subroutines an integral part of the current program. All parts of a program share the same data and symbol

§FORTRAN also provides a FUNCTION capability which will be described below.

table. Thus, we see that although two languages are outwardly similar, they can differ significantly in the way a program is translated and executed.

4.3.1.3. COBOL

The COmmon Business Oriented Language, COBOL, was developed in response to a 1959 Department of Defense initiative to produce a common language for the adaptation of electronic computers to data processing. Some 40 representatives from users, government institutions, computer manufacturers, and other interested groups combined to form a loosely organized COnference on DAta SYstems Languages (CODASYL) to develop such a language. By the mid-1960s the language had gone through several revisions, there was an established standard, and many manufacturers offered COBOL compilers. Today, COBOL remains the most widely used of all mainframe programming languages. This reflects the scope of business data processing applications.

There are several features of COBOL that set it apart from other programming languages. One of its objectives was to use natural language to produce self-documenting programs.[‡] It organized each program into four divisions.

IDENTIFICATION DIVISION: A description of the program.
ENVIRONMENT DIVISION: A description of the hardware and file names used.
DATA DIVISION: A description of the data structures to be processed.
PROCEDURE DIVISION: The processing logic.

Because the language was intended to be used by business programmers, the syntax favors explicitness over scientific conciseness. The following are statements that might appear in a PROCEDURE DIVISION.

```
SUBTRACT 7 FROM X GIVING Y.
DIVIDE 13 INTO X GIVING Q REMAINDER R.
DIVIDE X INTO Y ROUNDED.
```

The language also has many commands designed to facilitate the manipulation of files. For example.

```
OPEN INPUT TRANSACTION-FILE
```

will open the logical file called TRANSACTION-FILE as an input to this program; no program will be able to write to that file once it has been opened as INPUT. The linking of the logical file name with the physical data is done with a SELECT statement in the ENVIRONMENT DIVISION.

Although the use of natural language statements is now considered verbose and not favored by most language designers, COBOL did introduce a concept

[‡]Natural language, however, is of significant interest to designers of end user products. Here the goal is to provide a syntax that provides a natural bridge between the users' problem statements and the commands interpreted by the system. This approach is used in many Fourth Generation Languages.

that has become an integral parts of most modern languages: the data structure that establishes the relationships among individual elements and a larger whole. Up to this point, we have considered only individual data elements: e.g., A, B, and C. Both FORTRAN and BASIC support a data structure called the array. Vectors and matrices are examples of arrays. Arrays normally contain values of the same data type and are indexed using integers. For example, a vector that describes a point in three-dimensional space might use three floating point numbers to define the east-west position, the north-south position, and the altitude as:

V(1): the east-west position
V(2): the north-south position
V(3): the altitude

In this case, the array V is a data structure containing three elements. Next, assume that there were five objects that we desired to relate to their positions in space. We might define a matrix, M, as a 5 x 3 array where the first index specifies the object chosen and the second index specifies a spatial position. In FORTRAN we would define these array structures as follows:

```
DIMENSION V(3), M(5,3)
REAL V,M
```

The north-south position of object number 4 would be found in M(4,2). Since V and M are defined as real numbers (i.e., floating point), every element in the array is real.

Although the array is a powerful data structure for mathematical computation, it is not well suited for the complexities one encounters in business applications. Here one deals with both text and numbers. Further, there is a need to manage repeating groups. For example, a bill contains one heading and a set of one or more specific charges. This type of structure cannot be represented as a vector, matrix, or other type of array. To see how COBOL manages data structures, first consider the previous matrix example of five objects and their positions in space. Assume for the moment that we wish to give a name to each object and also save its position in space. One way to do this would be to include the following definition in the DATA DIVISION.

```
01 OBJECT-POSITIONS.
   05 OBJECT-NAME PICTURE X(10) OCCURS 5 TIMES.
      10 OBJECT-POSITION PICTURE 9999V99 OCCURS 3 TIMES.
```

The numbers 01, 05, and 10 indicate a hierarchical relationship among the elements. The PICTURE X(10) indicates that the object name is 10 characters long; the PICTURE 9999V99 indicates that each position is 6 digits in length with 2 digits after the decimal point. As in the FORTRAN example, the north-south position of object 4 is:

```
OBJECT-POSITION(4,2).
```

However, unlike in FORTRAN, one can also access the 10-character name of object 4 with

```
OBJECT-NAME(4).
```

This form for defining data structures may be used for very complex structures that are retained in either working or permanent storage. This can be illustrated by showing how COBOL data structures define repeating groups. To return to the example of a bill, there are two major components.

- The bill which identifies the customer, data, and salesman.
- The detail which identifies the name, quantity, and cost for each item entered.

A definition of this structure in the DATA DIVISION might be

```
01 BILL.
   02 HEADING.
      03 CUSTOMER-NUMBER PICTURE 9999.
      03 DATE
         04 MONTH        PICTURE 99.
         04 DAY          PICTURE 99.
         04 YEAR         PICTURE 99.
      03 SALESMAN-NUMBER    PICTURE 9999.
      03 ITEM-COUNT      PICTURE 99.
   02 ITEMS OCCURS 1 TO 99 TIMES DEPENDING ON ITEM-COUNT
      03 ITEM-NAME       PICTURE X(40).
      03 ITEM-QUANT      PICTURE 999.
      03 ITEM-COST       PICTURE 9999V99.
```

Again, the programmer assigns numbers (01, 02, 03, 04, . . .) to indicate the hierarchical relationship among elements in the data structures. The PICTURE phrase indicates the data type and is used in validating the data. The number 9 indicates numeric, X(40) in ITEM-NAME indicates a 40 character string of alphanumerics, and the V in the ITEM-COST definition indicates a decimal point. The number of repetitions of ITEMS is given by the value of ITEM-COUNT.

Surveys show that almost half of all programs are written in COBOL. The reasons for its extensive use are the investment in program libraries, the reliance on large data files essential to business operations, and the many programmers and analysts familiar with the language.

4.3.1.4. MUMPS

The Massachusetts General Hospital Utility Multi-Programming System, MUMPS, was developed in the late 1960s to provide interactive support for database applications. Implemented as an interpretive system, today's Standard MUMPS has many features in common with the more complete versions of BASIC. The differences are twofold:

- The syntaxes of the two languages are very different. BASIC was developed to teach students how to write programs as a precursor to learning FORTRAN. MUMPS was designed as a language to implement systems with relatively small computers. As a result, the MUMPS language is optimized for performance and conciseness (occasionally at the cost of clarity).
- MUMPS was designed for database applications. It therefore has a very powerful database manager with operators to facilitate data manipulation. Further, MUMPS was specifically designed for the data structures commonly encountered in medical applications.

Since a discussion of the language will contribute little of significance to this chapter, we shall focus the discussion on how MUMPS manages its data.

In the languages previously presented, we have defined the concepts of data type (e.g., real, integer) and array (e.g., vector, matrix). We have seen that languages such as FORTRAN have nonexecutable statements that define the data type (e.g., REAL) and the array dimensions (DIMENSION). MUMPS is a nondeclarative language; that is, it has no such statements. There is only one data type in MUMPS:

- Strings which are sequences of characters, e.g., "JOHN PAUL JONES," "CHF," "150 LBS." Numbers such as 1,789, -3.417, and 16.0 are examples of a special type of string.

Assignment uses a SET command. The following are valid MUMPS assignment statements:

```
SET NAME="JOHN PAUL JONES"
SET DX="CHF"
SET WEIGHT (NAME)="150 LBS"
```

The first two examples are clear. The third requires some explanation. In the previous discussion of data structures we introduced arrays with integer indices. In the case of MUMPS, we have only strings, so we must use a string as an index. In this case, we set

```
WEIGHT ("JOHN PAUL JONES") = "150 LBS"
```

Recall the discussion of symbol tables that was presented in the section describing BASIC. After the expression A + B was evaluated, if it was found that C did not exist in the symbol table, then it would be added. The same process is carried out with MUMPS. If not yet defined, WEIGHT ("JOHN PAUL JONES") will be added to the symbol table with a pointer to where the data are stored. In this case a pointer is necessary because the string "150 LBS" will not fit one word; it requires many words. In fact, the number of words required by the data will vary. For example, the assignment statement

```
SET WEIGHT ("JOHN PAUL JONES") = "150 POUNDS"
```

will require more space than the previous value of "150 LBS." To make the best use of working memory, MUMPS manages working storage dynamically, i.e., it makes adjustments as necessary.

Now assume that an individual has a series of weights recorded:

```
SET DATE = "84/03/17"
SET WEIGHT (NAME, DATE) = "148 LBS"
```

Here we have two index elements: NAME and then DATE. If WEIGHT were recorded on three different dates, then we might find:

```
WEIGHT ("JOHN PAUL JONES," "83/12/17") = "152 LBS"
WEIGHT ("JOHN PAUL JONES," "84/02/02") = "150 LBS"
WEIGHT ("JOHN PAUL JONES," "84/02/17") = "148 LBS"
```

All the indices will be sorted in their normal collating sequence order. Many index terms may be used; the length of the data string is arbitrary (but normally limited to 256 characters). This data structure is called a sparse array: array because it uses indices similar to a FORTRAN dimensioned array; sparse because it allocates space only for the entries it uses. By way of contrast, the FORTRAN matrix M(5,3) allocates (reserves) 15 words to hold all possible matrix elements; MUMPS allocates no space until an element is assigned to the array.

The sparse array structure is simply a hierarchy in a tree structure.

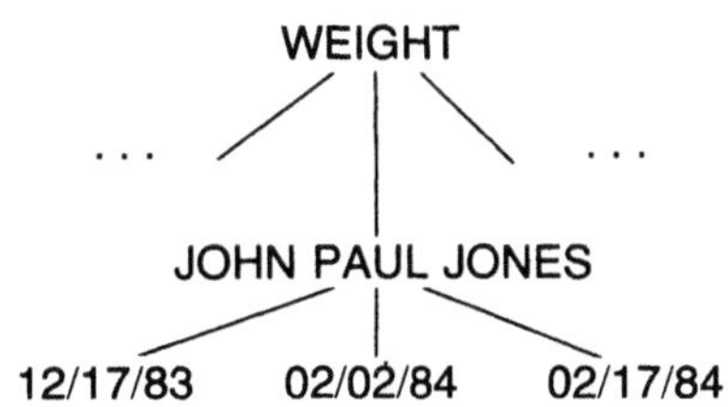

By use of a very simple rule, the same structure can be stored in permanent storage, e.g., on disk. The up arrow character (^) indicates that the associated label is to be found or stored on the disk. Any data stored on the disk is called a global. In effect, one can think of two symbol tables. The symbol table in working memory is used when the up arrow is not used; the symbol table on the disk is used when the up arrow is used. Thus,

```
WRITE "THE WEIGHT OF ", NAME, " ON ", DATE", IS ", ^WEIGHT (NAME,
DATE)
```

uses data stored on disk in an output statement. The data could be entered into the global with

```
SET ^WEIGHT(NAME, DATE) = "150 LBS "
```

From this very brief discussion, it can be seen why MUMPS has been effective for medical applications that process hierarchically structured text strings. Until quite recently, most MUMPS implementations required the MUMPS operating system as well. Thus, it was impossible to mix MUMPS and non-MUMPS applications in the same computer. This limitation is disappearing, and there is a possibility that MUMPS will find a broader audience in the near future.

4.3.1.5. ALGOL and Pascal

The languages ALGOL, Pascal, and Ada span some 25 years of experience with block structured languages. ALGOL 60 was the first language to introduce a block organization. Recall that FORTRAN, its contemporary, used subroutines for independent applications. Each subroutine was compiled separately and loaded into working storage with all its data before the program was initiated. The assignment of storage for programs and data, therefore, was static. Once the program was loaded, the addresses of all variables were known. ALGOL 60 was designed to be implemented using a stack. A stack is a data structure that can be accessed only at the top. One can put something on top of the stack (push) or—if it is not empty—take something from the top (pop). In this sense, the stack is like the cafeteria well that supplies saucers; as long as the well is not empty, one can replace or retrieve the top saucer.

All code in ALGOL 60 was written as blocks within a larger program rather than as independent subroutines. When a block was to be used, space was allocated for its data. Since the space was allocated dynamically, the system could determine how much storage space was required at the time it was requested. Thus, one could write programs that computed how much data storage they needed. (This is similar to the approach used later with interpretive implementations.) The process was managed through use of a stack.

To contrast the two approaches, the FORTRAN CALL statement transferred control to a fixed location that was already loaded in memory together with all the space required to store the program's data. The ALGOL 60 process, on the other hand, identified a program block (already in memory) and sent control to the operating system. The amount of space required for the block's data was computed, and that space was allocated for use by the block. The location from which the block was called was saved in the stack and execution of the new block began. When the block processes were complete, its storage would be released, and the stack would indicate where processing should resume. Of course, during execution, the block could initiate other blocks. In such cases, its processing state would be placed on the stack until the block it called was complete. In fact, a block could call itself; that is, ALGOL 60 supported recursive programming. Fig. 4.3 illustrates how the dynamic allocation of storage is used.

The use of block structures was quickly adopted by a large segment of the computer science community as the most natural way to describe algorithms. The selection of this format was reinforced in 1967 when it was proven that the flow charts for any program could be written using only three structures:

- Sequence: a block of one or more instructions, executed one after the other.
- Iteration: the DO (or FOR in BASIC) statement previously noted. This is generally written

This figure illustrates the dynamic allocation of storage for a program (Prog1) which calls
  Factorial (ANS,6)
where Factorial is a recursive program which, for N > 1 calls
  Factorial (ANS,N-1)
The machine state just before the Prog1 call to factorial is

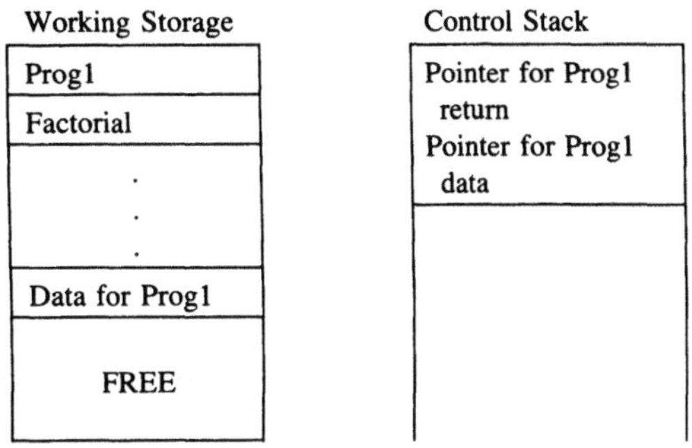

After the call to Factorial (ANS,6), the state is

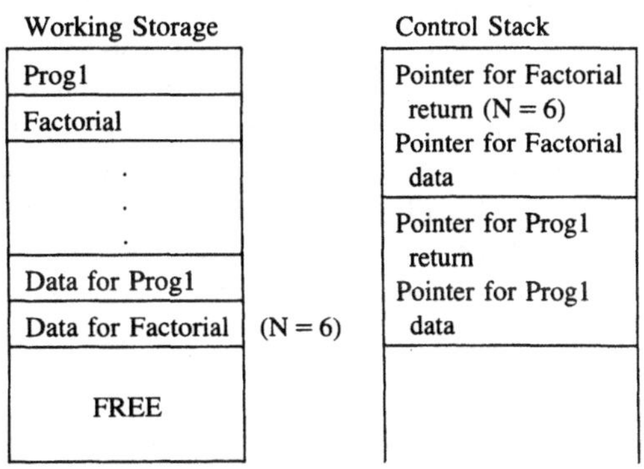

After the call from Factorial to Factorial (ANS,N-1) the state is

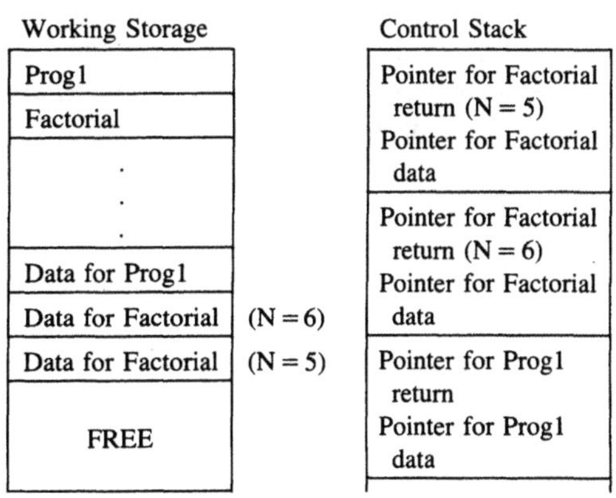

When the Factorial returns, the top of the stack indicates where control should be sent and which block of data be deallocated. Thus, after the initial call to Factorial has been completed, the state is as shown in the first case except that the value assigned to ANS may have been altered.

FIGURE 4.3. Illustration of dynamic allocation of storage.

```
DO WHILE(condition is true)
  block of code to be executed
  END;
```

- Selection: The IF statement. It is usually written to allow the execution of a block of code if the condition is true or false as follows

```
IF condition THEN DO
                 block of code
                 END
               ELSE DO
                 block of code
                 END
```

Of course, each block of code, in turn, could assume the form of one of these structures.

Given this emphasis on block structures, it was natural that the successors to ALGOL 60 would use this style. As we have seen earlier, the development took two directions. The first emphasized richness and functionality at the cost of complexity. ALGOL 68 and PL/1 are examples of this approach. In reaction, Wirth developed Pascal as a tool for teaching programming. This second direction, the Pascal design, emphasized conceptual simplicity and formal verifiability. It removed some of the features of ALGOL but added richer data structures. For example, Pascal expanded the data type to allow user definition of specialized data types. Suppose, by way of illustration, that it was desired to have a data type that represented the days of the week. One could define an enumerated data type as follows:

```
type days = (Sun,Mon,Tues,Wed,Thurs,Fri,Sat)
var start,stop:days
```

The "type" statement defines a data type called days, and the "var" statement indicates that start and stop are both variables of that type. (Pascal uses lowercase names for the variables.) This means that the statements

```
start := Sun; stop := Tues;
```

are valid and

```
start := 37.45
```

is not. Moreover, in this case.

```
start <= stop
```

can be evaluated; it is true. Notice how the enumerated data typing allows the program to build in tests for the validity of data.

The Pascal programming style is similar to that of ALGOL. We can examine the style in a simple program to compute the factorial of n.

```
i := 0; fact := 1;
while i < n do
  i := i + 1 ; fact := i * fact
  end
```

In contrast to FORTRAN, the symbol for assignment is := and not =. This avoids confusion between the use of the equal sign in X = Y as the logical condition (is X equal to Y?) and the assignment process (set the value of X equal to the value of Y). The semicolon separates statements that can be placed on a single line to facilitate understanding. There are no statement numbers. The "while" statement is a more powerful iteration construct than the DO of FORTRAN. Indentation is used to make the block structure more readable.

Pascal can also support recursion—a useful feature for the efficient definition of algorithms. Recall that we began with a formal definition of n! as

```
for n>0  n! =n  (n-1)!
for n=0  n! =1
```

We illustrate recursion with a function that we shall call "factorial." A function is identical to a procedure (subroutine) except that one does not call it; one uses it in an expression. The square root function is an example of a function normally included with a language, e.g.,

```
sd := sqrt (variance)
```

FORTRAN, BASIC, and most high order languages support the definition of functions. In this case we define a factorial to be a function used in an expression. To see how it would be used, consider

```
Y := 3;
X := 5 * factorial(Y)
```

In this case, X would be set to 5 * 3! or 5*3*2*1 or 30.

The recursive definition is as follows:

```
function factorial (n: integer): integer
begin If n > 0 then factorial := n * factorial(n-1)
  else factorial := 1
```

The (n: integer) indicates that the input n must be of data type integer; the final : integer on the definition line indicates that the function returns a result of data type integer. Notice how similar this function is to the formal definition.

As already noted, Pascal was initially developed as a teaching and research tool; it was not designed for the implementation of larger systems. It is firmly entrenched as a language for students and microcomputer applications. Its successor, MODULA-2, combines the basic syntax of Pascal with the modular structures better suited to more complex systems. Another block structured language of the 1980s is Ada. Both are designed to use the concepts of modularity and information hiding discussed in Chapter 6.

4.3.2. Functional (Applicative) Programming Languages

Each of the previous languages presented is an imperative language; each operates as a sequence of steps that have their primary effect by assigning values to variables. The functional or applicative languages, on the other hand, have their effect by applying functions. In this section we shall introduce four such languages.

4.3.2.1. APL

The first language to be considered is A Programming Language (APL). Introduced by Iverson in 1962, its popularity grew in the latter half of the decade with the release of an efficient implementation. The initial goal of APL was mathematical computation using matrices and vectors. As we have seen, programs such as FORTRAN require the user first to define an array in a DIMENSION statement and then to operate on the matrix one element at a time. APL was designed to operate on scalars, vectors, and matrices with minimal explicit housekeeping overhead. The result is a concise language that relies on a special character set to add richness to the language.

A box (□) is the symbol for both input and output; □ ← means to print the value of what follows; A ← □ means to request an input and bind it to the variable A. Thus, the user program

```
A ← □ Return
```

will cause the computer to display the prompt

```
□
```

this prompt, followed by a user entry of

```
1 2 3 4 5 6 Return
```

will define A to be a vector of dimensionality 6. Alternatively, the entry of

```
2 3ρ 1 2 3 4 5 6 Return
```

defines A to be a 2×3 matrix. (The ρ symbol indicates that the first inputs define the dimensions and not the values.) Note that the nature of A is determined only at the time its contents are entered.

A slightly more complex APL program computes an average:

```
(+/A) ÷ ρ A ← □
```

It is processed from right to left. A ← associates an input with A. The unary operator ρ counts the number of elements in A; the result is a scalar. The (+/A) is the sum of the element values in the vector A (also a scalar); the parentheses are used to indicate that the summation must be done first; otherwise APL will first divide each element of A and then sum the quantity. The final operation, division (÷), produces the mean. Thus, once the program is entered, an input of

```
10 12 14 16 18 20 RETURN
```

will produce an answer of 15. An equivalent FORTRAN program would require a DIMENSION statement, a read statement, a loop to produce the sum, division to produce the mean, and a write statement. The major difference, however, is not in the brevity of the notation. In the FORTRAN program, all storage must be allocated in advance, and thus the nature of the array must be defined before compilation begins. In the case of APL, the nature of A is determined only when it is used; moreover, no variables were assigned to represent the number of elements in the array, the sum of the element values, or even the resultant mean.

4.3.2.2. FORTH

A very different approach to functional programming can be illustrated with FORTH. This language was first developed by Charles Moore in the late 1960s for his personal use. He believed that it represented a fourth generation of languages, and so he adopted the name FORTH. The unusual spelling derived from the fact that the initial implementation required variable names to be five or fewer characters in length. FORTH has become popular among small computer users; it is compact, faster to code than assembly language, and generally efficient in operation.

We have selected FORTH to illustrate (a) how processing can be performed without assignments and (b) how recursion is supported using stacks. Recall that a stack is a list that allows one to add a new top element (push) or remove the top element (pop). The objects in FORTH are called words. Some words are already defined; the user may define new words by using existing words. The words are arranged in Polish postfix notation (e.g., AB+ for A + B) and processing begins with the first word and continues through the last.

We define a word to compute N! which we call FACT. The definition of a word begins with a colon and terminates with a semicolon. The definition of the word FACT is

```
:FACT DUP 1 - DUP 2 = NOT IF FACT THEN *;
```

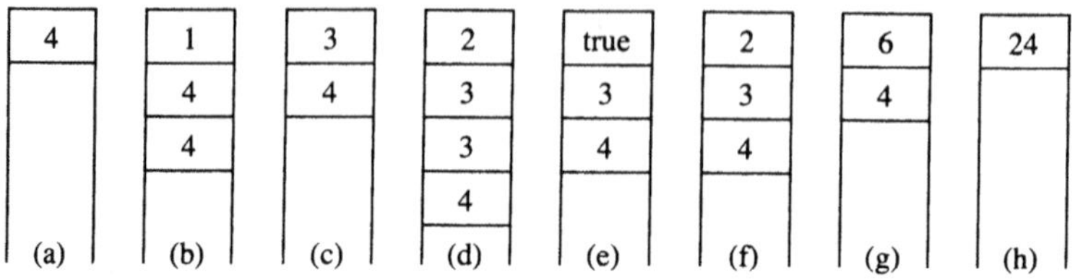

FIGURE 4.4. FORTH stack contents in the computation of 4! (From H. Katzen, *Invitation to FOURTH,* Petrocelli Books, Inc. Reprinted by permission.)

The processing for this definition is shown in Fig. 4.4. FACT is initiated with the number whose factorial is to be computed being placed on the stack (4a). There is also a separate stack that indicates where control should resume when FACT is complete. The first word in the FACT definition, DUP, causes the top of the stack to be duplicated; a word consisting of a number causes that number to be added to the top of the stack (4b). The word – is the binary operator for subtraction; it removes the top two numbers from the stack and replaces them with their difference (4c). DUP again duplicates the top of the stack and 2 places a 2 on the top (4d). The = is a binary operator that replaces the top two stack entries with a Boolean value that indicates whether they were equal. In this case it is false; the NOT replaces the top of the stack with its Boolean negation, i.e., true (4e). The IF word removes the top of the stack and, if true, executes the next word; otherwise it continues following the THEN. In this case, the top of the stack is true and the word FACT is again executed.

With each recursive execution of FACT, an entry is pushed into the control stack such that, on completion, it will resume starting with the word after FACT. Thus, after the next processing of FACT, the IF condition is false and the stack is as shown in 4f. The processing resumes after the THEN with the binary operator *. This removes the top two numbers in the stack and replaces them by their product (4g). FACT pops the top of the control stack and resumes processing following the last execution. In this case, the position is THEN * and the top two stack elements are replaced by their product (4h). Again, the control stack is popped and control returns to the flow with the top of the stack replaced by the factorial of the initial value.

4.3.2.3. LISP

The LISt Processing language LISP was developed by John McCarthy in 1959; it is the language most commonly used in artificial intelligence applications. Each of the languages that we have examined operates on a limited class of objects. FORTRAN operates on numbers in a variety of formats; APL operates on vectors and matrices; and MUMPS operates on character strings. LISP operates on lists.

The smallest element of a list is called an atom. The empty list (NIL) contains no atoms. This sentence is a list with eight atoms. A list may also contain lists as well as atoms. Lists are called symbolic or s-expressions and are normally encased in parentheses, thus:

```
(THIS SENTENCE IS A LIST WITH EIGHT ATOMS)
```

Operators in LISP are written in Polish prefix notation.

```
(PLUS A B).
```

will produce A + B. The "assignment" operator is SETQ. Thus

```
(SETQ C (PLUS A B))
```

will set the value of the atom C to the result of evaluation of the s-expression (PLUS A B), i.e., C = A + B.

Clearly, the power of LISP is not in its ability to compute FORTRAN-like statements. In most cases the LISP style makes little use of the assignment concept. Two of the most useful operators are those that extract portions of a list or construct new lists from existing atoms and lists. CAR is an operator that returns the first element in a list; CDR (pronounced "coulder") returns a list with the first element removed. In each case the R stands for "register"—a reflection of the techniques used in the earliest implementation. The apostrophe in the s-expression '(THIS IS A LIST) indicates that what follows is a literal, i.e., it takes on the value shown. (In other programming languages it is common to write literals with pairs of quotation marks, "THIS IS A LIST.") The s-expression

```
(CAR '(THIS IS A LIST))
```

returns the atom THIS while

```
(CDR '(THIS IS A LIST))
```

returns the list (IS A LIST). An atom is written without parentheses, a list is written in parentheses.

Notice that the lists we have shown are like a stack. The CAR gets the first element of the list; it is similar to a POP. To PUSH, one needs an operator to construct a list from atoms and lists.

```
(CONS 'THIS '(IS A LIST))
```

produces the list (THIS IS A LIST).

If one now adds a conditional operator (such as a form of IF . . . THEN . . . ELSE), two predicates to determine whether a list is an atom and whether two lists are equal, and some functions for binding labels and variables, then the definition of LISP is complete. The entire LISP language may be defined in terms of these constructs.

By way of illustration, we return to the n! problem. In LISP, the DEFINE function is used to define a new function. In this case, we define a function called FACTORIAL with an argument N as

(DEFINE (FACTORIAL N) (s-expression))

When FACTORIAL N is used in a LISP program, the s-expression will be substituted; if FACTORIAL M is used, the s-expression will be modified so that every occurrence of the atom N will be replaced by an occurrence of the atom M. Thus, the processing is simply replacement of equivalent symbol strings with a reduction to strings and functions already defined. In this example, the s-expression will be recursive. On the condition that N is equal to 0, it will return a 1. Otherwise, it will return the product of N and the factorial of N-1. Fig. 4.5a contains the LISP definition of FACTORIAL. Compare it with the Pascal function repeated in Fig. 4.5b. Note that there is no data typing or assignment in LISP. The "blocking" indention in both languages is not necessary; it is used to enhance readability and comprehension.

Not all LISP programs need to be expressed recursively. The same factorial function could be defined as a sequence of serially executed s-expressions. There is even a branching function GO as in (GO LOOP). Fig. 4.5c presents a more procedural definition of FACTORIAL; the equivalent FORTRAN flow is shown in Figure 4.5d.

One can gain an appreciation of LISP only by seeing how some more complex problem can be solved using functional programming. In what follows we illustrate how a LISP program can be used to solve simple algebra problems written as English language statements such as:

If the number of customers Tom gets is twice the square of 20 percent of the number of ads he runs, and the number of ads he runs is 45, what is the number of customers he gets? (From Patrick H. Winston, *Artificial Intelligence,* © 1973, Addison-Wesley, Reading, Massachusetts. Pgs. 335-340. Reprinted with permission.)

The system described was developed by Daniel Bobrow in the mid 1960s. The example we use was presented by Patrick Winston.[4]

The solution to the problem begins with the problem statement in the form of a s-expression. The punctuation marks are encoded to avoid confusion with special LISP symbols. The input, therefore, is:

(IF THE NUMBER OF CUSTOMERS TOM GETS IS TWICE THE SQUARE OF 20 PERCENT OF THE NUMBER OF ADS HE RUNS C AND THE NUMBER OF ADS HE RUNS IS 45 C WHAT IS THE NUMBER OF CUSTOMERS HE GETS Q)

The next task is to separate the problem statement into pieces that are the equivalent of the equations to be solved. In this case:

```
(DEFINE (FACTORIAL N)
    (COND ((ZERO N) 1)
          ((TIMES N (FACTORIAL (SUB1 N))))))
```

(a) LISP Definition Using Rrecursion

```
function factorial (n:integer) :interger
begin if n = 0 then factorial : = 1
    else factorial : = n * factorial (n – 1)
```

(b) Pascal Definition Using Recursion

```
(DEFINE (FACTORIAL N)
    (PROG (RESULT)
          (SETQ RESULT 1)
          LOOP
          (COND ((ZEROP N) (RETURN RESULT)))
          (SETQ RESULT (TIMES RESULT N))
          (SETQ N (SUB1 N))
          (GO LOOP)))
```

(c) LISP Definition Using Iteration or Branching

```
      INTEGER FACT (N)
      FACT = 1
10    IF (N .EQ.0) RETURN
      FACT = FACT * N
      N = N – 1
      GOTO 10
      END
```

(d) FORTRAN function following the flow of (c). Note that in both cases there is the side effect that N is set to zero on return; N is not altered in the first two examples.

FIGURE 4.5. Implementations of the factorial function.

```
((THE NUMBER OF CUSTOMERS TOM GETS IS TWICE THE
SQUARE OF 20 PERCENT OF THE NUMBER OF ADS HE RUNS)
(THE NUMBER OF ADS HE RUNS IS 45)
(UNKNOWN IS THE NUMBER OF CUSTOMERS HE GETS))
```

Once separated, the individual statements must be translated into statements which can be evaluated. This becomes

```
((EQUAL (THE NUMBER OF CUSTOMERS TOM GETS)
  (TIMES 2.
    (EXPT (TIMES 0.2
      (THE NUMBER OF ADS HE RUNS))
   2.)))
```

```
(EQUAL (THE NUMBER OF ADS HE RUNS) 45)
(EQUAL (UNKNOWN) (THE NUMBER OF CUSTOMERS HE GETS)))
```

At this point, the difference between the applicative language LISP and the imperative language Pascal becomes more clear. The EQUAL function returns a value of "true" if the two following s-expressions are identical. Thus to "solve" the problem, all of the EQUAL functions must return "true." This means that the list

```
(THE NUMBER OF ADS HE RUNS)
```

identical to the atom

```
45.
```

Thus the atom 45 replaces the list

```
(THE NUMBER OF ADS HE RUNS)
```

in the previous s-expression to produce

```
... (TIMES 0.2 45) ...
```

which can be evaluated to produce ultimately a numerical value that must be equal to the list

```
(THE NUMBER OF CUSTOMERS TOM GETS)
```

By pattern matching, it can be seen that this list is equivalent to the list with the atom TOM replaced by the atom HE. Thus, the solution is

```
(EQUAL (THE NUMBER OF CUSTOMERS HE GETS) 162)
```

which can be printed out as the answer:

```
(THE NUMBER OF CUSTOMERS HE GETS IS 162 P)
```

In an imperative language, the s-expression

```
(TIMES 2.
  (EXPT (TIMES 0.2
    (THE NUMBER OF ADS HE RUNS))
    2.))
```

could be written as the FORTRAN expression

```
2 * (.2 * (NAHR) ** 2)
```

But this expression could not be evaluated unless preceded by the assignment statement

```
NAHR = 45
```

The variable NAHR represents a storage location in working memory; it is bound to that location at the time of compilation. In LISP, on the other hand, NAHR is represented by the list

```
(THE NUMBER OF ADS HE RUNS).
```

This is bound to the value 45 at execution time. It is not associated with a specific storage location. In fact, given the pattern matching that will interchange TOM and HE, one would get the same solution with the two s-expressions:

```
(EQUAL (THE NUMBER OF ADS TOM RUNS) 45)
(EQUAL (THE NUMBER OF ADS HE RUNS) 45)
```

This little example gives some insight into why LISP is so popular for AI applications. Although the parentheses of the s-statements seem very strange at first, one can quickly develop the skills which make this a natural form for expressing nested functions. The power of the language, the large community of users with common interests, and the libraries of tools all combine to make LISP the language of choice for AI investigators in the United States.

4.3.2.4. PROLOG

The last of the languages to be presented here is the language PROLOG. This language has been chosen by the Japanese for their Fifth Generation Computer; its popularity in Europe and Japan justifies a cursory introduction. As its name implies, PROLOG applies PROgramming in LOGic. For example, if we have the two assertions

```
if A then B
A
```

then we deduce that B is true. To give a more concrete illustration,

```
if Gerry is the mother of Jane then Gerry is the parent of Jane.
Gerry is the mother of Jane.
```

Therefore, Gerry is the parent of Jane.

PROLOG provides a very simple structure for defining these logical relationships.

```
mother (gerry,jane).
```

is called a clause. In this case, the clause establishes the relationship "mother" between "gerry" and "jane." Mother is called a functor, gerry and jane are called arguments. Arguments with uppercase letters are variables; those with lower case letters are constants. (Some implementations prefix constants with an asterisk.) To establish that Gerry is Jane's mother, one would use the clause

```
assert(mother(gerry,jane)).
```

A sentence (consisting of one or more clauses) that shows the relationship between mother and parent might be

```
parent(X,Y) :- mother(X,Y).
```

In this case, the logical statement is written in the form

```
B if A
```

and the operator :- represents the if. An "and" is written as a comma, an "or" as a semicolon. The meaning of the following PROLOG "program" should now be clear:

```
parent(X,Y) :- mother(X,Y) ; father(X,Y).
grandmother(X,Y) :- mother(X,Z), parent(Z,Y).
```

The obvious question is, how is this program used? First we shall assume the following assertions:

```
father (john,jane).
mother (gerry,jane).
mother (mary,gerry).
```

To find Jane's grandmother using the rules in the previous sentences, we shall prove grandmother (X,jane). That is, we shall find a value for X such that grandmother (X,jane) is true. The actual proof, of course, is managed by PROLOG and the system either returns with a failure, or in this case, the binding X = mary. One could just as easily have asked the question, who are Mary's grandchildren?

```
grandmother (mary,X).
```

Programs can be written to have X contain either a single name or a list of names.

In a sense, PROLOG can be thought of as a language that searches a database of assertions. In fact, the functors of PROLOG are very similar to the relations of database theory which will be described in the following chapter. The objects processed here are symbolic strings and the language—like LISP—has powerful pattern matching capabilities. As in all of the applicative languages presented, the processing is not described procedurally and the binding of a variable to a data string is used instead of assigning a variable to a specific storage location.

4.4. Concluding Remarks

This chapter has introduced a variety of programming languages. The purpose of this presentation was to illustrate the diversity available and to suggest that there are many ways to write a program. Disregarding assembly languages, it is now possible to group the languages into three categories:

- *Folk languages*. These are languages which were initially implemented because (a) they reflected a natural way of expressing a class of problems and (b) they satisfied some specific language design objectives. Examples are FORTRAN, COBOL, BASIC and MUMPS. In each case there is an investment in education and program libraries. This investment will ensure the long term existence of these languages—hence the term "folk."
- *Structured languages*. These are languages which were designed to manage the description (i.e., programming) of formal processes. Derived from ALGOL, modern examples include Pascal, MODULA-2, and C. The most "modern" and complete language in this category is Ada. The structures provided by these languages include internal processing blocks for sequence, selection and iteration as well as intermodule facilities such as abstract data types and concurrency management. Hence the term "structured."
- *Functional languages*. These are languages that apply functions to data. The programs and data are one; processing is separated from the management of memory; and procedural description of processing is avoided. Examples include LISP and PROLOG. Because of their ability to express relationships concisely and to process symbolic data, these languages are used in artificial intelligence applications.

The above categorization, of course, is offered only as a guideline. FORTRAN 77 has many structured attributes; in some ways MUMPS is an applicative language; the enthusiasm of the FORTH users group suggests that its success is based upon its folk appeal. Nevertheless, one can expect languages in each of the three categories to flourish; however, academic training and research will be restricted to the last two classes.

Finally, we note that a fourth category of languages is just emerging: the user oriented languages. The languages are designed as tools for computer supported applications. Current examples are word processors, automated bank tellers, and natural language interfaces. By the end of this century, interaction with computer systems by using a combination of voice, graphics, and typing will be commonplace. The programs that support these systems may be written in languages of the above categories, or they may be written in the same language as the target product. And if this is the direction in which computers will be taking us, then it is important to recognize that there is more to programming than simply understanding BASIC.

For Further Reading

There are a large number of books about programming languages. They vary in projected audience from motivated novice to graduate student. Among the more general works are T. Pratt, *Programming Languages: Design and Implementation*, Prentice Hall, 1975, which provides a general overview and A. Tucker, *Programming Languages*, McGraw-Hill, 1977, which describes and compares six languages. (ALGOL, FORTRAN, COBOL, PL/1, RPG and SNOBOL). For persons with some computer science background, E. Horowitz, *Fundamentals of Programming Languages*, Computer Science Press, 1982, provides an excellent and readable overview of the principle issues.

With respect to specific programming languages, there are many books available. Experienced programmers may be satisfied with a reference manual; novice programmers may require considerably more support. Among the books I have examined are:

COBOL: D. D. McCracken, *A Simplified Guide to Structured COBOL Programming*, John Wiley, 1976. (McCracken has a clear, mature style and his books for any language are to be recommended.) Also, C. Sass, *COBOL Programming and Applications*, Allyn and Bacon, 1979.

FORTRAN: J. W. Crowley, C. E. Miller, *A Structured Approach to FORTRAN*, Prentice Hall, 1983, P. Chirlian, *Introduction to Structured Fortran*, Matrix Publishers, 1979, and A. Balfour, and D. H. Marwick, *Programming in Standard FORTRAN 77*, North Holland, 1982.

ALGOL: D. Brailsford, and A. Walker, *Introductory Algol-68 Programming*, Wiley, 1979.

PL/1: J. Hughes, *PL/1 Structured Programming*, 2nd ed., Wiley, 1979.

PASCAL: R. Conway, D. Gries, E. C. Zimmerman, *A Primer on Pascal*, Little, Brown, 1981, and P. Gregono, *Programming in PASCAL*, Addison-Wesley, 1980.

BASIC: There are a large number of introductory texts. Most systems come with one. A short and simple book is provided by K. Knecht, *Microsoft BASIC*, Dilithium Press, 1983.

MUMPS: A Primer and manuals are available from the MUMPS Users Group, College Park, MD 20740.

FORTH: H. Katzen, *Invitation to FORTH*, Petrocelli, 1981.

APL: R. P. Polivka and S. Pakin, *APL The Language and Its Usage*, Prentice-Hall, 1975.

Ada: P. Wegner, *Programming with Ada*, Prentice-Hall, 1980.

LISP: P. H. Winston, *LISP*, Addison-Wesley, 1981.

PROLOG: W. F. Clocksin and C. S. Mellish, *Programming in PROLOG*, Springer-Verlag, 1981.

Modula 2: N. Wirth, *Programming in Modula-2*, Springer-Verlag, 1983.

References

1. N. Wirth, On the Design of Programming Languages, *1974 IFIP Congress,* North Holland, 1974, pp 386-393. Copyright 1974, North Holland.
2. P. Wegner, Programming Languages—the First 25 Years, *IEEE Trans. Comp.*, (C-25,12) p 1209.
3. *Ibid* p 1219.
4. P. Winston, *Artificial Intelligence*, Addison-Wesley, Reading, MA, First Edition, 1973 pp 335-340.

5
Data Bases

5.1. Introduction

In Chapter 2 we identified three types of objects to be processed. These are data, information, and knowledge. Data were defined as the smallest elements that could be processed, information was described as sets of data organized to assist in decision-making, and knowledge was presented as the rules for creating information from data and information. Given this orientation, we now may define a database as a collection of data, organized as information, using a structure derived from a knowledge of its potential use. This implies that we must address how the data are stored physically, how they are organized to present useful information, and finally, what rules are used to establish a database design. These are the topics of the next three sections.

5.2. File Structures

A file is a collection of data that is stored outside the working storage. Files may be stored online, e.g., on a hard disk, or saved on some removable medium, e.g., a magnetic tape or floppy disk. To be useful, however, the file must be available online; therefore, in what follows we shall assume that all files of interest are loaded and available to the computer.

There are many types of files. Some files contain source programs; these represent data to a compiler. Other files contain the output from a compiler—the object programs; these represent data to the operating system's loader. Finally, there are files that contain application data. Databases are restricted to this last class of data. The operating system normally uses the same set of tools to manage all file types.

The computer term file is derived from the common word used to describe a collection of data or information. Frequently, we use the concept of a file drawer with folders to classify the materials stored. In the file cabinet model, we have random retrieval to the level of the folder. That is, we can select the file drawer and then select a folder in that file drawer. Our retrieval system will be as efficient as the filing system. If materials are not carefully associated with the correct folder, then retrieval of the folder may not produce the information we desire. Moreover, if the labels on the folders are cryptic, we may find it difficult to identify which folder we desire. Of course, both these problems have to do with how we use the file system and not its physical structure.

To continue with the file cabinet analogy, once a folder is identified, it must be removed and we must page through its contents to find what we are looking for. We expect the contents of the folder to have some order, e.g., correspondence filed in descending date order. This will help us find what we are looking for. There also may be visual clues: paper color, stationery type, coffee stains. The search may be for a complete document or an extract from it. When the desired material is found, the search is completed and the analysis begins. If the desired material is not found, additional searches (folders) are processed until either the materials are found or the fact that they cannot be found is accepted.

The contents of that file cabinet are a database; its organization, storage, and retrieval are the subject of this chapter. This section illustrates how the computer equipment models the file cabinet. In its simplest expression, the computer model provides access to a folder given its address. The address in the file cabinet analogy is: file cabinet, drawer, position in drawer. For a computer system it may be: disk unit, cylinder, track, block. In either case, the first step in retrieval or filing is complete once the desired folder (or block) is extracted and the document (or record) is removed or inserted.

Note that we have used two computer terms: The block is the smallest physical collection of data that can be retrieved as a single unit. The record is the smallest logical collection of data that may be stored in the database. A record normally contains many fields (or data elements); a block generally contains more than one record. (In some cases a record may extend over more than one block.) As an example, the record for an item list in a bill might consist of three fields as follows:

```
ITEM-NAME   (PICTURE X(40))
ITEM-QUANT  (PICTURE 999)
ITEM-COST   (PICTURE 9999V99)
```

This record is 49 characters long. A block of 1,000 characters could hold 20 such records.

To summarize, a file is a collection of records, each of which has a similar (if not identical) definition, and files are physically stored as blocks. A file access method is a technique for retrieving (or storing) records in a file. Access methods operate at the logical level; they do not require that the user have a knowledge of the physical location of a record, i.e., its address in permanent storage. There are three basic access methods.

- *Serial or sequential.* In this case all records are ordered and one can access only the the first record or the next record. The end of the file is indicated by a special record called the end of file (EOF). Magnetic tape, because of its physical organization, supports only serial files. However, it is common to use serial files with random access storage devices such as the disk. For example, a sorted output file is accessed serially.

- *Random*. In this case each record has a key (or index) that allows it to be accessed. Access to the record is determined only by the contents of the key. Each record is independent and records with similar keys are not "close" to each other; there is no concept of a "next" record or "end of file."
- *Indexed Sequential*. In this case the file is organized as a serial (or sequential) file, and each record has a key as in the case of the random access method. The index sequential access method (ISAM) provides tools for the user to read randomly any record and also read the next record. Thus, the user can start reading at any point in the file and then read serially from that point.

In the random and indexed sequential access methods each record must have a key (or index) that serves as an identifier for that record. The key is part of the record and generally contains one or more data elements (or fields) in the record. We shall assume that the key uniquely defines a record. (There are implementations that allow multiple records with the same key.) Limiting the discussion to the problems of retrieval, it can be seen that both the random and indexed sequential access methods require that the system be given a key and then either return the record that matches that key or a "not found" message. There are several ways of implementing this.

5.2.1. The Heap

The easiest—and most—inefficient technique is to organize the file as a heap (or pile). This has no structure and access is accomplished by reading a record, comparing it to the key, and returning if a match is found. The process continues until each record in the file has been tested; if it fails, then the "not found" message is returned. For a file of n records, an average n/2 tests will be required for a success and n matches will be required for each failure. For small values of n this technique can be considered; for the larger values that are typical in database applications, such an organization is unacceptable. Note that the access method described is valid only for random access. Since we assumed nothing about the organization of the heap, the selection of the "next" record returns a random record. Of course, the heap may be ordered in some way and used as a serial file.

5.2.2. Random Access with Hashing

We now consider more efficient techniques for implementing a random access method. Recall that records are relatively small and that the file is physically organized as blocks that contain one or more records. We now introduce the concept of a bucket that consists of one or more blocks in storage. A bucket contains a group of records that have some similar key property. Each bucket is identified by that key property. The random access method uses a record key that is logically linked to the bucket identifier. The bucket is retrieved and each record in the bucket is examined for the desired key. That is, within the bucket we use a heap organization. Since the input/output (I/O) operations are relatively slow, if we can minimize the number of transfers from the disk to working storage (i.e., the number of blocks or buckets that must be read or written), then we can maximize efficiency. Although the searching through a bucket in working storage may seem cumbersome, it can be performed very rapidly.

The most common technique for identifying the bucket is called hashing. The term comes from the accounting practice of adding a sequence of numbers—such as the last digits of each purchase order in a batch—to produce a meaningless hash total. If a subsequent addition does not produce the same hash total, then an error is present or a document has been lost or added to the batch. In the case of hashing for retrieval purposes, the record key is converted into a hash number that has no meaning with respect to the key. However, the hashed number serves as an identifier for the bucket containing the record.

To illustrate, assume that there will be a random file with 1,000 records such that 20 records will fit in a bucket. If, for some reason, we wish to keep each bucket half full (on the average), then we will need 100 buckets. We identify these buckets as 0, 1, 2, ... 99. If each record has a key in the form of a number from 1000 to 999999, then we can find the bucket identifier for any record by dividing the record key by 100 and using the remainder as the hash value. For this case, the hashing function is the record key modulo 100.

In this example, we assumed that the assigned record numbers were random. Thus, the modulus 100 value would be random, and there would be an equal probability of assigning a record to any bucket. If this is true, then retrieval of a record is very simple. Apply the hashing function to find the bucket address, retrieve the bucket, search through the bucket, and either return the record or the "not found" message. This requires the minimum of one I/O to get the bucket. However, what if the record keys were not randomly assigned? What if they were 1000, 1100, 1200, ... 999900? Then the hashing function we chose would map all records into a single bucket. The obvious solution would be to choose a different hashing function. Still, there will always be the problem of what to do when a bucket is full.

When a bucket is too full to hold another record, an overflow bucket is assigned to hold the record. Normally, this overflow bucket is considered an extension of the initial bucket. When this is the case, the initial bucket contains a pointer. If that pointer is null, then there is no overflow bucket; if that pointer is not null, then it contains the address of an overflow bucket. The overflow bucket, in turn, has a pointer that may point to its overflow bucket. As shown in Fig. 5.1, each bucket is a chain with an initial bucket and overflow buckets. Retrieval involves accessing the initial bucket, examining the records in it, and, if necessary, repeating the process with each overflow bucket. If there are n-1 overflow buckets, then, on the average, n/2 buckets will be examined when the desired record is

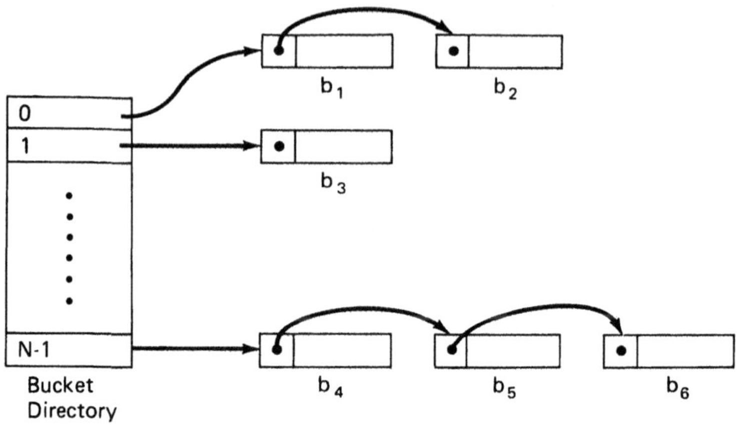

FIGURE 5.1. Hashed File Organization. The Bucket Directory translates the bucket identifier (0, 1, 2, . . ., N) into the physical address of the bucket. The period at the front of the bucket indicates the pointer. The N-1 bucket chain includes three buckets. The bucket b_6 has no arrow going from its pointer; thus, it is the end of the chain. The association of buckets in a chain bears no relationship to their physical location. Buckets b_2 b_6 could be physically adjacent.

found and n buckets must be examined to return a "not found" message. Consequently, the use of overflows slows processing.

Up to this point, we have considered only the task of record retrieval: apply the hash function, get the bucket, search for the desired record, if not found, get the chained overflow bucket, and continue until the record is found or the "not found" message can be sent. To replace (or modify) a record, one retrieves the record and places the modified record in the same position. However, if the records vary in length, then the replacement record may be longer than the record to be replaced. In this case, the old record is deleted and the new record is added.

To add (or insert) a new record, the system finds a space in the bucket large enough for the record. That space may never have been used or it may have been created when a record was deleted. If no space is available, an overflow bucket must be created. The system maintains a list of empty buckets that can be used for overflows. When an overflow is required, a bucket address is taken from bucket overflow list, and that address is used as a pointer at the end of the current bucket chain. The record is then added to the empty overflow bucket. If no overflow buckets are available, then the task aborts with a "file full" message.

The deletion of a record requires that the record be located and then removed. In practice, the deleted record is not removed but marked as deleted. The record is not removed because there is the possibility that it may be the only record in a bucket. Removing the record may then require the removal of the bucket, the adjustment of pointers in the bucket chain, the restoration of the empty bucket to the overflow list, etc. To avoid this processing, the record is flagged as deleted but retained. The actual removal of the record is normally done by a utility program; the process is sometimes called garbage collection.

5.2.3. The Use of Index Files

The use of hashed files is most efficient when random access is required and an efficient hashing function can be found. Retrieval of patient data by patient identifier is an ideal application. There is no logical connection between patients with "similar" identification numbers. Thus, each retrieval is independent and the user has no interest in the other records in the bucket. However, what if a patient's data are to be retrieved by the use of a name rather than an identifier. One may wish to look at similar names to select the desired patient. In this case there is a relationship among records and one would like the buckets to group records according to that relationship, e.g., one bucket chain would contain all last names with initial letters SMI through SN. To do this requires an index that is stored as an ordered file.

The index is similar to the index tabs found in a library catalog. The library catalog assumes that all the cards are sorted and that each tab indicates the first card with the initial letters shown on the tab. To find a specific card, one looks for the first tab that is larger than (i.e., lexically follows) the desired card. Then the card—if it exists—will be between that tab and the tab that precedes it. The index file is simply a collection of the tabs in the form of a sorted file; each tab entry has pointers to buckets in a file where the data for that index (tab) are stored. To use this file organization, at least two I/O accesses are required. The first retrieves the bucket in the index file to find the pointer to the bucket containing the data; the second I/O retrieves the bucket containing the records "close to" that index (or key).

As in the case of hashed files, individual buckets can grow too full and overflow buckets may be required. With indexed files there are two files: the index file and the data file. The index file is generally defined when the file is first created and it provides pointers to the bucket that contains records between that initial index and the next. When there are too many records within the given key range, overflow data buckets are added as shown in Fig. 5.2. There are several ways of searching through an index. The first is to start always at the top and search serially until the desired index pointer is found. This linear search is the least efficient. An alternative approach is to use a binary search. One selects the central index value and compares it with the desired key. If the key is smaller, then the program knows that the desired index is among the smaller indices; otherwise it must be among the larger indices. This half of the index is bisected again until an acceptable index is found. If there is no prior information about the distribution of the index, then the binary search is always the fastest technique. Where there is prior information, however, it can be used to calculate the index address for a more efficient search.

Selecting the proper index record points to the bucket chain that may contain the desired record. Records in the bucket chain may be sorted or random. Sorting

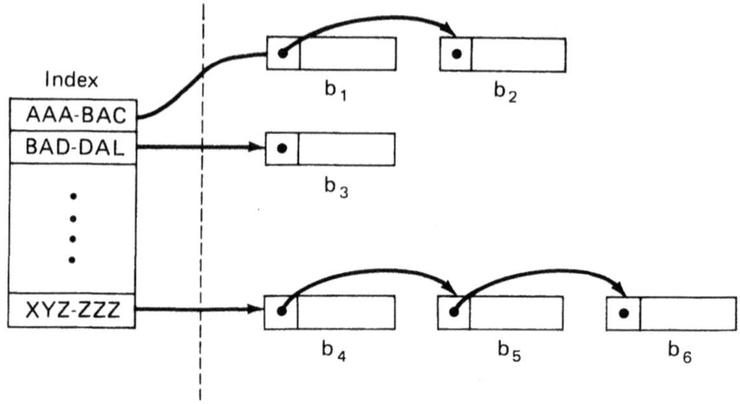

FIGURE 5.2. Indexed File Organization.

makes the retrieval easier; it adds complexity for inserting (adding) new records. Once the initial bucket has been retrieved, its processing is similar to that for hashed files. The major difference, of course, is that all records in the bucket have similar keys. One can sort the contents of the bucket to produce the "next" record. This allows one to read through the file sequentially. When one comes to the end of a bucket, one can return to the index file, find the "next" index record, and then get the next data bucket for the "next" record. When there is no next index record, one returns an end-of-file. This is the method most commonly used to implement the index sequential access method (ISAM).

The index just described is called a sparse index because there are index records only for the buckets; that is, there are more records than there are indices. The disadvantage of this organization is that all file maintenance requires that one identify the record in the bucket. An alternative approach is effective if the key is small and the record large. One treats the data file as a heap and the index file has one index for each record. This is called a dense index because every record has an index record pointing to it. The dense index is sorted, but because the index is small, the cost to maintain the index is less than the cost to maintain the data using a sparse index.

Finally, we note that it is possible for a file to have more than one index. For example, assume that we have a hospital system and we wish to retrieve inpatients by either ward or admitting physician. One could construct a secondary index called "ward" which—for each ward—provided pointers to the patients in that ward and a secondary index called "admitting physician" which contained—for each admitting physician—pointers to the patients he or she admitted. Sometimes a secondary index is called an inverted index. The latter term is derived from the library subject card index which is an inversion (reordering) of the cards by another key.

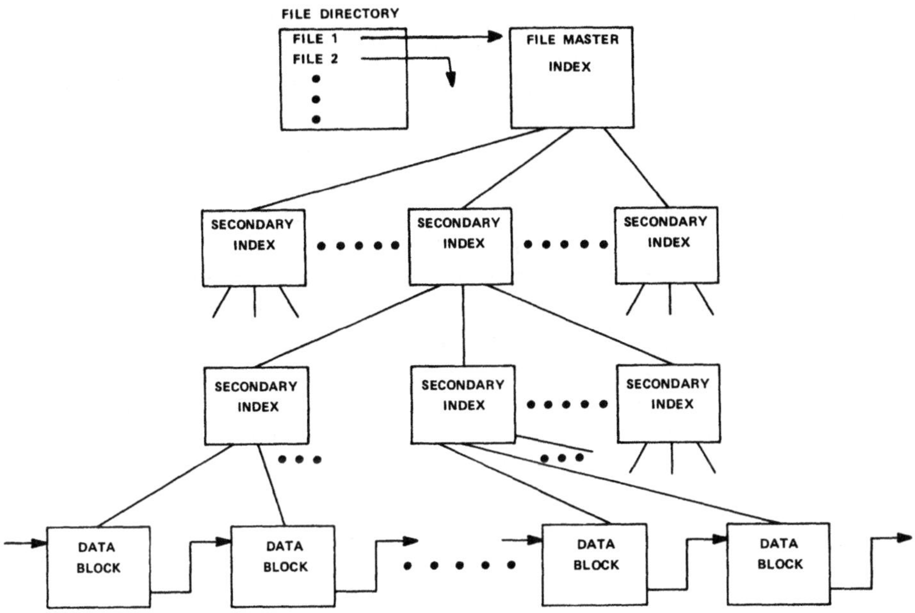

FIGURE 5.3. Sample B-Tree structure (typical of MUMPS implementations).

5.2.4. The B-Tree

In each of the previous organizations we have assumed some knowledge of the file to set up the file, its index, hashing functions, etc. When the knowledge is accurate, a more efficient file results. However, when the file grows in unexpected ways, there are overflow buckets with the associated additional processing. The B-tree (also called B* tree and M way tree) is a technique for producing efficient files by automatically adjusting the structure as data are entered. It does this by maintaining an index of its index.

As shown in Fig. 5.3, there is a tree structure of index buckets at the top and a chain of data buckets at the bottom. The search begins with the first index bucket for a given file. The index bucket either points to a data bucket that contains the data or to another index bucket. This process continues until a data bucket is pointed to. The records in the data bucket normally are sorted. Note that in the file shown, one traverses the same number of index buckets to locate any record. The index therefore is said to be balanced. The B-tree structure tends to remain in balance. Thus the cost to access a record is about the same for any record in the file.

Overflows occur when a data bucket is not large enough to hold all the records that are assigned to it. In this case, the data bucket splits into two buckets: the first with the lower keys, the second with the higher keys. After the split, each data bucket is half-empty. Since the index bucket pointing to the initial data bucket does not point to the new data bucket, an additional pointer must be added to it. If there is no room to hold an additional pointer, then the index bucket splits and the index bucket that pointed to it must be altered. This is, of course, an example of recursion. The index splitting can continue until the top node has split into two nodes and a new level of index buckets has been added. This process generally preserves the balance of the level of index buckets; there is also a simple algorithm that can rapidly reconstruct a balanced index. Note that, since the data buckets are chained together, sequential access can be supported without use of the index once an initial record has been defined.

Most MUMPS implementations use a B-tree. The index and data records are both variable in length. (This means that the search through the bucket requires some special indicator to signal the end of a record or key string. This may be done by using a special "end-of-string" character or by preceding the string with a character count.) In the case of MUMPS, the key is stored as a character string of up to 64 characters in length. The key may consist of more than one field, for example (from Chapter 4)

```
JOHN PAUL JONES#83/12/17
JOHN PAUL JONES#84/02/02
JOHN PAUL JONES#84/02/17
```

illustrates three keys with the "#" acting as a separator between the fields in a key. Since much of the same information is repeated, storage can be minimized by use of key compression techniques. In this case, the keys stored would be

```
 0 JOHN PAUL JONES#83/12/7
17 4/02/02
22 17
```

where the 0 indicates that this is a full key, the 17 indicates that what follows should be appended to the first 17 characters of the previous key, and the 22 indicates that what follows should be appended to the first 22 characters of the previous key. In this way, redundancy is eliminated and a bucket can represent more information than the number of characters it contains. This leading character compression is used in both the index and data buckets in the MUMPS B-tree. (Since the index is sparse, the records must be stored with their key.)

The IBM Virtual Storage Access Method (VSAM) is organized to use a different implementation of the B-tree algorithm. In this case, it provides facilities that were designed to take advantage of the characteristics of the IBM 360 type of computer. As in the case of most of the file access methods, even with the same algorithm, there are many local variations.

5.2.5. Using an Access Method

Each of the access methods described simply returns a record. The most common type of file processed is the sequential file. For example, the input data to be processed by a FORTRAN program is organized as a sequential file. The statement

```
READ ...
```

will read the first one or more records in the file depending on the argument list and format statement. Once read, a record can not be reread. Another example of sequential access is the printed output with a WRITE; this sequences one output record after the other as a serial file.

To read records in a random or index sequential file one must supply a key. Let us illustrate accessing an ISAM file using a COBOL program. The Environment Division would contain a statement such as

```
SELECT INDEX-SEQ-DISK-FILE ASSIGN TO (unit)
     ACCESS IS RANDOM
     NOMINAL KEY IS SEARCH-KEY
     RECORD KEY IS KEY-ITEM OF
          INDEX-SEQ-DISK-REC.
```

The Data Division would contain a definition of the file INDEX-SEQ-DISK-FILE which contained records whose contents were defined as INDEX-SEQ-DISK-REC. One of the fields in the record INDEX-SEQ-DISK-FILE must be KEY-ITEM which is used as the key to this record. SEARCH-KEY is a variable that will contain the desired key before a read; it must be defined with the same format as KEY-ITEM.

Given this set of definitions, it is now possible to read arbitrary records in the ISAM file. The following section of a Procedure Division sets a desired value into the key and then reads the record with that key. If no record with that key is found, an error flag is set.

```
MOVE DESIRED-KEY TO SEARCH-KEY.
READ INDEXED-SEQ-DISK-FILE
     INVALID KEY MOVE 'YES' TO ERROR-FLAG.
```

If ERROR-FLAG is not "YES," then one can process the data contained in the record.

In the COBOL example it was necessary to declare the file organization and the structure of its record before the file could be accessed. Some access methods do not require any such declarations. In MUMPS, the access method is implicit in the syntax of the language. For example, the statement

```
SET X=^WEIGHT("JOHN PAUL JONES","84/02/17")
```

will set X to the value of the record in the file WEIGHT with the key (index) of

```
"JOHN PAUL JONES","84/02/17"
```

The UNIX operating system offers a different file access method. Each file is a continuous stream of characters. There are no records. One may read one or a given number of characters from the file starting at the beginning, after the last read or at a given point in the file. Notice that in both MUMPS and UNIX, the contents of the "records" are never formally defined as it is in the case of the COBOL example. This provides flexibility; it also means that there is more processing that must be explicitly controlled by the program's logic.

Each of the access methods described in this section is designed to provide access to a given record. Most operating systems support several access methods. These are sufficient for most applications. In some circumstances, it is necessary to develop custom algorithms, but that is rarely necessary. In all cases, however, it should be noted that all access methods simply deliver records. The definition of the record contents and the logic for their use must be presented explicitly in the program. Where the files are independent and used separately, this is not a problem. Yet, where the files overlap and share elements, alternative techniques are suggested. They are the topic of the next section.

5.3. Data Base Management Systems

A database is a collection of files that contains related information about an organization. In a hospital information system (HIS) the database contains files describing the patients' demographics, diagnosis, insurance status, therapies, outstanding orders, payments, and so on. There are also many different files used to describe the staff, the hospital inventory, the third party payors, and so forth. Many data elements—such as the patient identification, name, and hospital location—are repeated in many files. Some files—for example, the clinical laboratory orders and results—are used for many different functions—in this case for charting, communication, laboratory management, and patient care.

Organizing this database as a series of separate physical files was a necessity in the early 1960s. At that time there were few disks, and those that existed were relatively small and expensive. Thus, most files were stored on magnetic tape and serial processing was used. By the mid-1960s, however, disk storage became more common, and the direct access techniques of random access and indexed sequential access were incorporated into the third-generation software systems. The hardware could now support an online, integrated database; the next step was to establish a conceptual framework and develop the software to implement one.

Because most database applications were associated with commercial applications, the leadership in the development of database standards was assumed by the Conference on Data Systems Languages (CODASYL)—the group responsible for the standardization of COBOL. The approach defined by their Data Base Task Group (DBTG) is commonly called the network model. It was established in the late 1960s and represents the first definition of a system to manage databases: or the Data Base Management System (DBMS). At about the same time, IBM produced its DL/1 (or IMS) DBMS which was based on hierarchical structures. Finally in 1970, Codd defined an alternative data model that used relations; commercial implementations of this model, however, did not appear until the late 1970s.

Today we speak of three types of DBMS: network, hierarchical, and relational. They differ in the way in which they structure the data; yet each shares a common organization. Every DBMS provides three views of the database:

- The system (or global) view considers the entire database from a system perspective. All data elements are defined in the context of natural groupings (records) and relationships among groupings. This definition is generally called the schema.
- The application (or external) view considers the database only from the perspective of a specific application. Only the data required by that application are presented; relationships outside the application are hidden. This definition is generally called the subschema. In the HIS example, the nursing station order entry and clinical laboratory internal management applications may share the same files but will use different subschemas to reflect their different data needs.
- The physical (or storage) view considers how and where the files are stored. All files used by a DBMS must be managed using an access method provided by the support system. The DBMS provides a tool to relieve the application programmer of having to know about the physical storage. Moreover, since the application can be written using only the subschema definitions, changes can be made in the physical organization without altering the application programs. (This is called physical data independence.)

The definition of the schema, the subschemas, and the physical storage assignments is the responsibility of the Data Base Administrator (DBA). Fig. 5.4 illustrates how these definitions are used by the DBMS. At the application level, each application has its own subschema. The programmer uses this subschema in the Data Division (for COBOL programs) and all references to the physical files and their data are managed through this subschema. As shown, each compiled program generally has a work area. Data from the database are moved to and from this work area and then moved to and from the storage assigned to variables for processing.

At the system level, the DBMS interfaces with the host computer's operating system. It uses the operating system and its access method services to move blocks of data to and from I/O buffers. The DBMS also has services to move data to and from application working areas. The DBMS has access to the application subschema plus the system schema. This allows the DBMS to map the application view into the global view for the system. From this view, the logical groupings can be translated into physical files and their locations; the physical database descriptions and directories support this function.

In general, most DBMSs operate in this manner. Some, such as that illustrated here, support application development; others are fully self-contained and simply provide access to the DBMS functions of query and file management. All DBMSs, however, are complete systems: they offer more than a file access service. Each provides tools to define the database; access the data and files by the given names (called symbolic referencing); and support system level functions such as security,

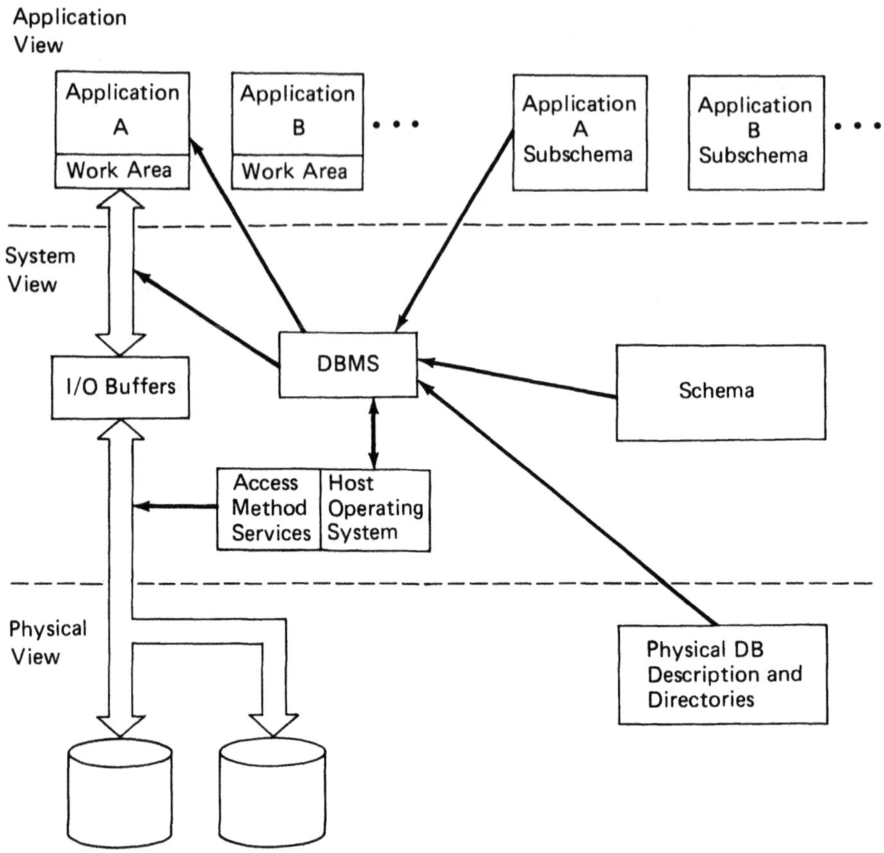

FIGURE 5.4. A database management system.

concurrency management, backup and recovery, and tuning. A DBMS is normally classified by the model used to define the database: network, hierarchy or relation. This affects only the schema and subschema. Physically, the storage of the data need not reflect the logical view of the schema. In fact, relational database systems normally do not store their data as relations; retrieval time would be too great to justify such an organization. The following subsections describe each of the three basic models. It should be noted that any model could be used for a given application. Thus, once a DBMS has been selected, it will be used for all applications.

5.3.1. The Network Model

The network (or plex or CODASYL) model was the first attempt to formalize a DBMS. It replaced the random and index sequential access methods described above with a more formal set of tools that allows the user to navigate through

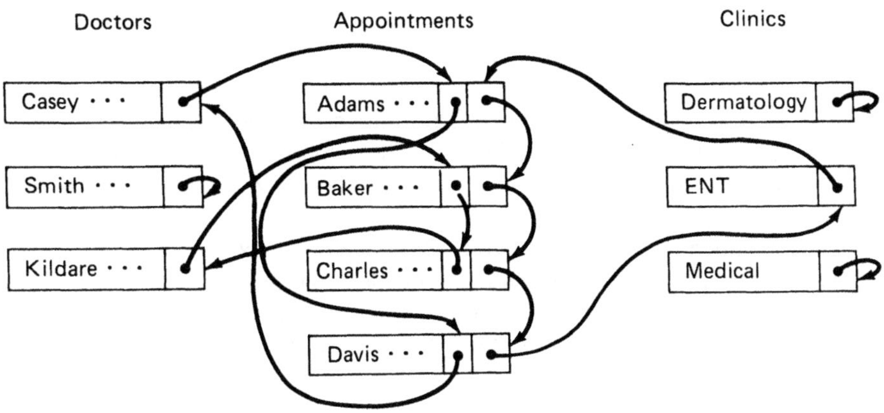

FIGURE 5.5. Multilist structure for the appointment database.

the database. There is no "standard" CODASYL DBMS, each is a proprietary product. In what follows we shall use a simple example to illustrate how a network DBMS is used. The commands are illustrated using a language in an abbreviated COBOL style.

Consider an appointment system. There are individual appointments consisting of the patient's name, date and time of appointment, and reason for the appointment plus lists of appointments by doctor and by clinic. Each individual appointment appears on each list. If we make the simplifying (and unrealistic) assumption that a patient never has more than one pending appointment, then the following schema models the database:

- A file of doctors in which each doctor record is limited to zero to n appointment records, i.e., each doctor record points to the appointment records containing information for patients he or she is to examine.
- A file of clinics in which each clinic record is linked to zero to n appointment records.
- A file of appointments each of which is linked to both a doctor and a clinic record.

With this model, we can produce a list of patients coming to a given clinic on a given day by (a) finding all appointment records linked to the given clinic, (b) extracting only those appointment records for the given date, and (c) printing those selected records.

The organization of the data can be thought of as shown in Fig. 5.5. This shows an instance (i.e., a set of sample entries) for the data base. The DOCTORS file has three entries, one each for Drs. Casey, Smith and Kildare. There are four patient appointment records, one each for Adams, Baker, Charles, and Davis. Finally, there are three clinics: Dermatology, Ear Nose and Throat, and Internal Medicine. Each record contains both data and pointers. To find the doctors in the DOCTORS file, simply read down the file. To find the appointments for a doctor, follow the pointers. In this instance, the pointer from Dr. Casey's record goes to the appointment for Adams. The (first) pointer for that record goes to Davis and the (first) pointer for that record returns to the Dr. Casey record, thereby completing the chain. Dr. Smith has no appointments. Dr. Kildare has appointments with Baker and Charles. The second pointer in the appointments record is used for clinics. It can be seen that all appointments are for the ENT clinic.

The implementation of this structure without a DBMS would be a considerable task. Each time a record was added or deleted, the pointers would have to be updated; searching through a list would require considerable programming to eliminate the housekeeping. The DBMS simplifies this by allowing the user to define the three basic files

- DOCTORS
- CLINICS
- APPOINTMENTS

and the two sets of links

- DR-APTS
- CLIN-APTS

These links are called SETs in the CODASL DBTG terminology. Each SET consists of an OWNER and a MEMBER. In this case, the OWNER for DR-APTS would be DOCTORS and the MEMBER would be APPOINTMENTS. This implies that for each record in the OWNER (DOCTORS) there is a chain of records in the MEMBER (APPOINTMENTS).

The introduction of the SET provides a tool for the definition of a schema that reflects the multilist organization shown in Fig. 5.4. One may now navigate through the database by reading a record. If that record is an OWNER in a SET, then one may read MEMBER records from that SET. While reading MEMBER records, one may begin to process OWNER records in another SET, and so on. In effect, as one processes a database using a CODASYL DBMS one has access to any of the records currently being pointed to.

A sample schema for the appointment system is shown in Fig. 5.6. The format will depend on the DBMS used; the figure includes several styles for pedagogical purposes. The definition of the DOCTORS and CLINICS records is clear. The APPOINTMENTS record introduces the concept of VIRTUAL. This implies that the elements DR-NAME and CLINIC-ID are to be considered logical parts of the record; however, they will not be stored with the record. The remainder of the VIRTUAL clause specifies how the system is to find the values for a given record, e.g., DOCTORS.DR-NAME (DR-NAME field from the DOCTORS record) as defined in the DR-APTS SET. The two SETs are defined by supplying their OWNER, MEMBER, and keys. Throughout this example, multiple records with the same key are invalid (DUPLICATES ARE NOT ALLOWED).

To see how this would be used in an application, consider a program to list out all patient appointments by doctor. The process first FINDs the record we

```
SCHEMA NAME IS APPOINTMENT-SYSTEM
RECORD NAME IS DOCTORS;
    DUPLICATES ARE NOT ALLOWED FOR DR-NAME IN DOCTORS.
        DR-NAME; TYPE IS CHARACTER (30).
        DR-SPECIALTY; TYPE IS CHARACTER (40).
RECORD NAME IS CLINICS;
    DUPLICATES ARE NOT ALLOWED FOR CLINIC-ID.
        CLINIC-ID; TYPE IS CHARACTER (10).
RECORD NAME IS APPOINTMENTS;
    DUPLICATES ARE NOT ALLOWED FOR PATIENT.
        PATIENT; TYPE IS CHARACTER (30).
        DATE; TYPE IS CHARACTER (8) TEST AS DATE.
        TIME; TYPE IS CHARACTER (8) TEST AS TIME.
        COMPLAINT; TYPE IS CHARACTER (30).
        DR-NAME; VIRTUAL
                  SOURCE IS DOCTORS.DR-NAME OF OWNER OF DR-APTS.
        CLINIC-ID; VIRTUAL
                  SOURCE IS CLINICS.CLINIC-ID OF OWNER OF CLIN-APTS.
SET NAME IS DR-APTS;
    OWNER IS DOCTORS;
    ORDER IS SORTED BY DEFINED KEYS
        DUPLICATES ARE NOT ALLOWED.
    MEMBER IS APPOINTMENTS;
        KEY IS ASCENDING PATIENT IN APPOINTMENTS;
        SET SELECTION IS BY VALUE OF DR-NAME IN DOCTORS.
SET NAME IS CLIN-APTS;
    OWNER IS CLINICS;
    ORDER IS SORTED BY DEFINED KEYS
        DUPLICATES ARE NOT ALLOWED.
    MEMBER IS APPOINTMENTS;
        KEY IS ASCENDING PATIENT IN APPOINTMENTS;
        SET SELECTION IS BY VALUE OF CLINIC-ID IN CLINICS.
```

FIGURE 5.6. Network appointment schema.

are seeking and then GETs the data from it for printing. The FIND, in effect, sets the keys and pointers and brings them and the record to the work area shown in Fig. 5.4; the GET will move data from the work area to the words assigned to the variables in the program. The term CURRENT refers to the current setting of the pointers in the context of the statement. The small example in Fig. 5.7 illustrates how the DBMS represents this. The access methods and housekeeping associated with navigating through the database are hidden. The program is simple and rather easy to read. An understanding of the processing, however,

```
FIND FIRST DR-NAME IN DOCTORS
PERFORM UNTIL end-of-doctors
    FIND FIRST PATIENT IN DR-APTS CURRENT
        USING DR-NAME IN DOCTORS
    WRITE new page and heading
    PERFORM UNTIL end-of-patients
        GET APPOINTMENTS
        WRITE ...
        FIND NEXT PATIENT WITHIN DR-APTS
        END-PERFORM
    END-PERFORM
```

FIGURE 5.7. Illustration of a program using a CODASYL DBMS.

requires a detailed understanding of the database structure. The program is highly procedural; that is, it details how the program is to go from record to record in the database. As we shall see, the relational data model provides tools for query and processing that are nonprocedural, and that is one of its advantages.

5.3.2. The Hierarchical Model

DBMSs that use the hierarchical model are very similar to those that use the network model. In a network there are nodes (records) and pointers. There may be more than one pointer to a record. In a hierarchy, on the other hand, every node must have exactly one pointer to it. (There is a single exception: the root node which has no pointers to it.) A hierarchy is also called a tree. Each branch may lead to other branches, but a branch cannot be reached from more than one branch. We also speak of parent and children nodes with each node having only one parent. Finally we note that an outline or table of contents is an example of a hierarchy and that the hierarchy is a special case of a network.

To illustrate how a hierarchical model may be used, consider an appointment problem in which there was only one clinic and each doctor scheduled a patient for many visits. This would suggest the following hierarchy:

DR-NAME	
PATIENT	(all patient appointments for a given doctor)
DATE	(all appointment dates for a given patient and doctor)
TIME	(data which are identified once the DR-NAME, PATIENT, DATE
COMPLAINT	are known.)

A schema for this hierarchy might be written as

```
TREE    DR-APTS
  RECORD    DOCTORS        ROOT
            DR-NAME        (KEY)
            DR-SPECIALTY
  RECORD    PATIENTS       PARENT IS DOCTORS
            PATIENT        (KEY)
            AGE
            SEX
  RECORD    APTS           PARENT IS PATIENTS
            DATE           (KEY)
            TIME
            COMPLAINT
```

The navigation language does not require both a FIND and GET. Since the structure of the database is established by the hierarchy, a GET can navigate from node to node in the hierarchy. For example, to list all patients for Dr. Casey, one might write the program shown in Fig. 5.8 (using a PL/1 type language). In this case, GET LEFTMOST (also called GET UNIQUE) will (conceptually) start to scan at the start of the database and continue to the level shown meeting the conditions shown. Thus, the first line of Fig. 5.8 causes the DBMS to scan from the start to the first entry in DOCTORS where DR-NAME is Casey. The next part of this command (the next line) causes the scan to continue at the next lower level and start at the beginning. After the scan, the DBMS is pointing to the first patient in the record PATIENT whose parent is a record in DOCTORS with DR-NAME equal to Casey. Within the WHILE loop, the GET NEXT WITHIN PARENT ensures that all PATIENT records returned have the same parent in the DOCTORS record. There is also a GET LEFTMOST WITHIN PARENT for initiating processing within a level, and a GET NEXT for reading serially through the hierarchy as if it were an outline. Fig. 5.9 illustrates how one could produce a report listing all patients for Dr. Casey between two dates. The first three lines define the path to the node in the hierarchy to be processed. Processing at this node is done WITHIN PARENT. The GET supplies the logical selection information which is not implied in the hierarchical structure.

The example we have chosen was very well suited to a hierarchical description; the model we chose was ideal for printing a report of appointments by doctor

```
GET LEFTMOST DOCTORS (DR-NAME = "Casey")
GET LEFTMOST WITHIN PARENT PATIENT
WHILE (data exists)
   PRINT ...
   GET NEXT WITHIN PARENT PATIENT
   END
```

FIGURE 5.8. Illustration of program using a hierarchical DBMS.

```
GET LEFTMOST     DOCTORS (DR-NAME="Casey")
                 PATIENTS
                 APTS (DATE > DATE1 & DATE < DATE2)
WHILE (not finished)
                 PRINT ...
                 GET NEXT WITHIN PARENT
                   APTS (DATE > DATE1 & DATE < DATE2)
                 END
```

FIGURE 5.9. Printing a doctor appointment list using a DBMS.

sorted by patient name. What if the report was to be sorted by date instead? There are two choices. First the output of the program shown in Fig. 5.9 could be used as the input to a sort. Alternatively, one may wish to define another tree that matched the output requirement better. Records can be defined as VIRTUAL so that the schema will indicate where the data will be found without introducing unnecessary redundancy. Note that we have made some conditional retrievals by placing some conditions in parentheses as WHERE clauses, e.g., (DATE > DATE1 & DATE < DATE2). This same facility is available with most network DBMSs as well.

5.3.3. The Relational Model

The term relation is a mathematical term for a set of ordered n-tuples with a property (predicate) that defines the membership of a set. For example, the successor relation consists of all pairs of integers such that the second is the successor to the first (greater by 1). Thus the elements

(1,2) (2,3) (3,4) (999,1000)

satisfy the relation and the elements

(1,5) (33,2) (4,3)

do not. The relations do not have to be restricted to numbers. For example, one can define a parent relationship (A, B) where A is the parent of B. A much easier way of viewing a relation, however, is to think of it as a table. In table form, the above relations are

Successor Relation		Parent Relation	
Number	Successor	Parent	Child
1	2	Mary	Jane
2	3	Jane	John
3	4	Jane	Henry
⋮		⋮	
999	1000	Jane	Sue
⋮		⋮	

DR	SPEC	PAT	DATE	TIME	COMP	CLINIC
Casey	ENT	Adams	4/17/84	9:00	Hearing	ENT
Kildare	Gen Med	Baker	4/17/84	9:30	New patient	ENT
Kildare	Gen Med	Charles	4/23/84	9:00	Return visit	ENT
Casey	ENT	Davis	4/17/84	9:30	Breathing	ENT

FIGURE 5.10. Appointment database as a table.

If a relation is as simple as a table, why use mathematical jargon? As it turns out, relations can be modeled as simple mathematical objects. We can develop an algebra for manipulating relations and can define a calculus for carrying out such manipulations. Since relations are sets, what we know about sets will be true for relations as well. Thus, by selecting a database model that is similar to a mathematical model that we already understand, we begin with a sound foundation and have a formal basis to test new theories. This understanding of the formal structures is a prerequisite to the transformation of high-level, nonprocedural database queries into navigational implementations.

Having now made the point, we shall use some commonly accepted, informal notations. The relations are called tables. Tables are composed of rows (or records; also called tuples as in 3-tuple, 4-tuple, etc.) Each row has one or more elements (attributes). Some of these may be keys to the row (also called the index elements or the key domain); there may be terms that are not keys (the data elements or the non-key domain). To illustrate, consider the instance presented in Fig. 5.5. It is shown in Fig. 5.10 as a table. Written in the standard format used to describe relational databases, this would be

APTS(DR,SPEC,PAT,DATE,TIME,COMP,CLINIC)

where APTS is the name of the table or relation. The key terms are normally underlined and written to the left. Thus, if the table used DR and PAT to uniquely identify a row, this would be written

APTS(<u>DR</u>,<u>PAT</u>,SPEC,DATE,TIME,COMP,CLINIC).

To reflect this description, the table in Fig. 5.10 would have to interchange its second and third columns. (Note that tables are not assumed to be in any sorted order.)

In this example, we have placed the entire database in one table. This means that we have items in one table that refer only to the doctor (SPEC or specialty) and other items that describe the appointment. It would be logical to divide these into two tables:

APT(<u>PAT</u>,<u>DATE</u>,TIME,COMP,DR,CLINIC)
DR(<u>DR</u>,SPEC)

(Both PAT and DATE have been defined as key terms in order to allow for more

Table T1

A	B	C
1	2	3
4	5	6
7	8	9

Table T2

A	B	D
1	2	10
1	2	11
4	5	12

Join of T1 and T2

A	B	C	D
1	2	3	10
1	2	3	11
4	5	6	12

Projections of T2 on A

A
1
4

Join of T1 and (Projection of T2 on A)

A	B	C
1	2	3
4	5	6

FIGURE 5.11. Projection and join.

than one appointment per patient.) With this simple data model we can now illustrate the relational algebra.

Because every row in a table has the same structure, one can apply all the usual set operations on a table. For example, given table A and B with the same format (definition), it is easy to create

- a set with rows that are in either (A B or union),
- a set with rows that are in both (A B or intersection).
- a set with rows in A but not in B (A − B or difference).

Such operations would be difficult to express with the structures and pointers of the network and hierarchical models. In addition to the standard set operations, there are two operations that are unique to relational databases. These are the join and projection.

Simply stated, the join of two tables with common elements creates a new table in which they are joined by the values of the common elements. As shown in Fig. 5.11, there is one row in T1 and two rows in T2 with identical values of A = 1 and B = 2. The join of T1 and T2 contains all combinations of C and

D from the rows with A = 1 and B = 2. Both tables also have rows with A = 4 and B = 5; one table has no rows with A = 7 and thus a row with A = 7 will not appear in the join.

The projection of a table is a table with only specified columns and no repetitions. The projection of table T2 on column A contains all unique values in column A. Since the results of a join and a projection are—in themselves—tables, they may be projected or joined. To return to the instance shown in Fig. 5.10, the set of all days on which patients have visits scheduled is

```
Projection of APT on DATE or
  DATE
  4/17/84
  4/23/84
```

The problems to be addressed by Dr. Casey are

```
Projection of APT on DR(="Casey") and COMP or
  COMP
  Hearing
  Breathing
```

The list of doctors with appointments in the ENT clinic who do not have the ENT specialty is

```
Projection of (join of DR and
  (Projection of (APT on DR and CLINIC (="ENT")))
  on DR and SPECIALTY (not = "ENT")
```

In this more complex query, we see that

```
Projection of (APT on DR and CLINIC(="ENT"))
```

is

DR	CLINIC
Casey	ENT
Kildare	ENT

Join with DR becomes

DR	CLINIC	SPEC
Casey	ENT	ENT
Kildare	ENT	Gen Med

When projected on DR and SPEC (not="ENT") we get the desired answer of Dr. Kildare whose specialty is General Medicine. This same query, written in the SQL (pronounced sequel) query language would be

```
SELECT   DR,SPEC
FROM     DR,APT
WHERE    DR.DR = APT.DR AND
         CLINIC = "ENT" AND
         SPEC not="ENT"
```

This more compact and natural presentation illustrates the power of the relational model. The SELECT specifies the fields to be contained in the join, the FROM identifies the tables and the WHERE establishes the selection criteria.

We conclude the section on the relational model with a brief description of the IBM Query-by-Example (QBE) system. Users of QBE interact at a terminal with tables. Thus, their view is that of the schema. For example, an EMPLOYEE table may define the following screen

EMPLOYEE	NAME	MANAGER	SALARY	DEPARTMENT

To print the entire table, one would enter the command P. in the column that contains the table name. Thus

EMPLOYEE	NAME	MANAGER	SALARY	DEPARTMENT
P.				

produces

EMPLOYEE	NAME	MANAGER	SALARY	DEPARTMENT
	ADAMS	JONES, A.	30000	TIN BENDING
	BACKER	SMITH	50000	PROGRAMMING
	CHARLES	TAYLOR	70000	SALES
	DAVIS	JONES, B	27450	PLANNING
	.	.	.	.
	.	.	.	.
	.	.	.	.

To list the names of employees who are in the TIN BENDING department and who make over $20,000 enter

EMPLOYEE	NAME	MANAGER	SALARY	DEPARTMENT
	P.		>20000	TIN BENDING

QBE also allows the user to create variables. For example, we can identify the manager of the TIN BENDING department as <u>FRED</u> with

EMPLOYEE	NAME	MANAGER	SALARY	DEPARTMENT
		FRED		TIN BENDING

FRED is an "example" of a manager. One could have used SMITH or 1234. The underlining is the key to indicating that it is an example. The use of this format for examples makes the system easier to learn and use. We can define FRED salary as 400 and then print out every one (independent of the department) who makes more than the manager of the TIN BENDING department with

EMPLOYEE	NAME	MANAGER	SALARY	DEPARTMENT
		FRED		TIN BENDING
		FRED	400	
	P.		$\geq$ 400	

Using the U. operator, one can update the database. The following update gives a 10 percent raise to the TIN BENDING department.

EMPLOYEE	NAME	MANAGER	SALARY	DEPARTMENT
U.			500 × 1.1	TIN BENDING

The ease with which these changes are made illustrates why the DBMS must have a comprehensive authority and security system.

The last illustration shows how one can list all employees who earn more than their managers:

EMPLOYEE	NAME	MANAGER	SALARY	DEPARTMENT
	P.	FRED	> 700	
	FRED		700	

This query will print (P.) all NAMEs where the manager is defined by FRED and the salary is greater than the salary defined by 700. From the first line, the system can select a value for FRED with each NAME tested. The value for 700 is defined in the second line as the salary for the FRED identified in the first line. Note how this query is nonprocedural. It states what is to be done without indicating how. Contrast this with the navigational approach of the other DBMS implementations. Because the relational model has a well defined mathematical analog, it is possible to create consistent systems to manage the database.

We conclude this subsection by drawing a parallel with the PROLOG language which uses relations called functors. The PROLOG example presented in Chapter 4 could have been implemented just as easily using a relational DBMS. The difference between PROLOG and systems like QBE is that PROLOG can process more complex structures (such as lists) and it has powerful pattern matching facilities. A relational database operates in very large sets of data that must be stored on disk in secondary (permanent) storage. AI applications, such as those implemented in PROLOG, have a limited number of assertions (i.e., a small database); operating efficiency requires that this database be kept in working storage whenever possible. Thus, the differences tend to be those of implementation and equipment limitations.

5.4. Database Design

A database is an integrated collection of data physically organized as files. These files may be managed independently using a variety of access methods, or they may be represented by a logical schema that interfaces to a DBMS. In either case, one must define and describe the contents of the database. The following chapter considers the general problem of design; this section presents some techniques that are used only in the design of databases.

There are two problems in the design of databases:

- What data are to be included in the database.
- How are the data to be organized within the database.

The first problem is addressed by modeling, the second by analysis. We begin with a discussion of modeling—the representation of some real world object designed to convey some information about the object. Some examples. A museum uses scale models of buildings and ships to present their external structure; a mathematical abstraction of a physiological phenomenon models the behavior of some part of that system; and a data model for a system presents the data elements and relationships used by the system to satisfy the needs of the user (organization or enterprise).

To develop a data model, one must first model the data needs of the organization—sometimes called the "real world." This real world model may then be transformed into a form that can be processed by a computer system. One common approach is the Entity-Relationship model (E-R model). This is constructed as follows. First, one identifies the things (entities) that are to be managed by the new system. For an appointment system, the entities may be patients, doctors, and appointments. Next, one defines the things that describe the entities, i.e., their attributes. For a patient this might be identification number, name, birthdate, sex; for an appointment it might be date, time, and complaint. Finally, the relationships among the entities are identified: Doctors schedule appointments, patients make appointments, etc.

The E-R approach collects this information and presents it in diagrammatic form. The entities are written in boxes, the attributes in ovals, and the relationships in diamonds. Nouns are used to describe the entities, and verbs are used for the relationships. Fig. 5.12 presents a simple E-R diagram for an appointment system. The diagrams may be extended to contain more information. For example, the

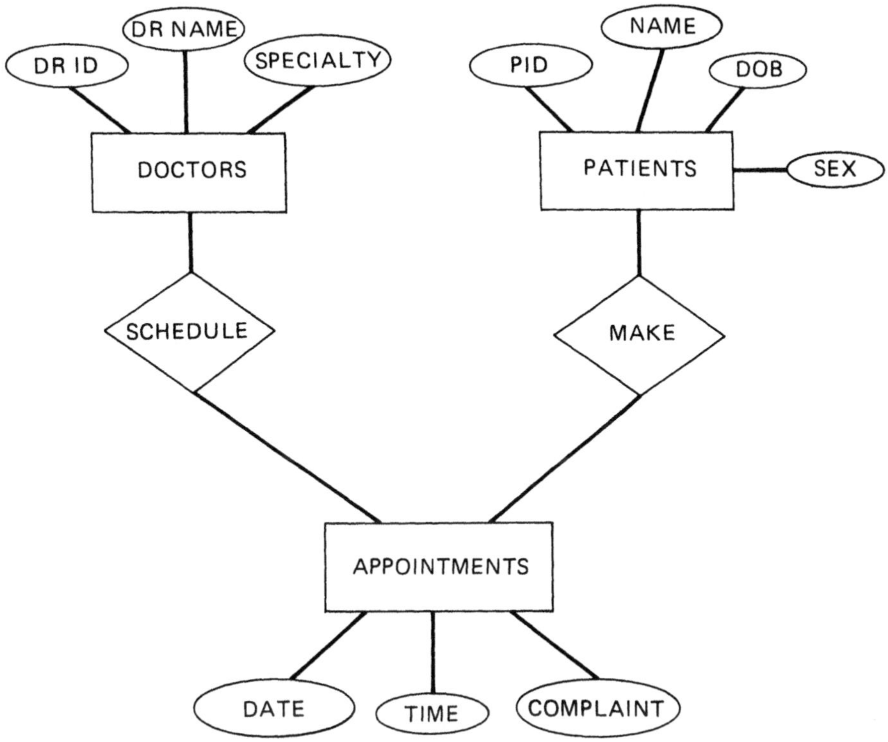

FIGURE 5.12. Simple E-R diagram.

appointments as defined in the diagram have no meaning unless there is a patient for the appointment in the database. This is called an existence dependency which is presented as a double box for appointments with an arrow from the patient's MAKE relationship. (It is also called a weak entity type.) Notice how similar the E-R diagram is to the records (entities) and sets (relationships) of the Fig. 5.6 Network Schema.

The E-R diagram can also be used to convey information about the type of relationship. Some relationships are one-to-one (1:1). For example, if we add the entity HOME ADDRESS and the relationship LIVES AT between it and PATIENTS, then the relationship will be 1:1 (assume that each patient has only one address). Since we allow patients to have more than one appointment, the patients MAKE appointments relationship is one-to-many (1:m). There is also a many to many-to-many (m:n) relationship. If we remove the attribute SPECIALTY from DOCTORS and make it an entity connected to DOCTORS by the relationship PRACTICES, then we have an example of a m:n relationship. Each doctor may have more than one specialty, and each specialty is practiced by more than one doctor. Fig. 5.13 displays the E-R diagram for this revised

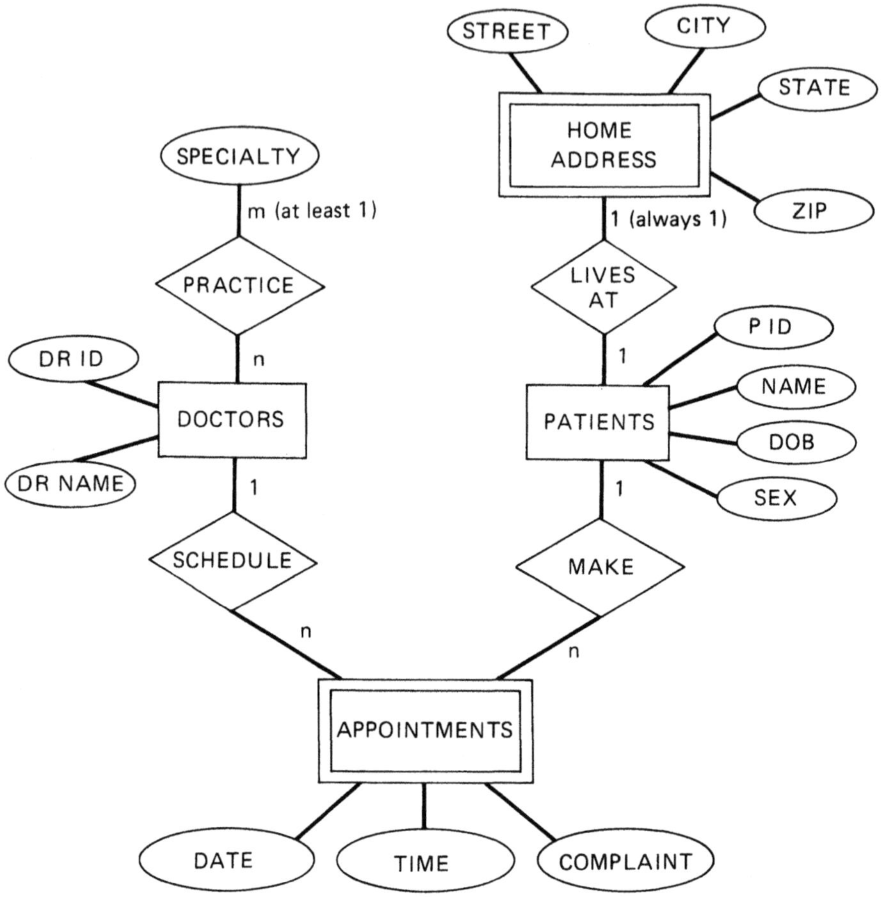

FIGURE 5.13. Expanded E-R diagram.

model. (Since the entity SPECIALTY has only one attribute, it is represented by the oval symbol for an attribute.)

It can be seen that, as in any diagramming technique, the diagrams can become more complex as the system grows and as the diagram is called on to represent more information. Nevertheless, the E-R diagram provides an easy to learn tool that helps to organize the real world environment in the form of a model. This, in turn, can be transformed into an implementable design. The entities suggest records with a field for each attribute. The relationships suggest some form of pointer or structural relationship. The type of mapping (1:1, 1:m, m:n) places a constraint in the relationship. A 1:1 mapping can be implemented by combining the entities in a single record. A 1:m mapping can be implemented with a hierarchy (or repeating groups); this is easily defined with COBOL type data structures.

A m:n mapping, on the other hand, must be decomposed into two files (one m:1 and the other 1:n) if indexing is to be supported for both entities.

We are now at the second step in database design: the definition of how the database is to be organized. Naturally, this process will be affected by the target environment. If a DBMS is used, the design must be for that DBMS. If there are tools such as a data dictionary, the analysis should rely heavily on its facilities. Ideally, one would like the database design to be:

- *Efficient*. The design should be decomposed into units that can be used for the high volume activities in an efficient manner.
- *Nonredundant*. Each element should be stored in the database just once. Thus, all activities that use that element will access the same value. For example, the patient's name should be stored in only one place so that changes to the name will be reflected in all functions that use the name.
- *Self consistent*. Whenever possible, knowledge of real world restrictions should be built into the database to ensure consistency. For example, if a home address is always required, the structure should not allow an appointment to be made if no address has been entered.
- *Flexible*. A database is a model of a larger system. Since the latter is bound to change, the database will change. This should be planned for by clarity of structure, avoidance of clever tricks, and good documentation.

These goals are not independent. Moreover, there are no formal rules to achieve them. In general, good database design requires a combination of careful thought and experience. For relational databases, however, there is a formal design process called normalization. Because data model can be first described as a relational model before implementation, it is useful to understand the normal forms for relations. The forms are based on the concept of functional dependency.

When we spoke of the key for a record, this was an example of a functional dependency. The patient identifier (PID) is a key to the patient record; given a value for a PID one can determine if a record with that key exists, and, if it does, which record it is. The key uniquely identifies only one record, and every record has a different key. Yet a record may have more than one key. For example, if the patient database is small and each patient has a different name, then NAME could be used as a key instead of PID. In this case, we say that the patient record has a functional dependency on NAME and a functional dependency on PID. NAME and PID are candidate keys. The fact that functional dependencies exist is determined by the analyst; the selection of which candidate key to use is also an analyst task. However, once the functional dependencies have been established, the formal normalization process can begin.

There are several normal forms. The first normal form requires that the data be written in the form of a table (relation). The appointment system (ignoring doctor specialty and patient address) might be defined as the following relation:

APTS(PID,DATE,TIME,COMPLAINT,NAME,DOB,SEX,DRID,DRNAME)

The key (PID,DATE) will uniquely define the appointment. Since this is clearly a table, it is in first normal form. But as we examine it, we note that it mixes several different types of things. It will be difficult to design clear programs to operate on this database.

In the above example, the elements PID and DATE serve as a key to the table. However, PID, by itself, serves as a key to NAME, DOB, and SEX. That is, for a given PID, the values of NAME, DOB and SEX will be the same for any value of DATE. That presents an update problem. If the patient's name changes, then that name must be changed in many records. It is best to separate this into two relations as follows:

APTS1(PID,DATE,TIME,COMPLAINT,DRID,DRNAME)
PATIENT(PID,NAME,DOB,SEX)

Now the underlined elements serve as keys for the table, and no element is functionally dependent on a (nontrivial) subset of the key. We say that this relation is in second normal form.

Nevertheless, there is still another functional dependency in the table APTS1. DRNAME is functionally dependent on DRID. Again, we decompose the table to remove the dependency:

APT(PID,DATE,TIME,COMPLAINT,DRID)
PATIENT(PID,NAME,DOB,SEX)
DOCTOR(DRID,DRNAME)

This is now in third normal form. There are other normal forms up to a fifth normal form. In most cases, when a table has only one or two elements in its key and is in third normal form, it is also in fifth normal form.

Notice how the third normal form reflects the structure shown in the E-R diagram (Figs. 5.12 and 5.13). The SCHEDULE relationship is expressed by having DRID in the APT table; the MAKE relationship causes PID to be in APT. Now that a normalized design exists, implementation decisions must be made. Should one expand APT to include NAME. There is a tradeoff between processing time and update efficiency. If APT is to be used very often, NAME changed very infrequently, and the application requires processing speed, then the analyst may choose to add a replication of NAME to APT. There is no requirement that the implementation be in a normal form; it simply is good practice to begin the detailed design from a normalized base. In that way, redundancy can be controlled and not introduced accidentally.

As the detailed design continues, the analyst must understand what the data mean and how they are to be used. Entries should not be made into APT unless there is already an entry in PATIENT with the same PID value. In some development environments, one can define this as a requirement, in others one must incorporate this into the program. To produce a list of appointments by doctor, APT must be accessed by DRID. This may be provided for automatically by the DBMS. Alternatively, one may create a secondary index

DRAPT(DRID,PID,DATE)

Finally, one may write a procedure that searches through APT, sorts and then prints.

In each case the goal is to produce a simple, easily maintained design. Wherever possible, use standard software tools rather than custom code. Let the definition of the database eliminate errors and database degradation. Just as strong data typing eliminates the entry of invalid data (e.g., "12AB" would be rejected as an integer), normalization eliminates inconsistencies (e.g., various spellings of NAME in APTS). Wherever possible, allow the development environment to filter out potential errors. Implement tests as procedural code only when there are no other alternatives. But when designing, always remember Murphy's law: If anything can go wrong, it will.

5.5. Concluding Remarks

The heart of any information system is the database. The database may be thought of as either a collection of independent files that are processed separately or as an integrated resource used to support an organization. Fragmentation into separate units facilitates development; the cost of decentralization may be manifested in the form of incompatibilities and reporting constraints. On the other hand, viewing the database as an organizational entity may result in excessive complexity and implementation delays. Fortunately modern DBMS technology and its associated tools provide avenues for managing the development process. In some cases, this involves trading efficiency for ease of use and maintainability. One would expect that, in time, improvements in technology will reduce the concerns about efficiency.

Three types of DBMSs were described. The first two—network and hierarchical—are based on the structure of the data. They navigate through the database, going from node to node and accessing records by use of pointers. The programs are highly procedural and relatively efficient. The third model—relational—has a mathematical foundation. Because of its mathematical roots, the relational model supports nonprocedural queries and offers a methodology for normalization of the data model. Moreover, the objects processed by a relational DBMS are very similar to those used by the Fifth Generation Computer language PROLOG. Consequently, there is considerable interest in relational DBMSs. However, there currently are no efficient physical organizations for storing a relation. Thus all relational DBMS translate the external model into one or more of the previously described access methods.

Finally, we note that a DBMS may not be available to or practical for all application environments. Nevertheless, the design of a data model can be treated as independent of its implementation. Two complementary design approaches were presented: E-R diagrams and relation normalization. Either (or both) techniques are recommended prior to the detailed design—an activity that will be discussed in considerable detail in the following chapter.

For Further Reading

The number of books dealing with databases is large. Most cover all of the material presented in this chapter. Among the most commonly used textbooks are G. Wiederhold, *Database Design*, (second edition) McGraw-Hill, 1983, J. D. Ullman, *Principles of Database Systems*, (second edition) Computer Science Press, 1982, and C. J. Date, *An Introduction to Database Systems* (third edition) Addison-Wesley, 1981. James Martin is a prolific author who has written extensively on information systems. Some of his earliest works include a brief introduction called *Principles of Data-Base Management* (1976) and a more complete discussion called *Computer Data-Base Organization* (second edition, 1977), both Prentice-Hall. G. Weiderhold has also written a short (75 page) monograph entitled *Databases for Health Care*, Springer-Verlag, 1981.

Readers interested in the Entity-Relationship model will be interested in P. Chen, "The Entity-Relationship Model—Toward a Unified View of Data," *ACM TODS* (1,1) 1976 pp 9-36. Since that paper, there have been several conferences which have discussed and enlarged the initial concepts and the literature is growing. Also of historical interest is E. F. Codd, "A Relational Model of Data for Large Shared Data Banks," *Comm ACM*, (13,6) 1970, pp 377-387; this introduced the relational model. Most DBMS vendors have both descriptive materials and user manuals which illustrate how their systems can be used.

6
System Implementation

6.1. Introduction

The implementation of software systems follows the pattern used in all development and research activities. We go through these steps when setting up a research project, when building a bridge, or when writing computer programs. One begins with a set of needs, goals, or objectives that describes what we intend the system or activity to accomplish. This is followed by analysis that determines how we are to achieve the desired outcome. Next, there is the doing of the task, e.g., collecting laboratory data, building a bridge, or writing computer programs. Finally, there is an evaluation of the product. Naturally, the specifics of the process will differ for each class of activity.

In the case of computer programs, the target product is not the program but the system of which it is a part. Thus, when we speak of System Implementation, we imply systems with software. The system itself consists of the programs and their documentation (the software), the equipment (the hardware), and the users of the system. In the case of an embedded application such as the CAT scanner, the computer is an integral part of the system and the user should have no perception of using a computer—only, (in this case) of using a CAT scanner. Information systems, on the other hand, are designed to be flexible so that they can accommodate the users' needs. For such systems it is important that the user helps define his role in the application use. In what follows, we shall restrict the discussion to this last type of application.

The implementation of an information system involves three different objects. First there is the system. It exists in the real world and—in general—predates the software system. That is, an operational environment normally is in place before the automated support is installed. The software system will modify the environment; therefore, although it may satisfy some needs, its application may create or uncover new deficiencies. Thus, system implementation is not a static process; it is dynamic and will proceed through many iterations. If one considers that the system operates within a changing organization using equipment that is continuously undergoing improvement, then the need for system evolution is obvious.

Within a system there is application software: the software portion. It is composed of a collection of programs with documentation for their use and maintenance. During the preliminary systems analysis, the equipment requirements are established and the functions to be supported by the application software are defined. There are many types of applications. They range from a large hospital information system to a small "throwaway" program. In part, the techniques used for managing the process will depend on the size, scope, projected lifetime, and use of the system. The task of organizing and managing the development of application software is called software engineering. This will be the main topic of this chapter.

The last of the three objects is the computer program. This is a realization of design as a set of instructions to the equipment. As we shall see, the activity of programming represents a very small portion of the total development time. Yet, because programming produces a "product," it often is considered to be the most important activity. Indeed, it is frequently equated with "computer literacy." However, the reason that we still write programs is a reflection of the inadequacies in our design definitions. Our goal is to produce a system. To do this, one must define the application software. If that definition were formal and complete, then the programming could be automated. In this context, computer programming is a necessary extra step. Perhaps by the end of this decade we will have systems in which programming is to software development as a knowledge of binary arithmetic is to FORTRAN programs. For the near term, however, it is essential that we understand the rules for effective program development.

The remainder of this chapter discusses each of the three objects.

6.2. System Level Activities

The system level activities are all associated with the system and not the application software or programs. The first step is to establish what the system is to do—that is, specify its requirements. Once this is done, the implementation path can be selected. If the information system is to be custom built, then the Requirements Specification becomes a contractual "build-to" document. Where an existing software product is to be purchased, the Requirements Specification acts as a guideline for selection. Finally, for in-house development, the Requirements Specification need be only as formal as the environment demands. The following sections discuss some of the system level activities.

6.2.1. Defining the Requirements

The need for an information system is motivated by a variety of factors. For example:

- *Barrier to operation*. Physical limitations may prohibit the support of a desired function using the current manual or automated system. Thus, a new system is required to enable operations at the desired levels. Examples are rapid reporting of laboratory results and the management of patient appointments in a decentralized setting.
- *Deficiency in operations*. The current system has faults that can be corrected by the implementation of a new system. Examples are access to correct patient identification and the reduction of errors in pharmacy orders.
- *Reduction in cost*. Automation may be used to reduce costs through integration or labor reduction. Examples are automated billing systems and the use of integrated databases.
- *Status*. The presence of an automated system (or links to one) frequently are motivated in part by a simple desire to have the system. For example, a hospital information system may help in recruiting staff or attracting patients.

These causes are relatively independent of each other. Often, the true motivations are not recognized. It is common for an analysis activity to begin as an exploratory exercise designed to find out how an operation may be "computerized" to solve its problems.

Whatever the reason for initiating a study, it is important to recognize that an information system can process only the data it stores. If an organization's problems are associated with the people in the system (e.g., management, improper staffing), then the installation of computer systems may aggravate the situation. However, where the problems and their technical solutions can be identified, the use of an automated system should meet the desired objectives.

Unfortunately, there are no simple rules for conducting the preliminary analysis. Much is based on experience and local variability. If the staff does not have experience, the use of a consultant is advisable. The focus of the analysis should be on those parts of the system that can be assisted by the use of an information system. The scope should be limited to what is practical in the time frame under consideration.

At the conclusion of the first stage of analysis, there should be two things:

- A high-level description of what functions are to be supported by an information system.
- A general budget for the implementation, operation, and cost savings associated with the information system.

The statement of objectives should not be too specific; however, it must identify all essential attributes of any new system. It must be remembered that there are many candidate systems, and over-specificity at an early stage may rule out otherwise acceptable choices. The cost constraints, on the other hand, ought to be specific and not biased by optimism. (One approach to estimating software costs is to double a reasonable estimate and hope.)

The requirements definition process concludes when there is a Requirement

Specification (or statement of objectives) that indicates *what* the new system is to do. There is also a budget to constrain the solution. The next step is to determine *how* the new system is to be implemented and to plan for its use.

6.2.2. Selecting the Implementation Approach

As a general rule, if a system exists that fully satisfies the organization's needs, then buy it. This will always be less expensive than custom development because the product vendor prorates his development costs among his many customers. In general, however, the "perfect" system does not exist: it doesn't do everything, it does some unnecessary things, it can't interface with other systems, it doesn't fit into the long-range plan, etc. The organization must come to a make or buy decision.

The first step in determining if an existing application is available is to survey the existing applications. Some organizations produce excellent evaluations of products, there are several software catalogs, and many of the computer magazines print periodic reviews. The more general a need, the more the potential purchasers, and the wider the range of products. For specialized needs, on the other hand, it is less likely that a desirable product exists. For example, appointment processing, health insurance management, and patient registration systems have a broad market; many systems are offered. This is not true for systems that support clinical decision making. Users of specialized systems have their choices: adopt one's needs to conform to the features offered by an existing system, develop a system for one's specific needs, or wait. Although the last option may seem facetious, it should be recognized that the development process may take years and the user will have to wait in either case.

Some things to consider in selecting an application package are:

- Will the system meet the organization's minimal needs? Most packages use parameters that allow them to adjust to the users' requirements. A hospital information system, for example, is designed to allow the nursing units to design (within limits) the screen and report formats.
- If program modifications are made, who will make, warrant, and maintain them? For some applications, program code changes will be necessary. There are questions of who will do this, what will be the cost, and how will the changes be integrated into subsequent versions of the package.
- What support is available for training and maintenance? Is the documentation adequate?
- Will the package fit in with the organization's plans for DBMS or networking?
- Will the vendor be in business over the life of the product's use? What is his reputation and that of the product? Contacts with other users are invaluable here.

At some point in time, the organization will determine that the functionality described in the preliminary Requirements Specification justifies the budgeted expenditures and a decision to proceed follows. A plan for the project should then be drawn up. The purpose of this plan is to set out how the project should be conducted. It helps to organize the project and also provides a source for reference. In general, it describes the following activities:

- *Initiating development activity*. This includes the selection of the development team, the formalization of budgets and schedules, the establishment of requirements, etc.
- *Monitoring development*. This includes review of the budget and scheduling; it also includes consultation regarding the intent of the requirements.
- *Management of the installation, training, and conversion to operational status*. Operational use, in turn, will initiate new requirements to be met by changes to the system.

Finally, there should also be a pragmatic appraisal of how specific the Requirements Specification actually are. Where a turnkey system is to be purchased, i.e., one that will be installed in finished form ready to "turn the key" and start, it is essential to begin with a firm understanding of what will be delivered. For internal development, a less formal statement of requirements may be advantageous. Finally, in some cases, the delivery of a product includes support in adapting it to meet the users' needs. In both of the last cases, knowledge gained during system development or as the result of working with the product may alter the initial Requirements Specification. Therefore, it is important not to overspecify at the preliminary stages.

6.2.3. Managing the Implementation

Systems level involvement continues until the system is finally replaced. Key activities include

- Review of the product with respect to the organization's needs. This entails active participation in design decisions.
- Training of users. This may include preparation of training materials, user documentation, or revised procedure manuals.
- Operational evaluation before the product is accepted for routine use.
- Management of product evolution. (This is also called maintenance; it will cost more than the initial development.)

Very little of the system level activity described here has to do with computer technology. Most tasks involve "classical" systems analysis and management. For example, it may take from 6 to 24 months to install a hospital information system (without any special program development). This time is required to establish what is useful for a particular organization and how it may be connected to (interfaced with) existing systems. The fact that the information system is managed by a computer is only a secondary consideration.

The development plan will identify the schedule, budget, and organization responsible for each activity. It should be recognized that the plan will be dynamic.

It should be kept up to date and used. Repeated failures to meet the planned objectives should be reviewed by management.

6.3. Application Software Development

In this section we assume that a software application is to be developed and we describe software engineering.

The field of software engineering has been defined as

> . . . the set of disciplines, tools and techniques (both technical and nontechnical) needed (and/or used) to produce efficient, correct, reliable . . . < any adjective denoting good > software in a manner which is timely, and is cost effective over the entire life cycle of the software.[1]

Software engineering was introduced as a popular term in the title of the 1969 NATO Conference on Software Engineering. After less than 25 years of experience with digital computers, the critical path was no longer how to write complex programs—it had become: how to develop complex systems. As suggested by the conference title, the initial emphasis was on the implementation of hardware-software systems: aerospace applications, computer operating systems, communication networks. In time, the scope has broadened, and software engineering now provides guidance to implementors of information systems as well as other classes of product. In the following subsections we present some of the major findings of this discipline as they relate to information system development.

6.3.1. The Software Life Cycle

The history of any organism proceeds from conception to death. This is called its life cycle. The software life cycle is similarly defined. It proceeds from project initiation through final retirement. A key event in the process is installation (or delivery). This separates the development phase from the operational and maintenance phase.

The basic software life cycle is modeled after the hardware life cycle. It is generally depicted as a sequence of activities that leads from one process to the next in a cascading arrangement as shown in Fig. 6.1. This also is called a waterfall chart. The labels on the boxes will vary from chart to chart. Some diagrams begin with a box representing the systems level requirements analysis described in the previous section. All diagrams show the basic direction of flow (solid lines) and the feedback or iteration (dashed lines). In each case, the life cycle is represented as a sequence of serial activities where one step cannot begin until the previous step is complete.

The activities depicted in Fig. 6.1 are as follows:

- *Analysis, also called Software Requirements*. This is the preliminary understanding of the problem which results in the definition of the requirements for the software component of the system.

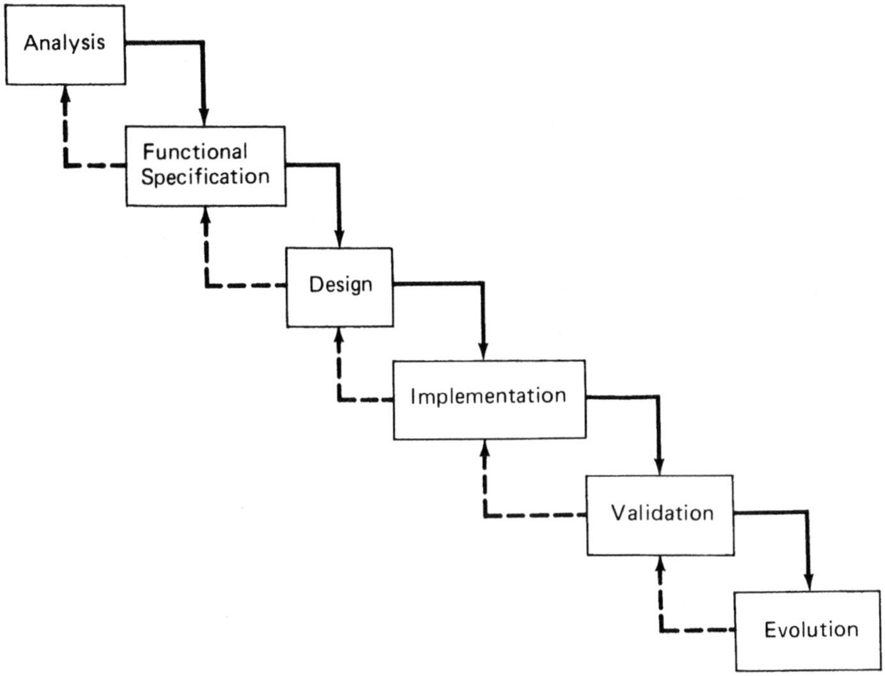

FIGURE 6.1. The software life cycle.

- *Functional Specification, also called Preliminary Design*. This is a transformation of the requirements (what is to be done) into an external design of how it should be done.
- *Design, also called Detailed Design*. This is a translation of the functional specification into a set of structures that can be implemented as computer programs.
- *Implementation, also called Code and Debug*. This is the translation of the design into executable code.
- *Validation, also called Test and Preoperations*. This is the process of ensuring that each unit or set of units satisfies its functional requirements. This actually is performed in several steps culminating in an operational acceptance of the entire product.
- *Evolution, also called Operations and Maintenance*. This consists of defect removal and modifications in response to new requirements. (New in the sense that they were not defined in the initial analysis.)

The model just presented is identical to the hardware life cycle model from which it was derived. (Replace Software with Hardware in the Analysis activity and change the Implementation activity to Fabrication and you will have the standard hardware life cycle). Yet there are obvious differences between software and hardware.

- Hardware engineering has a long history. Disciplines are in place to support the process. Many of the rules have been cataloged, and handbooks exist to guide its methods. Software engineering is only in its second decade; there are few empirically established principles.
- Hardware normally deals with multiple copies. Thus the effort to design the first copy will be prorated over the many copies produced. Most of this design activity is spent on drawings and instructions that detail how the product is to be manufactured. With software, on the other hand, the documentation is the product. There is virtually no cost beyond the first copy. Thus, a hardware prototype may be redesigned to reduce manufacturing costs whereas a "software prototype" may be delivered as the final product.
- Hardware is expensive to modify. Once a production line is in operation, it is difficult to make changes. Consequently there is a discipline of maintaining engineering drawings, carefully controlling changes, and thorough testing before the implementation (fabrication) begins. Software, on the other hand, is easily changed; it is also very difficult to test before the implementation (code and debug) begins. Indeed, with some embedded systems, management relies on software changes to correct for errors in the hardware.
- Hardware reliability is a measuring of how parts wear out. As such, it is a probability function. Software does not wear out; its reliability predicts when previously undetected errors will be found.
- Hardware builds on previous experience. Products are constructed from independently developed components and modules. Thus, although the hardware products are very complex, they are actually composed of smaller, complex modules whose behavior is well understood. There is little reuse of software at this time. In many cases, however, the need for new programs can be avoided by the use of existing application packages and program libraries.

Given these differences between hardware and software, it can be asked, why model the software life cycle after that used for hardware? There are several valid reasons. First, the process shown in Fig. 6.1 is an expression of the necessary three-step flow of (a) describe what is to be done, (b) do it, and (c) test and evaluate the result. Next, software frequently is developed for embedded applications, and management is accustomed to use similar tools for controlling both the hardware and software activities. Finally, the model shown in Fig. 6.1 has been studied extensively, and there are data that help to quantify the process. Therefore, it is useful to consider the classic software life cycle first and then consider alternative models.

6.3.1.1. The Standard Development Process

The distribution of effort among the activities leading to the delivered product is generally allocated using a 40-20-40 rule:

Analysis through Design—40% of the effort
Implementation—20% of the effort
Validation—40% of the effort.

Note that programming (implementation) comprises a very small portion of the total development cost.

The analysis produces the Requirements Specification. This is the most complete definition of what the delivered system is to do. For some projects it is the contractual description for what the developer will produce. Acceptance of the product implies that it satisfies all criteria laid out in the Requirements Specification. In theory, the requirements describe only *what* the software should do; it does not imply *how* this should be implemented. This is also sometimes called the behavior (*what*) and the structure (*how*) of the system. In practice it is impossible to separate the behavior from the structure. Nevertheless, we try.

When the Requirements Specification is complete, it is delivered to the development team. Everything they must know about the specific application must be contained in that specification; the designers are assumed to have a general knowledge of the application area so they can fill in what is implied by the specification. This is where experience is important. Some organizations specialize in hospital systems, others in business systems, others in compilers. An excellence in one area may not imply competence in another.

The design process typically goes through two stages. The first is a review of the requirements and their grouping into similar functions to be implemented. The functions are organized as modules. Once the modules have been defined, they are in turn decomposed into smaller units called programs. The behavior of the programs is fully defined before implementation (programming) begins. The two steps can be viewed as the continuous breaking down of the design into smaller and smaller units until the pieces are small enough to convert into code. In a large project, there are several reviews. After the functions have been allocated among the modules and the Functional Specification has been written, there is a review. If, at this point, the design seems satisfactory, the Functional Specification is used as the baseline document for the detailed design. For each program (or module) a design specification is prepared. It, too, is reviewed before coding can begin.

The process involves many iterations of taking a unit, breaking it into smaller units, and adding detail. The result is a document (or specification). This document is reviewed, approved, and then used as an input for the next iteration. The purpose of the review is to reduce the chance of errors being passed on to the next step. The use of a specification to initiate each new step ensures that the product will be consistent with the system design. At some point in time, all the necessary detail is in the specification. Now coding translates this into an executable program.

Each program is tested by the programmer after it is written—this is called unit testing or, sometimes, debugging. It is tested against the specification from which it was developed. Once the individual programs have been tested, they

Maintenance Categories		**Perfective Categories**		**User Enhancement Distribution**	
Corrective	20%	User Enhancements	42%	More Information	70%
Adaptive	25%	Documentation	6%	Reformation	10%
Perfective	55%	Efficiency	4%	Consolidation	10%
	100%	Other	3%	Other	10%
			55%		100%

FIGURE 6.2. Maintenance effort by category. Data from B. Lientz and E. Swanson, Software Maintenance Management, © 1980, Addison-Wesley, Reading, Massachusetts. Pgs. 151–157. Reprinted with permission.)

are combined as modules and tested. When all the modules have been tested, they are combined as a system and tested. Finally, when the system has been tested, it is placed in an operational setting and tested against the initial Requirements Specification to see if it meets the intended objectives. Notice that the testing is the inverse of the design process. Where the design decomposes the system into smaller and smaller units, the testing composes the system from these smaller units with tests at each step of the way. All tests are performed against the initial design criteria. That is, the test establishes that the product does what the design document states that it should. The program is tested against the Detailed Design Specification and the modules are tested against the Design Specification (or Functional Specification).

Once the system is accepted, operations begin. Most systems operate in a changing environment. Many systems also will change the environment. Therefore maintenance (or evolution) is a positive sign that the system is being used. Over half the total lifetime cost for a system is for maintenance; some estimates place this number as high as 80%. Thus, the ability to maintain a system should be considered as important as the initial cost to implement. In most commercial organizations, less than half the staff are available to begin new projects; the remainder are assigned to the maintenance of existing systems.

Maintenance activities are generally subdivided into three categories:

- *Corrective maintenance*. The identification and elimination of errors (defects)
- *Adaptive maintenance*. The accommodation to changes in hardware, software, or other external features of the system
- *Perfective maintenance*. The modification of the system to meet new or changed needs

As shown in Fig. 6.2, most of the effort goes to perfective maintenance. The process of making these changes will alter the structure of the system so that—in time—it will be less expensive to replace the old system than to alter it. In practice, however, there is often a decision to do neither: the system is frozen and no new modifications are approved. When this occurs, the system no longer meets the users' needs and alternative solutions are chosen. This, in part, explains the rising popularity of personal computers in institutions with powerful centralized facilities.

6.3.1.2. Evaluating the Standard Development Process

What we describe here as the standard development process was first initiated by large software and engineering organizations. The process of analysis, documentation, formal reviews, and implementation of a specification was an extension of their manufacturing experience. Many of the projects were quite large—100 or more programmers—and formal methods were required to manage communications. It is generally accepted that the above process is necessary to control large-scale software development. However, most software development is of a more modest size. Few projects in a health care or commercial setting require a staff of more than 10 persons. (Of course, many independent projects may be conducted in parallel.) Consequently, alternative development cycles are under review.

Before describing other approaches to managing the software life cycle, it is useful to summarize what we know about software development.

- Individual productivity, when measured in terms of lines of code produced, ranges from 10 to 30 lines per day. This is computed by dividing the size of the total product (less comments) by the effort days. The number includes analysis, documentation, testing, etc. Since coding is a small part of the total implementation effort (20%), productivity during that period is considerably higher.
- Individual productivity varies with the size of the project. For a small task that one can implement in about a month, 30 or more lines per day is common. For a task requiring several programmers over several months, the average is closer to 20 lines per day. For large programs that require tens of programmers over years, productivity falls to nine lines per day, and for very large projects, productivity averages of five lines per day are common. In part, the variation is due to project complexity; the reduction in productivity is also the result of the need to manage communications among the workers.
- Productivity, when measured in lines of code, is about the same independent of the language used. That is, a programmer can produce approximately the same number of tested assembly language or high-order language (HOL) statements in a given period. Since the HOL statements are more powerful, the effectiveness of the HOL will be greater. Indeed, the same problem will produce a smaller program with fewer lines. Because both programs will require the same effort for initial analysis and documentation, the assembly language lines of code per day may paradoxically suggest higher productivity than the HOL approach (i.e., the assembly language will produce a larger numerator for the lines per day computation). However, the HOL system will be less expensive to develop and maintain. The higher the level of the HOL, in general, the less expensive this system will be.
- The cost to repair a defect (error) increases with the delay in its recognition. To correct an error after a product has been installed may be 100 times more costly than its correction during the initial design. Most errors, by the way,

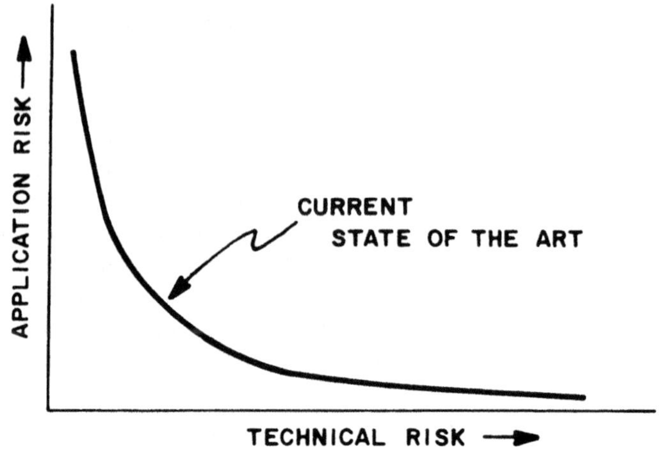

FIGURE 6.3. Two dimensions of risk.

are design errors; only about one-third of the errors result from the improper coding of a specification.

- A high proportion of the design activity is for housekeeping—the necessary support tasks that allow the system to perform the desired functions. In one small application it was found that > 95% of the code was for housekeeping. The use of a HOL, of course, reduces the amount of housekeeping.

Each of the above attributes of software development seems to be true for all application classes. When one narrows the focus to information systems, one finds that few perceive the standard production cycle to be satisfactory. Most commercial organizations report backlogs of 2—3 years for new applications; that is, it will take that long before requests can be transformed into implemented systems. One side effect of this delay is that the "invisible backlog" is generally greater than the formal backlog; people don't even bother to submit requests. Finally, in many cases the final product does not meet the users' needs. In one survey, 75% of the projects started were either never completed or never used, and—of those delivered—almost half were never used.

Clearly, there is a need to improve the process of developing information systems. Yet the application of the standard development process may not be the appropriate solution. To understand why this is so, consider Fig. 6.3. This describes the state-of-the-art in the context of two dimensions of risk:

- *Technical risk.* This is the risk that the technology will not support the application, i.e., the technology base and/or the knowledge base are not sufficiently broad to guarantee an implementation.
- *Application risk.* This is the risk that the completed product will not meet the needs it was intended to satisfy.

Note that projects high in application risk must be low in technical risk and vice versa. Where a project is high in both areas of risk it will be beyond the state-of-the-art and simplifying assumptions must be made. Using this figure as a guideline, we can make the following generalizations. Where the technical risk is high, preliminary analysis and formal specifications are mandatory and the standard development process is recommended. On the other hand, where the application risk is high, there is little certainty that the initial Requirements Specification will reflect the organization's true needs accurately; in such situations, a process designed simply to implement these specifications may be inappropriate.

As a result of this mismatch between the needs of a high application risk project and the formalisms employed in the standard development process, new life cycle models are being considered. This reexamination is going on at the time of writing, and it is not clear what the outcome will be. Several alternatives are being tested:

- *Use of higher level languages such as the Fourth-Generation Languages.* In some cases this allows development by the end users, thereby reducing the uncertainties in and reliance upon Requirement Specification. Higher level languages also are more compact and easier to use; thus the cost to develop and maintain will be lower. This approach is sometimes called programmerless development.
- *Use of different design techniques.* Rather than starting from a specification, one may build a simple model—called a prototype—and use that to define what the system is to do. The development may also proceed incrementally, with a small part developed, installed, tested, and used. The next increment will be built on the previous deliveries. Finally, there is an artificial intelligence-based view of "operational development" in which one specifies the system requirements and from them derives a working implementation.
- *Availability of off-the-shelf products that can be networked to provide the user with all the tools necessary to access and manage information.* Many of the tools are implemented as work stations that require little, if any, internal support.

By way of concluding the discussion about the software life cycle, note that we have gone through three historic stages.

Stage 1. Pragmatic attempts to translate a problem into an executable program using experience and cleverness.

Stage 2. Formalized structuring of the development process so that it could produce large and complex systems that perform as intended and are delivered on time and within cost.

Stage 3. Modifications to the standard development process to meet the special needs of selected application classes.

The failures of Stage 1 initiated Stage 2. The limitations of Stage 2 have introduced Stage 3. However, Stage 3 is not a reversion to Stage 1. One must understand what is intended and must consider how it is to be implemented. Programming remains a very small part of the activity. (With executable specifications, everything is done at the analysis level and programming disappears.) The removal of errors continues as a major activity, and the operational (maintenance) cost of a system normally exceeds its development cost. Thus, even if there is no consensus on the best way to develop a system, there certainly is a clear agreement about the unacceptable approaches.

6.3.2. Design Methods

The software life cycle consists of three activities: design, implementation, and test. A knowledge of the first and last are essential to anyone with a responsibility in the management of a software development project. A knowledge of implementation techniques is essential only to those with a responsibility for programming. Therefore, we close this section with a brief discussion of design methods and testing techniques. Section 6.4 is devoted to implementation issues.

As we have seen from the previous discussion, a requirements document tells what is to be done and the design describes how it is to be done. In high-application-risk projects one may not have a complete understanding of what is to be done; thus the requirements will not be an accurate statement of needs. In almost all projects it is impossible to separate the "what" from the "how" (the behavior from the structure) and therefore the requirements will generally imply some design. In particular, this is true where the requirements are written as a hierarchical collection of functions to be performed. All of this is to suggest that although we speak of formal specifications, they represent idealized models that may be achieved only imperfectly for a specific project. Human judgment is required and critical.

For an information system, the design flow is as shown in Fig. 6.4. There are two levels of design. The first is descriptive; it collects and documents information about the system, analyzes it, and presents it in a manner that should be understandable to users, analysts, and programmers. It is relatively implementation independent; that is the description will be essentially the same for systems implemented in COBOL or PL/1, on an IBM or a CDC machine. The second level details how the design should be translated into code; it is implementation-specific.

The descriptive design begins with the Requirements Specification which is derived from an analysis of the application domain. This is then translated into a functional design. For information systems the functions can be organized as data or as processes. That is, one can allow the structure of the data to determine how the processes are to be defined, or one can allow an analysis of the processes to identify what data are necessary. (The dotted lines imply that the requirements are not complete and some design activities involve further analysis of the application domain.) There are methods that favor each approach. It is important to recognize that each represents a different view of the same system. Once the functions have been allocated among the processes and data, the detailed design may begin. The processes are implemented as programs, the data defined in a

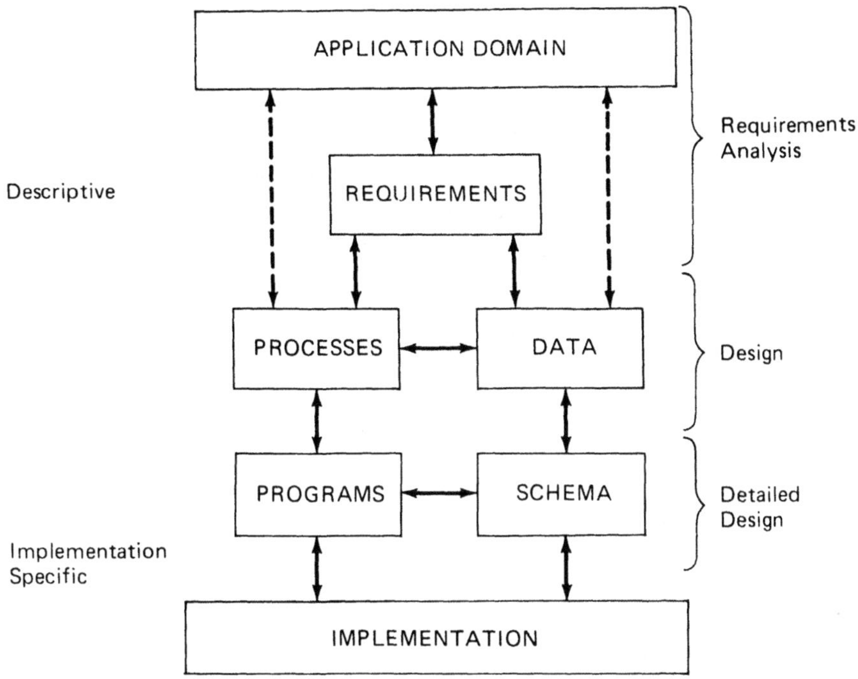

FIGURE 6.4. Information system design flow.

schema. (The term schema implies a DBMS. Where one is not used, the schema definition is distributed among the individual programs. Naturally, this introduces a potential for inconsistency.) Finally, the detailed design is implemented.

There are many methods in use for completing a design. This suggests that there is no "right way" to do the design—only wrong ways. The design process should be thought of as a modeling exercise. One builds a model, analyzes it, and then transforms it to another—generally more detailed—model. The process stops when there is a final design that can be converted into code. The code itself is a model of the operational program. In this modeling activity, each model may support several different equivalent transformations. There are many different functional allocations that can satisfy a single requirement; there are also many different detailed designs that can satisfy a given functional design. Thus, each step in the design process requires judgment and selection. Although there are some rules that guide the choice of alternative models (see Section 6.4), the experience and talent of the design team is critical. The transformation of the code, on the other hand, is invariant for a fixed compiler and machine.

A standard approach to deriving the requirements for a system is first to build a model of the organization that will use the system. Each organizational entity—billing department, personnel department, etc.—is drawn as a box with lines between boxes for their key interactions. Once this is done, a line is drawn

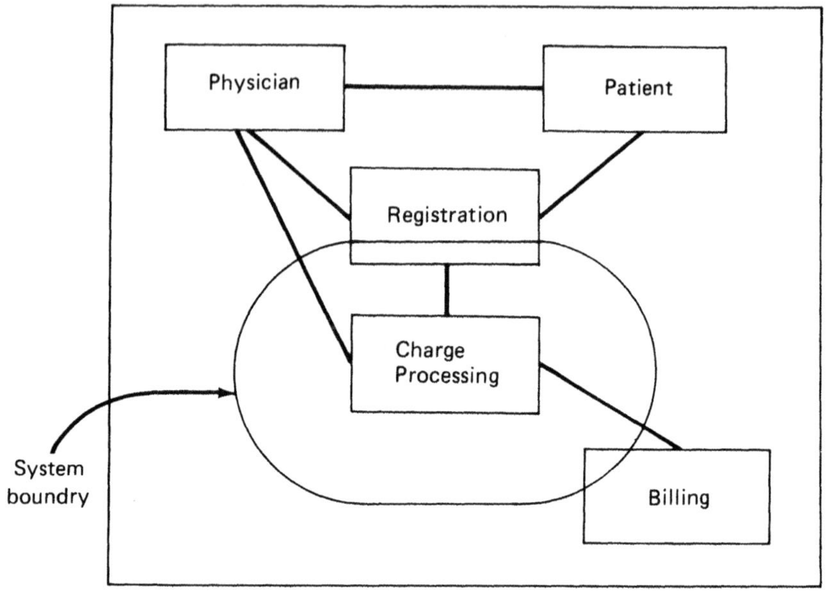

FIGURE 6.5. System boundary in an entity diagram (After K. Orr, *Structured Requirements Definition*. Ken Orr and Assoc., 1981.)

around those entities that are to be supported by the system. This is the system boundary. Everything inside will be automated; everything outside is manual. Fig. 6.5 illustrates such an entity diagram in the style of Orr. In general, this first modeling step is not very formal. The goal is to go from "fuzzy thinking" to "clear thinking." The diagram is a tool that helps the process. The objective is to define the system boundary and describe what the system should do for the entities within the boundary. Once the boundary exists, it is not too difficult to identify the functions to be performed.

As shown in Fig. 6.4, the design involves two basic entities: processes and data. This division is reflected in the two basic approaches to design: process flow analysis and data structure analysis. The method developed by Yourdon (and Constantine, DeMarco, *et al.*) is the most widely used implementation of the former. It is called Structured Analysis and uses data flow diagrams (DFD) to model the system. Processes are shown as bubbles, and the data that flow into and from each process are shown as lines. Each process (bubble) in the DFD is numbered; processes can be decomposed into more detailed DFDs until the design is complete, i.e., further detail is superfluous (see Fig. 6.6). The lowest level processes are then documented in minispecs that describe the functions to be performed by the process bubbles; the data inputs/outputs are described in a data dictionary. This is followed by detailed design which uses a different tool (Structured Design). For each minispec, an implementation design is prepared in the form of a hierarchical structure chart. Each box (program) is described in

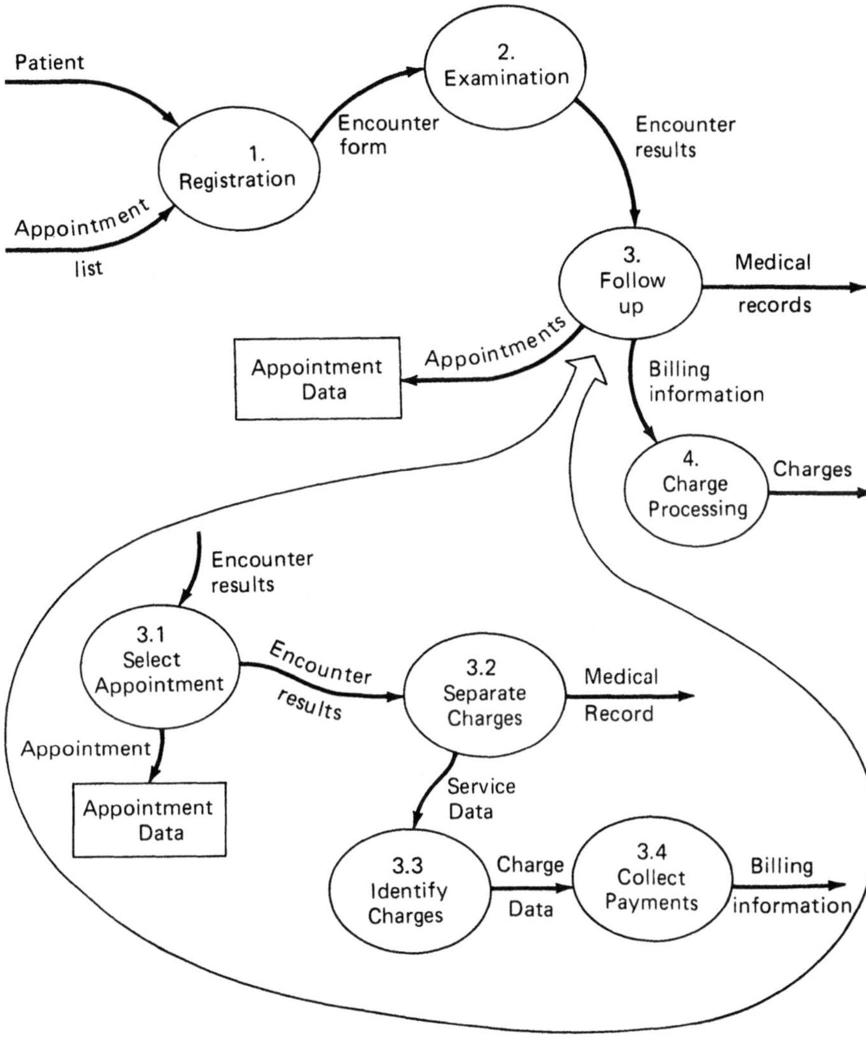

FIGURE 6.6. Data flow diagram (After E. Yourdon, *Classics in Software Engineering,* 1979 and *Writings of the Revolution,* 1982, Yourdon Press; and T. DeMarco, *Structured Analysis and System Specification,* Prentice Hall, 1979.

a module spec that lays out what the program is to do. (The concept of a module is discussed in Section 6.4.3.) Further detail is added to the data dictionary. Finally, the process of coding is simply the transformation into code of the model presented in the module spec. The function of the analysis is to structure the design activity and simplify the programming activity.

There are also variations to the above approach. The Hierarchy Input Process Output (HIPO) begins with a hierarchy of all programs in the system. For each implemented node in the hierarchy there is an Input Process Output diagram that describes the data input to each step in a process, the steps in a process, and the data output from each process step. Once the diagrams are drawn, they are converted to code. The use of a hierarchy assumes that there is a top to the system; thus, this general approach is called "top down." There is an alternative design approach in which one first searches for the generally used functions, designs them, and then designs the remaining programs in the context of these functions. This is sometimes called "bottom up." In actual practice, both top down (decomposition) and bottom up (abstraction) are used together. Both techniques generally imply emphasis on process definition.

Several methods are based on the belief that the structure of the system is best modeled by the data it uses. Jackson, Orr, and Warnier subscribe to this view. Jackson has developed two systems. The Jackson System Development (JSD) method provides an approach to the development of complex systems. It is not top down. Jackson believes that one knows the least about an application at the start of the design activity. Thus a top down approach—which superimposes a structure on the solution—is inappropriate; the top down description, however, is an ideal way to convey the design once it is understood. Thus JSD begins with model of the real world environment, and through constructive refinements produces a model of the final programs. Although the previous sentence is obscure, it should be clear that this approach is quite different from that of identifying the functions to be performed and then allocating them to modules. The technique is new, and there is limited experience with it. Nevertheless, many feel that the concepts used in JSD offer significant improvements over other approaches.

Jackson also has a method for program design (JSP) that has been in use since the mid 1970s. He begins by modeling the data used by the system and then designs the programs so that they reflect the data structures. The goal is to get a correct and maintainable system quickly. Both the data and program are modeled using identical notations. A brief example is shown in Fig. 6.7. It shows an appointment file with more than one patient and more than one date-time per patient. The iteration (or presence of more than one entry) is indicated by the asterisk in the upper right corner. Each appointment will be with either a doctor or a nurse. The doctor visits indicate the anticipated duration of the visit; the nurse visits indicate the procedures to be performed. The selection (one of the two) is indicated by the circle in the upper right corner. A program to list out the appointments is shown on the right. Notice how it reflects the structure of the data and the output. When the output does not match the data, there is a structure clash and JSP has a technique for accommodation. Once the diagrams are complete, they can be transformed into pseudocode, which is then translated into a program. The pseudocode provides the general form of the final program while suppressing detail (housekeeping). The Structured Analysis module spec is a form of pseudocode. A Program Design Language (PDL) is another example of pseudocode.

Although there are many different approaches to the design of an information

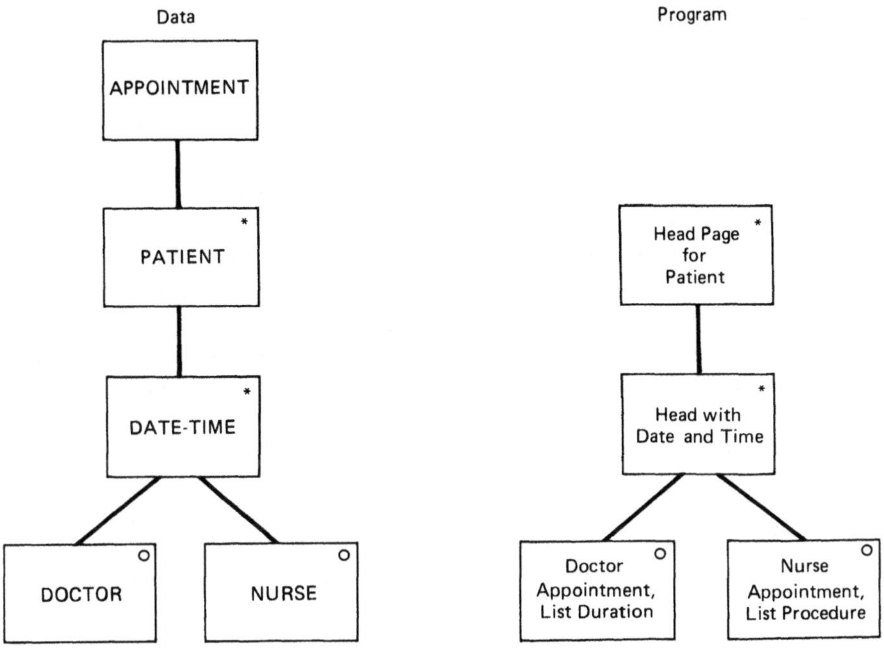

FIGURE 6.7. Illustration of Jackson JSP Diagrams.

system, there are advantages to accepting a single method. It provides guidance in the modeling process, it produces descriptions that are clear to those familiar with the method, it leads to early and consistent documentation, it affords management a view of project status, and it even introduces a Hawthorn effect. Where methods are used, productivity generally improves. However, as with any tool, there are examples of methods being misapplied so that energy is devoted to abstract design activities rather than to design. Pragmatism must temper the role of the formalisms.

6.3.3. Verification and Validation

Forty percent of the preoperational activity is normally spent on testing that the product is correct (has no errors) and corresponds to the environment's needs. These attributes are evaluated by two similar sounding, but very different, activities.

Verification (from the Latin *versus* meaning true) tests to see if the product is a "true" implementation of the specification. Errors are deviations from the specification.

Validation (from the Latin *validus* meaning strength or worth) tests to see if the product conforms to the needs of the users' environment.

As Boehm states it,

Verification is getting the system right,
Validation is getting the right system.

In the development of large systems there is usually an independent test team. During the period that the designers are producing their documentation, the testers use the design to produce test plans and scenarios. The separation between the design and test teams minimizes the testing bias. That is, the designer will produce a test for a product that reflects his view of what the product should do based on his understanding of the specifications. An independent tester, on the other hand, will have a different perspective. In this way errors and misconceptions can be resolved before system release.

Formal testing can begin only after there is a product—code—to be tested. The test plans detail the tests to be performed and the outputs to be expected. Each test is of the form: set up, run test, and evaluate results. Note that this is quite different from the sequence employed by casual programmers: set up, run test, accept if no pathological failures.

Testing is a process designed to detect errors. A test succeeds only when an error is found. Failure to find an error does not imply that the product is correct (with respect to its specification). It may be that the test case was poorly selected. There are two basic ways of testing programs:

White box testing in which one has a knowledge of how the program works. The test is designed to verify that implementation is correct.

Black box testing in which one ignores how a program (or collection of programs) works. The test is designed to verify the processing of its inputs and outputs—its interfaces.

An example of white box testing is path testing. In this case, one starts with a flow chart of the system and defines test cases that will cause every instruction and path in the test to be exercised at least once. An example of black box testing is a test driver (or harness) that feeds inputs to a program and then collects and evaluates the outputs.

Testing, like most of the development activities, is an art. Because testing comes at the end of the development cycle, there is frequently pressure to reduce the effort to meet schedule or cost commitments. It is difficult to say how much testing is enough. There are some models that project the number of errors expected to be present at the start of testing. Some suggest that testing continue until a given percent of the projected errors is found or until a budgeted amount of time has elapsed. As previously stated, the cost of repairing errors after release is quite expensive, thus the greater the number of corrections made prior to release, the lower the life cycle cost.

In the standard development process validation is the last step before operational use. The validation considers how the product operates in the real world. The product, by this time, is a set of correct programs. The evaluation relates to how those programs are used in the environment for which they were developed. Thus, the persons responsible for conducting the validation should be analysts and not programmers. The acceptance of the product is independent of how it was programmed. Once the system is accepted, it is put into operational use and maintenance (evolution) begins. Of course, the process is dynamic. If development takes several years, the requirements will have changed over that time. Thus the design and test plans will have to be changed as well. One way of minimizing the impact of these changes is to use a phased implementation. The system is broken into phases (or builds) that are incrementally produced, tested, and installed. Successive phases take advantage of the experience with the previous phases. This is also called evolutionary development.

In the case of high-application-risk projects it must be recognized that the initial Requirements Specification may not reflect accurately the organization's needs. Thus, the risk implies a high probability that a correct (verified) system will not correspond (be validated). In this situation, extreme care must be taken to avoid a project plan that too rigorously follows the standard development process and ignores the areas of risk. Some suggestions for these types of applications are:

- *Rapid prototyping*. Build a sample model of the application to test the ideas with greatest uncertainty, for example, the user interfaces. Do this quickly and plan to throw the prototype away once the analysis is complete.
- *High productivity tools*. Use Fourth-Generation Languages, DBMS, report generators, or other tools to reduce the effort. With less effort comes a greater willingness to make changes.
- *Conduct risk assessments*. Periodically, and especially in the early stages, review the project and try to identify the areas of greatest potential risk. Determine what actions are necessary to reduce the risk. Evaluate and monitor these key tasks.

6.3.4. Reviews and Proofs

The discussion of verification and validation was limited to activities that involved programs and completed products. It has been pointed out that the earlier a problem is found, the less expensive it is to correct it. Thus, it would be imprudent to begin some testing of the design until a program product was produced. The process of certifying the design before the code is created is variously called verification and validation, quality assurance, and product management. It is generally an intellectual exercise; there is no program that can be tested. This subsection presents some experience with the acceptance of preimplementation products.

In the 1960s, much of programming was considered to be an art—an extension of one's intellect and personality. As a result, the program was treated as a personal product and frequently held as a private object. In the early 1970s new approaches to organizing program activity altered this view. In a book called *The Psychology of Computer Programming (1971)*, Weinberg introduced the term egoless programming. The program should be seen as an open document that contributes to the team effort. Review of the program by other members of the team should be encouraged. Program examination is both a teaching and a learning activity, and all team members should be included.

At about the same time Mills and Baker introduced the concept of the chief programmer team. In this organization there was a chief programmer, an assistant, and several programmers who followed the chief programmer's direction. Because batch development was used, there was a program librarian responsible for managing computer runs, filing compilations and test outputs, and retaining a historical audit. Again, the idea of public code prevailed. The records were maintained by the program librarian and were open to all; no code was independently (or privately) maintained. In each of these cases, the public nature of the program invited review by peers.

The idea of reviews always has been an integral part of the standard development process. For hardware manufacture, nothing exists before production except for documentation and—perhaps—prototypes. Therefore, in both the hardware and software life cycles, two types of reviews are identified: the Preliminary Design Review (PDR) which reviews higher level specifications to determine if detailed design should proceed, and Critical Design Review (CDR) which considers the detailed design and authorizes the initiation of implementation. Note that these reviews are associated with management actions to proceed; they are not (like testing) designed to find errors. Nevertheless, the review process does detect errors, and in the early 1970s the interest in software engineering, openness of code, and the need for early problem identification all led to experimentation with software oriented reviews called walkthroughs or inspections.

Walkthroughs typically occur at two points in the development cycle that roughly correspond to the preliminary and critical design reviews. The key to quality and cost control is the early identification of errors. Where software tools are available, some errors can be uncovered automatically. For example, the Problem Statement Language/Problem Statement Analyzer (PSL/PSA) tests many of the requirements definitions for consistency and produces lists of missing information. Where such tools are not available or are incomplete, manual processes are required. The walkthrough generally implies that the producer of a design (or even code) will walk through the processing before a group of peers. The description process will formalize his concepts. The peer review will subject the product to external examination, and the developer will benefit from the experience of others. Walkthroughs may be managed with varying degrees of formality. They provide an excellent way to introduce new members of a team (or organization) to the standards and conventions currently in use.

A more formal approach—called inspection or structured walkthroughs—has been developed by Fagan. In this case there are two formal inspections: to evaluate the design before coding (called I_1) and after the first clean compilation (I_2). The inspection teams contain a moderator (who acts as a leader and coach), plus the designers, coder/implementations, and testers. The process includes an overview (by the entire team), preparation for the inspection (by the designer or implementer), the inspection (by the entire team again), with rework and follow-up for all identified problems. Checklists of potential errors are used, and records of errors and error types are retained. The process is relatively expensive to support, but the number of errors found suggests that the savings in testing and maintenance justify the investment.

TABLE 6.1. Some techniques for defect identification.

	Design reviews	Machine testing	Correctness proofs	Models or prototypes
Ommited functions	Good	Fair	Poor	Good
Added functions	Good	Poor	Poor	Fair
Structrual problems	Good	Fair	Poor	Fair
Algorithm problems	Fair	Fair	Good	Good
Human-factor problems	Fair	Poor	Poor	Good

The inspection technique is designed to ensure that the design and implemented code are correct. Recall that correctness is an attribute of verification; it implies that the product is correct with respect to its specification. As we have seen, for projects in which we have a poor understanding of the requirements, we may use modeling, analysis, or prototyping to establish the requirements and the best design approach to implementation. When, on the other hand, we have a well-defined process that is to be implemented as an algorithm, there is a logical technique called proof of correctness that allows one to prove that the algorithm is correct. Informal use of this technique can be applied to virtually any program. However, formal application remains a cumbersome and time-consuming exercise for any but the smallest programs. The technique involves establishing the conditions that are true before each statement is executed and then after each statement is completed. These assertions are then generalized to blocks and finally to the algorithm. The proof also requires the developer to demonstrate that the algorithm always terminates (i.e., no infinite loops). When the proof is completed, the algorithm may then be described by assertions about the algorithm's input and output states. It is believed that such a formal approach will allow us to build complex systems (such as compilers) that are correct. Less rigorous application of the concepts also seems to produce higher quality products.

Table 6.1 provides a cross-reference for the types of problems frequently encountered and the techniques used to identify defects.[3] There is no universal or automatic solution. Many of the benefits are derived simply by looking at the problem in a new way or with different people. Because of the need for reliability in health care applications and the high cost of later error repair, the use of early reviews and testing cannot be overemphasized.

6.4. Programming Heuristics

Programming is the translation of some design specification into computer instructions. Programming is also one of the nation's fastest growing hobbies. It is interesting, challenging, and sometimes exciting fun. When we measure productivity in lines of code, we are measuring only the product of programming activity. When we write a program, it performs a function, can be measured, and is an essential part of the delivered system. Thus, programming is a key part of application development. But it represents only 20% of the development cycle cost. Further, if we could implement the executable instructions from higher level specifications, then we wouldn't even need programming.

Since we have been writing computer programs for some four decades, we have a great deal of experience with and understanding of the process. Some aspects of programming can be formally stated and tested with mathematical rigor; others rely on informal rules: heuristics. In what follows we shall summarize much of what is agreed on regarding the implementation of computer applications. Before we begin, however, it is useful to make a distinction between what Orr calls "toy" systems and "commercial grade" systems. Toy systems (usually) work for (most of) the situations they are intended to support. There is generally a personal bond between the product and its developer, and the developer frequently has difficulty in distinguishing between what the system does and what it can do with just a few more weeks' time. A commercial grade system, on the other hand, does not suffer from these defects; it even includes good documentation.

Brooks points out that it may cost twice as much to produce a system for use by external users than it does to produce a system for internal use. The cost is for more complete testing, more complete error recovery, more complete documentation, etc. In both cases, he is speaking about commercial grade systems; the difference between toy and commercial grade systems is even greater. Thus, we begin with a few warnings:

- Experience based on the development of personal computer toy systems may be misleading in the development of commercial grade systems.
- Programming is deceptively complex. The result is that programmers are unrealistically optimistic.
- Programs are frequently reported to be 95% complete; this achievement may represent only half the task. Such programs are incomplete and ought not to be used.

6.4.1. Structured Programming

The term Structured Programming first became popular following a 1968 letter that Dijkstra wrote to the *Communications of the ACM* entitled "Go To Statement Considered Harmful." It began:

EDITOR:

For a number of years I have been familiar with the observation that the quality of programmers is a decreasing function of the density of **go to** statements in the programs they produce. More recently I discovered why the use of the **go to** statement has such disastrous effects, and I became convinced that the **go to** statement should be abolished

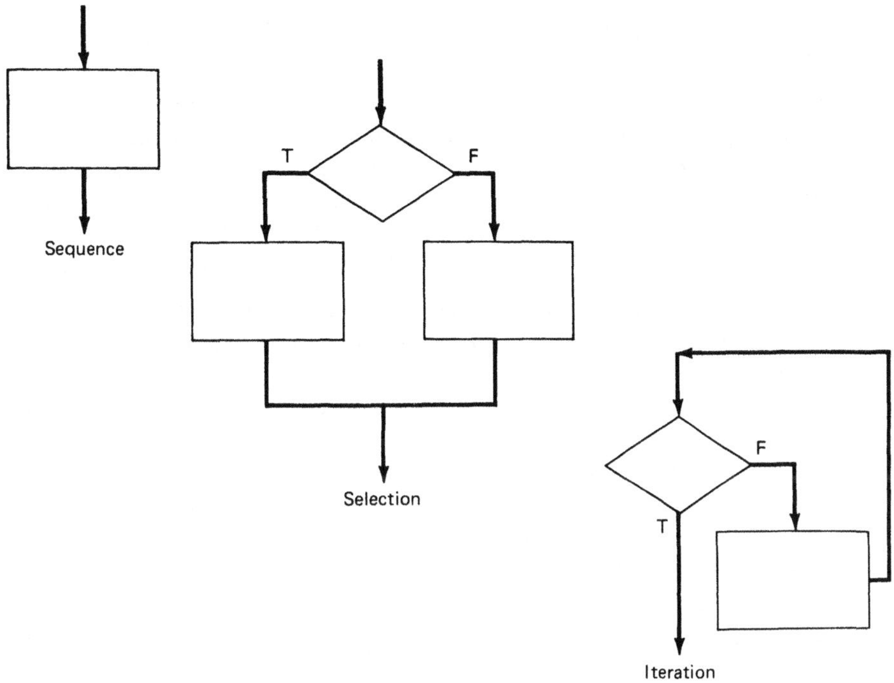

FIGURE 6.8. The Basic Flow Chart Constructs.

from all "higher level" programming languages (i.e., everything except, perhaps, plain machine code). At that time I did not attach too much importance to this discovery; I now submit my considerations for publication because in very recent discussions in which the subject turned up, I have been urged to do so. (From Dijkstra EW. *Commun ACM* (11,3):147-148, 1968. Copyright 1968, Association for Computing Machinery, Inc., reprinted by permission.)

He went on to note that the production of a program was complete after it was written and tested. Yet, the use of the program really depends on the control (i.e., branching behavior) of the program in a dynamic operational setting. "[O]ur intellectual powers are rather geared to master static relations and . . . our powers to visualize processes evolving in time are relatively poorly developed." This led him to conclude, "The **go to** statement as it stands is just too primitive; it is too much an invitation to make a mess of one's program."

Several years before this letter was written, Bohm and Jacopini had shown that all flow charts could be constructed using only sequences of instruction plus two formation rules: selection (**if . . . then . . . else**) and iteration (**do while**). The flow chart primitives are shown in Fig. 6.8. Each block can consist of either a sequence of instructions, a selection, or iteration. The **go to** was unnecessary and, in Dijkstra's view, harmful. Naturally, the use of these simple formal constructs played a major role in the development of the block structured languages of ALGOL 68, PL/1, and Pascal in the late 1960s and MODULA-2 and Ada in the late 1970s (see Chapter 5).

By the early 1970s Structured Programming was firmly entrenched. It was frequently equated with "**go to-less**" programming, and minor arguments arose over where and when **go tos** would be acceptable. However, the most popular languages, FORTRAN and COBOL, did not support the constructs. Therefore, the purity of the concept had to be compromised to meet the pragmatic needs of the users. What resulted was the following generally accepted practice:

- Wherever possible, organize the program as a nested set of the three basic constructs. Use indentation to suggest the structure of the program. Use **go tos** sparingly.
- Break the program into units, each approximately one listing page in length. Keep all the control (e.g., **go tos**, loops) on the page. Use a single point of entry and a single point for return (or exit).
- Abstract more complex processes as algorithms (procedures, subroutines) that can be accessed from the programs that use them. This is also sometimes referred to as stepwise refinement.

The result of this activity was small, easy-to-read programs, with levels of complexity relegated to lower level programs that, in turn, were small, easy-to-read, etc.

This is the essence of structured programming. The early 1960s produced systems that were longer and more complex than any that had been previously known. The programs became large, and an understanding required leafing through many pages of instructions. **Go tos** sent control from page to page with a logic that defied comprehension. Spaghetti code was the result. Structured programming cleaned up the chaos. Productivity improvements of about 25% were immediately recorded, and the style of structured programs is evident in the FORTRAN, Pascal, and LISP examples in Chapter 5. Most new programmers are taught only structured programming. One reason for the educational popularity of Pascal is that it has a command structure for these constructs. BASIC, on the other hand, requires the GOTO for both control and subroutine calls (procedure evocation); nevertheless, most BASIC programmers are taught to write code with structural indentation.

6.4.2. Algorithms

Much of any programming activity is the recoding of what has been coded before. HOLs eliminate the recoding of assembly language sequences; thus, we write READ . . . and need not worry about the assembly language statements that might be required to implement the function. In the same way generalized packages, DBMSs, and 4GLs provide general functions that can be used (or reused) with minimal effort. Where such features are not available in the development environment, the programmer may access a library of routines to select the desired function. Most vendor-supplied packages come with libraries.

Large transportable libraries for scientific and engineering applications have made FORTRAN the standard for this class of computing.

Where a program is not available, an existing program may be adopted. Many large organizations have program libraries that they routinely modify to produce new products for different customers. The modification of an existing program is less expensive than a completely new program; it also has the advantage of being well understood. (One caveat: Recall that modification degrades the structure of a program so that at some point it is better to discard the product than to alter it. Program modification assumes the existence of a well-structured initial product.)

In many cases the user will have to write a completely new program. This subsection serves as a reminder that the logic for part of that program may have been worked out already; only the recoding of an algorithm is necessary. The advantages of using an existing algorithm are enhanced performance and reduced development time. There are many books that describe algorithms and detail how to construct them. In what follows, we shall briefly address the problem of sorting values in an array. We describe several algorithms, i.e., sequences of computer steps to perform a process that terminate with a desired output. The descriptions are brief, informal, and conceptual. To be more precise would require a knowledge of some specific programming language.

We begin with an array of numbers in some unknown sequence. Our goal is to end with the contents of the array sorted in ascending order with duplicates. For example:

Before	*After*
A(1) = 6	A(1) = 3
A(2) = 12	A(2) = 6
A(3) = 3	A(3) = 7
A(4) = 7	A(4) = 7
A(5) = 14	A(5) = 12
A(6) = 17	A(6) = 14
A(7) = 23	A(7) = 17
A(8) = 7	A(8) = 23

There are many ways to perform this sort. The one that is most easily remembered (and also the most frequently used) is called the bubble sort. In this algorithm, adjacent pairs in the array are compared and the larger of the two is set as the second. This process repeats until all pairs have been tested. After the pass, the largest value has "bubbled" to the bottom. The process is repeated again, but this time excluding the last element; the next largest value "bubbles" down. This continues until there is only the top element in the array and the sort is completed. Fig. 6.9a describes the algorithm and Fig. 6.9b provides an instance using the first four elements A(1) through A(4) as input.

Although the algorithm is very simple, it is also very slow. To see why, consider the processing. It steps through the inner loop $N - 1$ times, then $N - 2$ times, and so on. That is, $(N - 1) + (N - 2) + \ldots + 1$ which is a

```
For I from N to 2 decrementing by -1
    For J from 1 to I
        If A(J)<A(J-1) then exchange them
        End of inner loop
    End of outer loop
```

FIGURE 6.9a. Buble Sort for array of A of length N.

Actual Values Stored					Computer Program in Array
Pass 1	6	12	3	7	Compare 6 and 12, no change
	6	12	3	7	Compare 12 and 3, exchange
	6	3	12	7	Compare 12 and 7, exchange
	6	3	7	12	End of Pass 1
Pass 2	6	3	7	12	Compare 6 and 3, exchange
	3	6	7	12	Compare 6 and 7, no change
	3	6	7	12	End of Pass 2
Pass 3	3	6	7	12	Compare 3 and 6, no change
	3	6	7	12	End of sort

FIGURE 6.9b. Sequence of operations for three passes using a Buble Sort. (Both a and b from B. Blum, *M.D. Computing* (1, 1). Copyright 1984 by Springer-Verlag. Reprinted with permission).

total of 1/2 (N^2 − N) comparisons. Assuming the numbers are randomly distributed, half of the adjacent numbers will be out of order and will have to be interchanged. Since each exchange involves three moves, there are 3/2 moves per comparison. So the average number of steps is

$$1/2\ (N^2 - N) \text{ compares plus}$$
$$3/4\ (N^2 - N) \text{ moves}$$

Thus, the time it takes to complete a bubblesort is roughly proportional to the square of the number of items to be sorted. For small arrays (N = 10) the sort is easy to code and the processing time is not consequential. However, for larger arrays (N = 1000) it is unsatisfactory.

A somewhat faster algorithm is modeled after the way we sort a deck of playing cards. We start with a sequence that is sorted and take a new card. We find where the new card belongs in the sequence and insert it. We then get another new card and continue until all the cards have been inserted in the proper place. This is what the insertion sort does. It starts with a sorted sequence (the first element in the array) and the next element in the array. It saves that next element in a temporary location, thus leaving a "space" in the array. It compares the element in the temporary location with the highest element in the sorted sequence. If it is greater, then it is inserted and the pass is complete; otherwise the tested element is moved up to the "space" and the next higher element is tested. The process is shown in Fig. 6.10a with an instance given in Fig. 6.10b.

```
For I from 2 to N
    Save A(I) as TEMP
    For J from I to 2 decrementing by -1
        If A(I-1)>TEMP
            Them move A(I-1) to A(J)
            Else move TEMP to A(J) and end the inner loop
        End of inner looop
    End of outer loop
```

FIGURE 6.10a. Insert Sort for arrary A of length N.

Actual Values Stored in Array					Copmuter Program Action
Pass 1	6	12	3	7	Remove 12 for compare
	6	12	3	7	Since 6<12, put 12 in empty space
Pass 2	6	12	3	7	Remove 3 for compare
	6		12	7	Since 12>3, move 12 to the empty space
		6	12	7	Since 6>3, move 6 to the empty space
	3	6	12	7	Finished, put 3 in empty space
Pass 3	3	6	12	7	Remove 7 for compare
	3	6		12	Since 12>7, move 12 to empty space
	3	6		12	Since 6<7, insert 7 into empty space

FIGURE 6.10b. Sequence of operations for three passes using an Insert Sort. (Both a and b from B. Blum, *M.D. Computing* (1, 1). Copyright 1984 by Springer-Verlag. Reprinted with permission).

Is the insert sort better than the bubble sort? The program is a bit more complicated but it is faster. Instead of doing an exchange (with three moves) it does a single move. Also it stops each pass as soon as it has done an insert. On the average, it will do

$$1/4\ (N^2 + N - 2) \text{ compares and}$$
$$1/4\ (N^2 + 9N - 10) \text{ moves}$$

This provides little advantage over the bubblesort for small Ns, but the insert sort is twice as fast for large Ns.

Are there better algorithms? In 1959, Shell came up with an approach requiring approximately $N^{1.2}$ processing steps compared with bubble sort's N^2. It is called the Shellsort and is only slightly more complex than bubble sort. However, since 1959, even better algorithms have come along that are based on two concepts:

- *Divide-and-conquer*: Break large arrays into partially sorted, smaller arrays that can be quickly merged.
- *Recursion*: The ability of a procedure to call itself or call another procedure that calls the first one again. This allows each division step to call the divide-and-conquer program.

TABLE 6.2. Comparison of sorting times for five different sort implementations on randomly sorted arrays of size 256 and 512.

Type of sort	Time in milliseconds N = 256	N = 512
Bubble sort	1,026	4,054
Insertion	366	1,444
Shellsort	127	349
Mergesort	102	242
Quicksort	60	146

(From N. Wirth, *Algorithms + Data Structures = Programs*. Prentice-Hall, Inc., Englewood Cliffs, N.J. 1976)

Two easy-to-learn and easy to reconstruct sorts are Mergesort and Quicksort. Each is effective for large sorting operations. Mergesort starts by making small strings, sorting them, then merging them together. This requires only N log N moves and even fewer comparisons. The prize goes to Quicksort, first defined in 1962 by Hoare. Quicksort requires only one-sixth the number of Mergesort's moves for a randomly sorted input. Descriptions of the Mergesort and Quicksort are beyond the scope of this subsection. Table 6.2 illustrates some timing comparisons among the algorithms mentioned here. There are more sort algorithms, and the relationships in the table will vary with the input state of the array. Nevertheless, the messages are obvious:

- There is much more to programming than a simple program that works.
- A great deal of knowledge already exists about algorithms; it should be applied to new applications.

6.4.3. Modularization

The term module comes from hardware engineering. A module is a physically separable unit with clearly defined interfaces, i.e., definitions of the inputs and outputs. A product can be fabricated by combining modules. One major advantage of a module is that it can be used without knowing how it works; it is treated as a "black box" that is defined solely in terms of its interface. A software module attempts to echo this property. It is a unit of code that can be thought of only in terms of its inputs and outputs. Parnas popularized the term "information hiding" to describe what a module should do. If all modules did only what was defined by their interfaces, then the coding and maintenance of modules would be vastly simplified. Unfortunately, this is not always the case as we shall explain.

There is no generally accepted definition of a module. It may be a term used for a major function, for example, the appointment module of an ambulatory care system. Others define a module as a unit of program code that can be listed on a single page, i.e., a structured program as defined above. Although there are vast differences in these concepts of a module, the heuristics we shall discuss are valid for both concepts.

Structured programming emphasizes presenting each unit so one can fully comprehend what that unit does. The objective of modularization is to minimize interactions (side effects) among units. We have seen, for example, where stepwise refinement identifies complex processes of a larger program and isolates them as a separate procedure called from the first. The rules of information hiding require that one not try to take advantage of any special knowledge of how the new module works beyond what is specified in its interface (e.g., calling sequence). However, where both modules share a common symbol table, that may not be possible. Changing the value of a variable in the first may inadvertently impact the second module. To illustrate, consider this flow:

```
MODULE1
        .
        .
        .
        I := 10
        .
        .
        .
        Call MODULE2
        .
        .
        .
END MODULE1
MODULE2
        .
        .
        .
        I := 20
        .
        .
        .
END MODULE2
```

What is the value of I in MODULE1 after the call to MODULE2? The answer could be either 10 or 20; it depends on the environment.

The interconnection among modules is called coupling. It ranges from low (with no direct coupling because of no interaction) to high (where one module takes advantage of knowledge of the internal structure of a second). The most common low coupling interaction uses a calling sequence to pass data from one module to another. When the data passed include "flags" that indicate what the second module should do, it is called control coupling. Sharing the same data is called external or common coupling. Content coupling is the highest (tightest) coupling; it should be avoided. The higher the coupling, the greater the probability that changes in one module will have an impact on other modules.

A second characteristic of modules describes its internal relationships. It is called cohesion. Low cohesion suggests that the module is a collection of independent tasks, e.g., a utility module that groups broadly used utility tasks. High cohesion is called functional cohesion; it is a single algorithm. This is most desirable. As with coupling, there are intermediate stages. Both coupling and cohesion are concepts. They cannot be measured, yet an awareness of each will enhance module independence and facilitate development, testing, and maintenance.

6.5. Concluding Remarks

System implementation invokes two separate activities. The user of the system must determine what the new system is to do and how it will be produced, i.e., make or buy. The user must then participate in the development or procurement process, prepare for the installation, train the new users, and operate and maintain the new system. Although the user should expect expert help in this activity, the primary responsibility is his. Management plans and ongoing reviews are essential; monitoring the progress as defined by the plan will help management determine how realistic the target objectives are.

The development of a system is a very different activity. There are some standard rules for development that have been proven to be effective for certain classes of large systems. For information systems there are also new tools that can be used to facilitate and speed development. Although there is no single path for effective development, it is known that an undisciplined, poorly directed, or excessively dogmatic approach will yield poor results. Experience, good judgment, and pragmatism here—as elsewhere—improve the chance for a successful project.

Programming is the briefest part of the development cycle. The skills used by programmers are different from those used by analysts. Although some individuals may possess both sets of skills, this is not always the case. The program development process is well understood. The concepts of structured programming and modularization can be applied to all environments, even where the language does not support block structures.

The differences between programming and system development can be seen in the following observation. When Knuth chose a title for his encyclopedic collection of algorithms, he called it *The Art of Computer Programming*. Although much of the art remains, Gries' new book, *The Science of Programming*, presents a view that emphasizes a vigorous, formal construction of programs. However, it may be decades before a science of system implementation emerges. System development (as opposed to programming) is—and for some time will remain—an art.

For Further Reading

There are a large number of books that describe the process of software engineering. Two recent texts that cover the field are R. S. Pressman, *Software*

Engineering: A Practitioner's Approach, McGraw-Hill, 1982, and R. W. Jensen and C. C. Tonies, *Software Engineering*, Prentice-Hall, 1979. The more general works on the subject are the very enjoyable F. P. Brooks, Jr., *The Mythical Man-Month*, Addison-Wesley, 1975, the equally engaging G. M. Weinberg, *The Psychology of Computer Programming*, Van Nostrand, 1971, the first software psychology text by B. Schneiderman, *Software Psychology: Human Factors and Information Systems*, Winthrop Press, 1980, the management text by P. J. Metzer, *Managing a Programming Project* (second edition) Prentice-Hall, 1980 and the comprehensive survey by B. W. Boehm, *Software Engineering Economics*, Prentice Hall, 1981.

There are a large number of collections of papers. The IEEE Computer Society has quite a few excellent tutorials on topics such as design methodologies, programming productivity, testing techniques, etc. Each contains introductory material plus reprints of key papers. Some titles of particular interest are: P. Freeman and A. Wasserman, *Software Design Techniques*, 1980, G. Bergland and R. Gordon, *Software Design Strategies*, 1979, C. Jones, *Programming Productivity*, 1981, E. Miller, *Automated Tools for Software Engineering*, 1979, D. Reifer, *Software Management*, 1979, E. Miller, *Program Testing Techniques*, 1977, and G. Parikh and N. Zvegintzov, *Software Maintenance*, 1982. E. Yourdan also has edited two collections, *Classics in Software Engineering* and *Writings of the Revolution*, Yourdan Press, 1979 and 1982.

Among the books on design methodologies are M. Jackson, *System Development*, Prentice Hall 1983, K. Orr, *Structured Requirements Definition*, Ken Orr and Assoc., 1981, T. DeMarco, *Structured Analysis and System Specification*, Prentice-Hall, 1979, and J. D. Warnier, *Logical Construction of Systems*, Van-Nostrand, 1981. An excellent book on testing is G. J. Myers, *The Art of Software Testing*, Wiley, 1979. D. Gries, *The Science of Programming*, Springer-Verlag, 1981 provides a readable introduction to the concepts of proofs of correctness. The first three volumes of D. Knuth, *The Art of Computer Programming*, Addison-Wesley, 1969-1973, deal with algorithms. Another, less complete treatment, is in N. Wirth, *Algorithms + Data Structures = Programs*, Prentice-Hall, 1976.

References

1. J. E. Sammet, Language Aspects of Software Engineering, in H. Freeman and P. M. Lewis II (eds), *Software Engineering*, Academic Press, New York, 1980, p 181.
2. B. Lientz and E. Swanson, *Software Maintenance Management*, Addison-Wesley Publishing Co., Reading, MA, 1980, pp 151-157.
3. C. Jones, A Survey of Programming Design and Specification Techniques, *Proceedings, Specifications of Reliable Software*, IEEE, 1979, p 98.

Part III. Clinical Applications

7
Hospital Information Systems

7.1. Introduction

This is the first of four chapters that describe clinical information systems (CIS). In Chapter 2 medical systems were organized by the objects they processed:

- *Data*. The uninterpreted items
- *Information*. Interpreted sets of data
- *Knowledge*. The rules, relationships, experience, etc. by which data become information.

Data applications were defined as those that (a) produced information by processing limited amounts of data and (b) do not maintain long-term databases. Examples are signal processing, imaging, and modeling. Such applications are generally considered to be the domain of biomedical engineering.

Information applications, on the other hand, imply the presence of a long-term database. Although data applications rely on computational processing, information applications are built on storage, retrieval, and communication concepts. The CIS is an information system that manages clinical data and is used in patient care. These systems are the topic of the next four chapters.

Finally, there are knowledge applications. As discussed in Chapter 2, all applications use knowledge. In data applications the knowledge is in the form of an algorithm that transforms the data into information. In expert systems, there is a database containing knowledge that is used to produce recommendations and explanations. In the CIS, knowledge is in algorithms, the database, *and* the users' environment.

The distinctions among data, information, and knowledge are somewhat artificial. However, they do provide a useful focus for identifying the objectives and structure of a system. Machlup presents some further insight into the distinction.

Information is acquired by being told, whereas knowledge can be acquired by thinking. Information in the sense of telling and being told is always different from knowledge in the sense of knowing: The former is a process, the latter a state. Information in the sense of that which is being told *may* be the same knowledge in the sense of that which is known, but *need not* be the same. That even in everyday parlance people sense a difference can be seen from the fact that in railroad stations, airports, department stores, and large public buildings we expect to find a booth or counter marked *Information* but never one marked *Knowledge*. Similarly, in our modern economy we find many firms selling information services, not knowledge services. On the other hand, we would frown on education programs that fill the student's head with loads of information: We want them to disseminate knowledge of enduring value and to develop a taste or thirst for more knowledge, not just information. (From F. Machlup, U. Mansfield (eds), Semantic Quirks in Studies of Information, in *The Study of Information*. John Wiley, New York, 1983, pp. 644-645. Reprinted with permission.)

Using this description of information, one expects the CIS to *tell* the user what he wants (or needs) to know. What and how the CIS tells will depend on the *knowledge* of the designer, user, and database. At one end of the spectrum, the CIS may be considered a passive information source; it merely retrieves answers to queries. At the other end of the spectrum, however, the CIS can play a very active role in the health care process. It can use the knowledge in its algorithms and database to "tell" the user both requested and unsolicited information necessary for clinical decision-making. As will be discussed in Chapter 9, there are differences between an Artificial Intelligence (AI) expert system and an "intelligent" CIS. For the purposes of this and the next chapter, we shall view the CIS as a tool that reports to the user using rules and conventions that the user fully understands. This information reported by the CIS then is integrated with other data to determine an action. Unlike a process control system, the user is the essential part of the decision system. Unlike an AI system, all reasoning is done by the user.

In what follows we shall describe and evaluate some major CISs—first in a hospital setting (this chapter) and then in an ambulatory care setting (Chapter 8). The technology used is mature, and our experience in a health care setting is significant. As will be shown, the CIS can be an effective tool in improving care and controlling costs. In Chapter 9 we review how the CIS may be expanded to provide further support in clinical decision-making; here the focus is on the use of medical knowledge, and both AI and non-AI approaches are presented. A final chapter presents a case study of a tertiary care CIS that integrates much of what already has been presented.

7.2. Information Processing

It is natural that some of the earliest clinical systems were implemented for hospitals. The computers of the 1960s were large and expensive. They required considerable financial, programming, and operational support. Thus, only larger organizations could afford to maintain them; further, only large operations would present the economy of size to benefit from their use. As we have noted, some of the first hospital applications were limited to the business office. However, by the mid-1960s, there were several admission and discharge systems in op-

TABLE 7.1. Cost of information handling expressed as a percentage of total hospital operating cost.

Department	Three hospital average (%)
Departments supervised by the director of nursing	
Nursing, dept. (units and office)	7.71
Other departments	1.30
Total	9.01
Administrative departments	
Accounting, including business office, etc.	2.72
Telephone (salaries and expense)	1.58
Other administrative departments	2.00
Total	6.30
Radiology department	2.91
Laboratories	1.66
Medical records department	1.32
Medical & surgical care (house staff)	0.99
Dietary department	0.71
Other:	0.99
Total Hospital Cost	23.89

eration. Most were locally developed, and few were interactive. A primary objective was to identify patients for the purposes of maintaining a census for accounting and billing.

Because hospitals were so labor-intensive, it seemed clear that automation could reduce costs. In 1966, Jydstrup and Gross carefully documented the cost of hospital information processing in a study of three Rochester, New York hospitals.[1] In this classic work they defined information as "knowledge of any phase of a hospital operation that is put into writing and paid for by the hospital," and information handling as "the recording, copying, summarizing, computing, transmitting, disseminating, storing, and retrieving of information." What they found was that approximately 25% of the total hospital operating cost was spent on information handling. The distributions by department and employee category are summarized in Tables 7.1 and 7.2.

When they reviewed how the data were recorded, they were able to identify 860 different documents of which 317 (37%) dealt with specific patients. Half of the patient-oriented documents were related to medical or nursing care. Of the total number of documents, some 5% were identified that accounted for 50% of the total cost of information handling. Of these, two thirds involved nursing personnel. Based on this analysis, they found that the nursing staff spent some 30% of their time in information handling (Table 7.3) which represented 25% of their paid time (Table 7.4).

TABLE 7.2. Time spent on information handling by types of employees (Rochester General Hospital).

Department and type of employee	Percentage of employee's available useful time spent on information handling
Nursing	
One medical-surgical unit	
Head nurse and assistant head nurse	64
Registered nurses	36
Practical nurses	22
Nursing aides	9
Ward clerks	85
Total (except students)	34
All units—North and Westside	28
Operating, labor, and delivery rooms	14
Central supply and I.V. service	6
Emergency department	28
Nursing offices	40
Total	25
Administrative departments	
Accounting, etc.	95
Other—administrative office, admitting, telephone, purchasing, personnel, health office, etc.	66
Total	73
Radiology (Diagnostic, Therapeutic, Isotopic)	
Radiologists	35
Technicians	28
Others—secretaries, clerks, orderlies	70
Total	42
Laboratories	
Bacteriology (including prorated part of clerical)	17
Hematology	20
Chemistry	30
Pathology	37
Total (including photography)	28
Other	
Medical records	95
Interns and residents	30
Dietary (10 dieticians—35%, 75 other—3%)	7
Physical medicine (1 director—50%; 3 clerks—80%; 11 other—5%)	22
Outpatient department	35
Pharmacy	26
EKG, BMR, EEG	36
Social service	45
Maintenance (chief and assistant—37%; 42 others, including secretary—4%)	6
Housekeeping and Laundry	<3
Total hospital (958 equivalent full-time employees)	26

TABLE 7.3. Amount of information handling on nursing units expressed as a percentage of available useful time and hours per patient day (three-hospital average).

	%	Hours pt. day
One medical-surgical unit		
Head nurse and assistant head nurse	58	0.15
Registered nurses	36	0.42
Practical nurses	22	0.13
Nursing aides	7	0.05
Ward clerks	73	0.15
Total for this unit	31	0.90
Total for all nursing units	27	0.83

Their analysis had clearly demonstrated that a large portion of a hospital's budget was devoted to information handling. However, they concluded:

It is believed that real improvement is going to require a comprehensive and organized effort involving the whole gamut of management skills. Conversely, real improvement is not likely to be obtained by any one activity alone—be it automation, the hiring of a methods engineer, or the development of better standards—desirable as it may be. This belief is based partly on what has been learned and partly on what is known about the experience of other organizations. Others have found that in making change there is no substitute for hard work, from administration on down, and with the drive coming from the top.[2]

Both their analysis and final observation are as valid today as they were in 1966.

Since such a large proportion of a nursing unit's activity goes into information handling, it is reasonable to examine the function of this handling. The primary reason for information handling is communications. For example, Jydstrup and Gross found that 20% of the patient forms were for charge processing. Every test and procedure requires information handling to transmit both the order and the result. Supplies, housekeeping, and all other hospital services require similar written orders. In addition to communication with other departments, there is also information handling that is directed to workers within the same unit. For example, in the nursing unit there are instructions passed from one shift to the next, orders from the physician to the nursing staff, vital signs and other records for providers,* an audit trail for medical/quality/legal purposes, etc.

Today, with modern computer systems, we are quick to recognize this as a natural application for a communication system. The advantages are obvious:

*The term health care provider (or simply provider) includes all those health care professionals who provide care, e.g., physicians and nurses.

TABLE 7.4. Analysis of total time paid for on a hypothetical medical-surgical nursing unit.

Activity	Hours/year per full-time employee	Percentage of time on duty	Remarks
Information handling	470	25	Based on our studies. Note that 25% = 30% of useful time.
Walking	300	16	Based on limited data from our studies.
Other indirect patient care, housekeeping supervision, education, etc.	220	12	A guess.
Direct patient care (other than information handling)	560	30	A guess.
Total available useful time	1,550	83	
Standby time (because of staffing for peak loads)	190	10	
Personal time	132	7	Assumes an average of 35 minutes per day for coffee breaks, rest room visits, etc.
Total time on duty	1,872	100	
Holidays	56	3	Assume 7 holidays per year.
Vacation	80	4	Assume 0-15 days, avg. 10.
Sickness and other	72	4	Assume 9 days avg.
Total time paid for	2,080	111	

- Communications will be speeded up. Once the information is recorded, it is available to all who need to read it.
- Redundancy can be reduced or eliminated. The same data can be shared among many reports.
- Error rates will be lowered. Invalid patient identification and misspelled names can be avoided and unrealistic data eliminated.

Thus, the primary function of a Hospital Information System (HIS) is to support communications; both among hospital departments and within a department.

Of course, much of the information is passed to "tell" what is to be done, for example, order a test, post a charge, etc. From the clinical perspective, most of the information is used to help the provider make a decision about a diagnosis, therapy, etc. What can be said of the flow of information within a nursing unit to the providers? Johns has constructed a model based on some studies at Johns Hopkins.[3] He defines this model in the context of clinical resource use, that is, those goods and services involved in the direct care of patients. These resources are expended either to get information (e.g., laboratory tests) or to act on information received (e.g., pharmacy services).

He begins by noting that clinical resources represent the largest items of hospital expense. For example, at Hopkins in 1978, they represented 34% of the total hospital expense, or $43.6 million. The magnitude of clinical resources was even more impressive when he considered a typical 31-bed medical inpatient unit. Half of the total expense, or approximately $1 million, was spent on ancillary services—laboratory studies, radiographic studies, and pharmacy services. Another 20% was expended on salaries of personnel on that nursing unit. Thus, some 70% of the expense of a nursing unit related directly to clinical resources. Looked at in another way, this implies that a 1978 Johns Hopkins Hospital nursing unit represented a $2 million a year operation in which 70% of the budget was largely controlled by the medical staff.

How were these clinical resources managed? Johns found that they were allocated in small units, often less than $20 each. For example, chest radiographs (one of the most inexpensive radiographic studies) represented 32% of the dollar volume of all radiographic studies. This is in contrast to the (then) much-maligned CAT scan which represented only 6% of the dollar volume. Similarly, in clinical chemistry the SMA 6 and SMA 12 together accounted for 28% of the total. In hematology the automated HEME 7 represented 32% of the dollar volume.

Thus, the relatively low-cost, high-volume items accounted for most of the costs of clinical resources. The management problem would have been much simpler if there were but a few high-cost resources that required surveillance. Such a strategy, unfortunately, would leave the major resources uncontrolled. Put another way, a 10% reduction in the number of chest radiographs was equivalent to a 50% reduction in CAT scans.

Johns concluded that, given an annual expenditure of $44 million in units that average some $20 each, there must be 2.2 million clinical decisions per year. This works out to 6,000 per day or some half-dozen per patient per day. Each of these decisions will impact both patient care and cost; each will produce data that affect future decisions. Thus, if the data can be managed to convey information better and improve medical decision-making, then the quality of care should improve and the cost of operations should go down. In what follows, we shall examine how the HIS manages data and shall see if, indeed, quality improves and costs are controlled.

7.2.2. An HIS Model

In the previous subsection it was established that hospitals are labor intensive; they require a great deal of information handling to communicate among departments; most of these communications involve expenditures of clinical resources; and, finally, there are many clinical decisions that must be made. Thus, one would expect an HIS to perform two primary functions:

1. Support communications
2. Organize data to facilitate decision making.

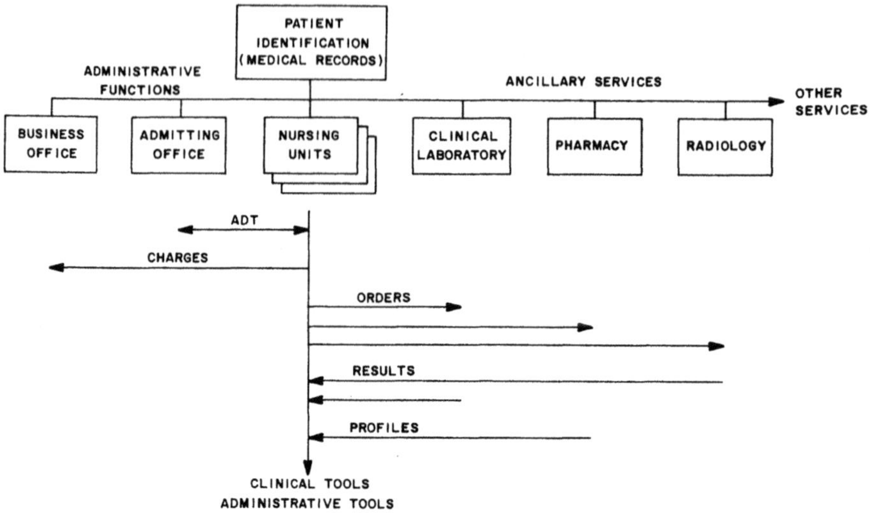

FIGURE 7.1. Hospital Information System (HIS) block diagram showing nursing unit interfaces.

That is, the HIS should provide tools for each operational unit to (a) communicate with other units and (b) support its internal operations.

Figure 7.1 contains a block diagram of a typical HIS. Since virtually all clinical activities are linked to the patient, a central function is that of patient identification. In some hospitals a unit record is retained that combines all medical information for a patient in a single record. When this type of record is used, it is essential that the proper identification be established so that a prior history is available. Other hospitals assign an identifier with each admission; in this case a separate link to other records for the same patients will be necessary. In either case, the patient identification function establishes an identifier for the patient that will be used for all clinical and financial activities during that admission.

Generally, the patient identification function is the responsibility of the Medical Records Department. The HIS may support this department with tools to look up names using phonetic indices, display data to resolve identification in the event of similar or identical names, and perform some administrative reporting. The HIS may also have a medical record locator system that can trace the location of all records not in the record room. In summary, the Medical Records Department views the HIS as a set of tools that they use to perform their function. When a call is received to find an identifier for a patient, they use the HIS to do this. If a medical record is to be logged out, they use the HIS to do this. Their perception of the scope, value, and speed of the HIS is always in the context of their application. Every other hospital department has a similar perspective.

The Admitting Office uses the HIS to admit, discharge, or transfer inpatients (the ADT function). Normally, they request a patient identifier from Medical Records. (In some institutions admitting registrars may be authorized to assign identifiers; identifiers may also be assigned automatically. This is an administrative rather than technical decision.) The ADT function includes:

- Patient registration including demographics, insurance information, next of kin, religious preference
- Assignment of a patient to a nursing unit. This implies a patient locator system as well
- Management of discharges and transfers
- Preparation of the midnight census and other activity reports. The midnight census typically is used to generate bed charges
- Admission scheduling including pre-admission processing, rescheduling and cancellations, and preparation of projected census reports
- Management reports.

Since the ADT function assigns location, it must communicate that assignment to the nursing units and the ancillary services. In many institutions, some of the transfer, discharge, and bed assignment functions are initiated in the nursing unit. In this case, the nursing unit must also communicate with the other departments.

The Business Office receives inputs from each of the services that generates charges. In most institutions the HIS is used to collect the data; the actual processing of bills and accounts receivables is performed by a separate system. Because the time when bills are processed is not critical, bills are frequently batched and run during periods of low utilization. (The period of highest HIS utilization is in the morning, after rounds, when the new orders are processed.)

Once a patient has been admitted, coordination of all care activities is managed from the nursing unit. Each unit typically has a "home screen" that displays the current unit census. In some cases, different nursing units will support different functions, e.g., surgery-specific applications. The HIS is used for communications and for information management. The communications involve:

- Administrative actions such as ADT changes and the generation of bed charges
- Order entry such as requests for tests and procedures or the ordering of drugs
- Result reporting such as the display of a test result or a drug profile.

The information management functions will be discussed in greater detail in subsequent sections.

Fig. 7.1 shows the three ancillary units most commonly integrated with an HIS. This does not imply that all HISs will support each such service or that additional services—such as dietary services, social services, or central supplies—will not be included. However, wherever an ancillary service is supported, the HIS performs in one of three modes:

- Acts as a complete system that supports the service's operation. In this

context, the system is viewed as an ancillary system that communicates with the nursing unit to receive orders and send results.
- Acts as an interface to a standalone ancillary service unit. This mode of integration is most common in the clinical laboratory where many of the process control functions require additional automation. Functionally, it is identical to the first mode.
- Acts simply as a communication link between the nursing unit and the service. Many dietary service units provide this limited capability.

The following discussion assumes that each ancillary service operates in the first or second mode.

The clinical laboratory component of the HIS receives the patient registration data and the patient orders and sends the results and charge information. Within the clinical laboratory, it supports the following operations:

- *Preparation of specimen collection lists*. These include work sheets, printed labels, and follow up-lists for samples not collected.
- *Work document preparation*. Each analysis step requires controls to associate a requisition with each sample analyzed. In low volume processes, this is relatively simple to do; where an autoanalyzer is used more detailed work lists and controls are required.
- *Results entry*. Results may be hand written on collection sheets for keystroke into the computer or they may be electronically transferred from the autoanalyzer. In each of these cases a data entry and verification step is required. For tests other than chemistries and hematology, the results frequently are entered manually on the final report.
- *Report preparation*. All tests that have their data in machine sensible form normally are processed by the Laboratory System. They may be printed as individual reports or cumulative reports. Abnormal results may be flagged and special comments added during the preparation process.
- *Internal reporting*. Management and quality assurance reports may be used to support planning and day-to-day operation of the laboratory.

The view of the HIS from the pharmacy is similar to that of the clinical laboratory. It also receives registration and order data and sends drug profiles and charges. Within an inpatient pharmacy, the following support is generally provided by the HIS.

- *Process orders*. Each order must be verified by a pharmacist. This requires a verification that a reasonable drug dose has been ordered, that the drug is appropriate and compatible with the existing medications, and that there are no known allergic reactions. Parts of this process may be automated; in any case, there is a requirement for a review and acceptance by the pharmacist.
- *Preparations of drugs for administration*. Work lists and labels are printed from the pharmacy database to guide in the preparation of drugs for administration. If a unit dose system is used, cart loading lists may be compiled. For bulk distribution systems, work lists are printed. For intravenous prep-

aration, labels and instructions are produced. If outpatient orders are also serviced, labels are also printed.

- *Inventory control.* The system maintains a formulary that identifies each drug available for dispensing in the hospital and contains information about key attributes of the drug such as units available, control category, and possibly inventory levels and shelf life. This may be used to validate orders and also maintain an inventory. Where an inventory control system is implemented, the HIS must automatically maintain the inventory controls and produce reorder lists.
- *Management Reports.* There are a variety of reports that are unique to a pharmacy that can be produced by the HIS. For example, there are requirements for an audit trail of controlled substances and an identification of authorized prescribers. In addition, other reports can be produced for planning and management.

The last of the ancillary services to be discussed, radiology, uses the same interfaces as the other services: reads in registration and orders, sends out reports, and charges. It also supports:

- *Preparation of the report.* This may be done directly by the radiologist. A more common approach is to have the radiologist dictate the report and then review and sign the completed report. The transcription of the dictation is typically done using word processing techniques with the use of special codes for standard normal reports. In some cases, a study is required at once and the film is read out and an oral report is communicated. Of course, where the radiologist directly enters the report, there is no need for an oral communication since the results are available as soon as they are reported.
- *Assembly of materials for use in preparing the final report.* This includes the original requisition, the current radiograph, and any radiographs from the film file. There are also tools to maintain a film file that identifies and locates all radiographs retained by the Department.
- *Scheduling.* In many institutions, the Radiology Department services both inpatients and outpatients. In such cases it may be desirable to schedule examination rooms and support registration.
- *Management Reports* are valuable to assist in planning and operations.

Note that the HIS model we have presented is open-ended and modular. More ancillary services or hospital functions may be added; each set of users views the system as a tool that supports its operations. The value of the HIS, however, lies in its ability to communicate among services. The amount of information transferred is relatively limited: key patient data, orders, results, and charges. Most of the HIS benefits can be traced to this communication (i.e., database sharing) function: consistent patient identification, elimination of transcription errors, automatic rejection of unreasonable data, improved availability of results, reduction in nursing clerical tasks, etc. As will be shown, when the communicated data are expanded to include diagnostic or therapeutic information, even greater benefits result.

7.2.3. HIS Implementation

In his study of the growth of medical information systems, Lindberg presents two system philosophies:

First is the concept that a reasonable system can only result from a holistic concept of the final product: the machine and procedures applied to the total problem area. One big system, according to this view, should be designed, built, and installed in a setting such as a hospital. The second philosophy is that the ultimate system should result from a sum of the successful subsystems that would have been directed toward parts of the overall problem of medical information processing. The parties to these disputes were not merely sophomoric debaters. Their beliefs derived from good and bad experiences with problems of receptivity of the medical settings, the sources and magnitude of funding available for the research, and good and bad experiences with large and small computers.[4] (Reprinted by permission of the publisher, from D.A.B. Lindberg, *The Growth of Medical Information Systems in the United States,* 1979.

The context of the debate between the holistic and cumulative approaches was the limited knowledge of and experience with the HIS. As the previous subsection clearly illustrates, the benefits of an HIS are derived from its ability to communicate, that is, its "wholeness." This "wholeness" also increases the development risk. If one produces a poor system, then nothing works well. Conversely, if one uses the cumulative approach to produce one component—say a laboratory system—then even though the potential benefits are fewer, the risk is clearly lower. Consequently, for well understood problems, the holistic approach is recommended. High-risk projects, on the other hand, may favor cumulative development.

Today, the context of the debate has changed. Information system technology has matured, communication systems are easier to implement, costs for computer equipment are falling, there is considerable experience with HIS applications, and users are more familiar (and comfortable) with computer systems. This might suggest that the need for a cumulative approach is no longer necessary. Unfortunately, it is also true that—at the time of writing—there are few commercially available systems that use modern, low cost equipment and implement all the desired clinical functions. The costs for developing an HIS still are so great that the systems with 10 years of field experience are also those that use the technology of 10 (or 15) years ago. Thus, an institution is faced with one of three choices: build, buy, or integrate.

The local implementation of an HIS is an expensive process that is not to be recommended. It requires a skilled and experienced staff. Development costs will run into the millions of dollars. Once the system has been installed, it will be difficult to retain the staff. Finally, few noncommercial developers will be successful in marketing their products to recover a portion of their investment. Thus, the building of an HIS is seldom desirable. Of course, where there are unique needs, the local development of an HIS component (or CIS) may be the only viable alternative.

The purchase and installation of an HIS also is not a simple process. It typically takes from 6 months to 2 years to implement a system. In effect, the installation of an HIS is similar to the development of one except that (a) an experienced vendor will supply consultation and support and (b) virtually no programming is required. The reason so much time is required is obvious: every hospital has its own set of procedures, forms, conventions, and staffing patterns. The installation of an HIS requires an analysis of the current flow, a tailoring of the system to meet the hospital's needs, training of the users, and the testing and validation of the system. All commercial systems are designed to facilitate modifications to accommodate to a specific hospital's requirements. All have display screen and report generators, data dictionary facilities, external system interfaces (for example, for processing by a billing system), etc. Most vendors also will provide custom programming, training, and continuing consultation.

One problem with the purchase of a complete HIS is that it represents a major investment that locks the institution to the facilities of a specific system. Since the role of the CIS is still undergoing change and the cost of equipment is falling, there is a danger that the purchase of an holistic HIS may limit flexibility in implementing new clinical functions. Fortunately, networking technology offers a third alternative: integration of existing systems.

As we have seen, the HIS model is composed of a series of relatively independent modules that are linked by communications. The volume of the data that is shared and communicated is relatively small when compared to the data required by only one module. For example, only the clinical laboratory requires the processing work lists and only the radiology system needs access to the film file records. Given this modularity, there are two design alternatives: have all modules share a single database or have each module manage its own database and coordinate changes to the shared data elements. The first approach requires a single integrated system; the second alternative can be implemented by integrating independent systems. This integration concept allows each ancillary service, for example, to select the system that best meets its internal needs. As newer, better, or less expensive systems become available, older modules can be replaced. In this way, new functions can be installed with minimal risk, the decentralized needs of the various hospital departments can be locally controlled, and there is a limited danger of an irreversible investment in obsolescence.

Although the integration approach has major advantages and probably represents the primary mode of future development, it should be recognized that this is still a new concept and we have limited experience. On the positive side, a demonstration system operates at the University of California, San Francisco Hospital; most standalone ancillary systems are designed to facilitate integration; local area networks are reliable and easy to install; and there are consulting companies with experience in hospital networks. However, the number of such systems is small; the range of available patient care functions is narrow; and application level programming is required to produce an integrated system.

Thus, the final conclusion is that no matter what type of HIS one installs, implementation will not be a simple process. (Recall Jydstrup and Gross' remarks cited earlier.) Nevertheless, it would seem that the integration (or networking) approach provides the greatest potential for the dynamic accommodation of new clinical tools.

7.3. Some Hospital Information Systems

At the present time there are some 20 HIS vendors. It would be beyond the scope of this book to attempt to survey or describe their offerings. In what follows, four systems have been selected for brief presentation. Their choice was based on their place in the history of medical informatics, the availabiity of references in the technical literature, and/or their ability to illustrate certain system characteristics. The discussion of each system is very incomplete; much of the power and use of each HIS is suggested in the figures that accompany the text. The following subsections describe two commercial systems that implement the previously described communications model and two systems that were developed as systems to assist in the care process. They are:

- *The Technicon Medical Information System.* This is the oldest and most studied system in use. It applies the holistic philosophy.
- *The IBM Patient Care System.* This is actually a general-purpose software package with some HIS functions already defined. It is generally implemented cumulatively.
- *The HELP System.* This was developed at the Latter Day Saints Hospital as an outgrowth of 15 years of research in the implementation of medical logic.
- *The PROMIS System.* This was—at the time of its implementation—the most technologically advanced of all systems. It was designed to manage a fully automated problem oriented medical record.

Again, it must be pointed out, these four systems are not necessarily representative of the HISs that are commercially available today.

7.3.1. The Technicon System

The first comprehensive HIS was developed for the El Camino Hospital, a 450-bed public, community hospital serving a middle class area around Sunnyvale, California. Collaboration began in 1965 between Lockheed and El Camino and some 2 years later a first phase of implementation was complete and a business office system was installed. The problems of expanding the system to a more complete HIS proved to be more difficult than had been anticipated, and in 1971 Lockheed sold the system to Technicon. At the same time, El Camino bought the system and the National Center for Health Services Research awarded contracts to evaluate the system's impact on (a) the organization and administration of health care delivery and (b) cost.

It is estimated that by 1977 some $20,000,000 had been invested in the system and its evaluation. Today, Technicon Medical Information System (TMIS) has been installed in about 40 hospitals. It generally operates from remotely located mainframe computers and supports light pen CRTs and two-color printers at each of the user stations. (In the personal computer era, we have become quite accustomed to seeing such terminals. However, in the context of the equipment and user attitudes of the mid-1970s, this was both technologically advanced and innovative.) The results of the evaluation will be presented in the next section. In what follows we shall limit the description to how TMIS is used in the nursing unit.

TMIS was one of the first systems designed to allow the physician to enter all of his or her orders and review the results. In the early stages of implementation, there was physician alienation toward the system. It was incomplete, there were operational difficulties, and there were few physician-oriented applications. As a result, much of the order entry function was relegated to the nursing staff. In time, the problems were corrected and new users were introduced to the system. As a result, it is estimated that at El Camino Hospital some 90% of all orders now are entered by the physicians. However, the TMIS system that is installed in Davis has a lower physician entry rate. This is because most of those physicians treat patients in several hospitals, and they are reluctant to modify their habits to accommodate a single hospital. Thus, the lesson seems to be that (a) if the HIS does something useful and is easy to use, then it will be used, but (b) what is perceived to be useful in one hospital may not be effective in another.

Figure 7.2 illustrates two of the physician screens. The first identifies and locates his or her patients in the hospital. It also provides a bulletin board function (announcements) plus access to medical information and the current antibiotic survey. The second screen provides an index to the patient record. One may enter, review, or delete orders, review results, define standard groups of therapy (personal orders), and initiate administrative actions. Listing of information on the small screen makes the display of information difficult. Consequently most information is printed and distributed as reports. Figure 7.3 illustrates two such reports. They are printed in red and black. (The ORD in the upper right, for example is in red. Letters printed using circles represent temporary reports; ORD spelled out in blocks would indicate the final report for the day that should be filed in the medical record.)

Since TMIS has access to all orders and clinical data, it can organize and print the data in a variety of formats for use by different people. In this case, Fig. 7.3A contains a list of current orders and Fig. 7.3B contains a patient care plan. Each shares some of the same information presented in a different order. Also note that the two reports are for different "hospitals." This illustrates how the system can be modified to produce different types of outputs that satisfy local requirements.

In addition to listing orders, TMIS presents results. The radiology reports are in the form of text, the laboratory results are shown as either results from a single test or in the form of a flow sheet; abnormal values are printed in red. Pharmacy distribution lists are printed for use in the ward. Other reports can be

A

B

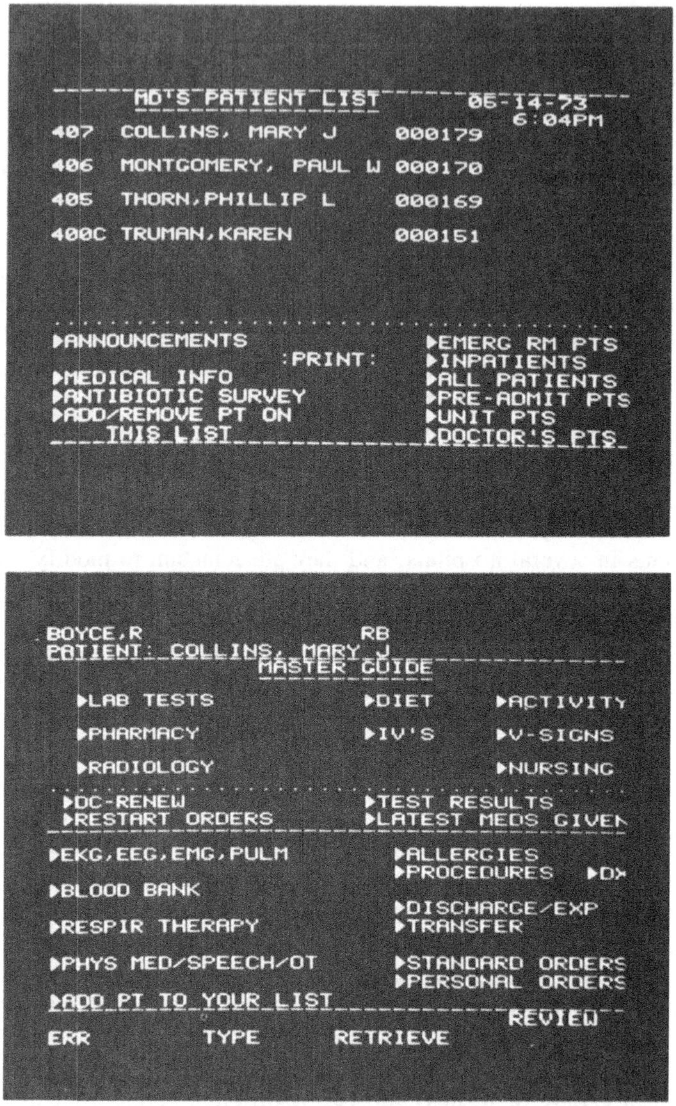

FIGURE 7.2. Technician Medical Information System (TMIS) screens for physician use. A: Sample patient list. B: Sample physician master guide. (Early 1970s formats). © 1985, an unpublished work by TECHNION DATA SYSTEMS CORP. All names are fictional.

prepared for social workers, dieticians, rehabilitation therapy, the blood bank, etc. In short, TMIS is an example of a holistic environment that (a) collects and manages much of the clinical data and (b) organizes and presents the data in forms that assist in the administration of care.

```
EAST-4898-01
3/14/73  5:23 PM                    PAGE 001                CARE
==========================================        ========================
SMITH, SAM                          F 34 532B
  228429        ADM: 03/10/73
  JONES, JOSEPH J. MD      SERV: ORTH              PATIENT CARE PLAN
==========================================        ========================

            FROM  3:00 PM  3/14/73 TO 11:30 PM  3/14/73
==========================================================================

DX:
  FRAC SACRUM W NERVE RT COMPRESSION
VITAL SIGNS:
   3/10  12.  V-SIGNS, T-P-R, Q6H
   3/13  27.  V-SIGNS, BP-LYING--AND, BP-SITTING, TID
DIET AND FLUID BALANCE:
   3/10   5.  DIET, REGULAR
HYGIENE/ACTIVITY/SAFETY:
   3/10  22.  TRACTION: START TRACTION, PELVIC, SINGLE STRAP, 15-POUNDS
   3/13  49.  ACTIVITY, BEDREST-BRP
PROCEDURES:
   3/10  13.  SUPPORTS, BINDERS: ANTI-EMBOLISM STOCKING, BILATERAL
   3/10  20.  AQUA K-PAD, CONTINUOUS, PRN LOWER BACK
   3/13  44.  NURSING:*TAKE ALL TEMPS RECTALLY
   3/13  47.  BL CULTURE, L&R ARMS, IF TEMP OVER 102R (PREP #39), EACH
              SPEC'M X2
MEDICATIONS:
*  3/10  11.  D.S.S. CAP-250 MG, #1, PO, QD, (03/11 09AM-..)
   3/11  26.  ASPIRIN, TAB-300 MG, #2, PO, PRN FOR TEMP ABOVE 102
   3/13  48.  DULCOLAX-SUPP., #1, PR, PRN
   3/14  53.  DRUG:*SALINE 2CC IM, Q3, TO, Q4H, PRN--PAIN--TELL HER IT IS
              STRONGER THAN YESTERDAYS SHOTS
*  3/14  54.  DRUG:*PLACEBO 1, QID--AND TELL HER IT IS A MUSCLE
              RELAXANT, (03/14 09AM-..)      5  9
*  3/14  55.  BENADRYL, CAP-50 MG, #2, PO, QHS, PRN INSOMNIA, (03/14
              09PM-..)     9
   3/14  56.  BENADRYL, CAP-50 MG, #2, PO, MR X1
OTHER DEPT.:
#  3/11  25.  (IN PROCESS) BL CULTURE, ONE ARM, STAT
#  3/13  40.  (IN PROCESS) THROAT CULT, TODAY , (03/13)
   3/14  57.  FANA, TODAY .(THIS 1 TEST ONLY)--TELL LAB TO DRAW WHILE
              OBTAINING ONE OF GTT SPECIMENS, (03/14)
PT CARE PLANNING:
   3/10       ALLERGIC TO CODEINE
   3/10       ALLERGIC TO PENICILLIN
   3/10       --PT DISCHARGED 1 WEEK AGO WITH SAME COMPLAINTS
   3/11       --OLD CHART HERE
   3/13       --STILL NEED STOOL FOR O&P X-3---HOWEVER ORDER THE--TEST

                              CONTINUED
```

FIGURE 7.3A. Technician Medical Information System (TMIS) printed report. Sample patient care plan. © 1985, an unpublished work by TECHNION DATA SYSTEMS CORP. All names are fictional.

7.3.2. The Patient Care System

The Patient Care System (PCS) was first implemented by the Duke University Medical Center as a replacement for an older HIS. Since the Duke system operated on IBM equipment and used the standard IBM DBMS, IBM elected to market the system as an Installed User Program. Some 50 systems have been installed,

```
1WEST-8694                 TECHNICON HOSPITAL
                                    PAGE 001
======================================
MOSS NANCY C                      F 32  208
 357078            ADM: 03/05/78
======================================

        ORDERS CURRENT AS OF:                                    9:02 AM    4/19
==========================================================================

     MEDICATIONS:
R    3/10 124.   VALIUM INJ: DIAZEPAM-10MG, IM, QHS, (03/10 09PM-..),
                 (HJK).
R    3/31 249.   MEPERIDINE-50 MG,TO,75 MG, IM, Q3H, PRN PAIN, (HJK).
R    4/6  272.   AMPICILLIN LIQ 250MG/5ML, 2 TSP(10ML),PO, Q6H, (04/06
                 12NN-..), (HJK).
     4/13 289.   TIGAN,SUPP-200 MG., #1,PR, Q4H, PRN NAUSEA, (HJK).
     4/14 298.   PHENERGAN-INJ: PROMETHAZINE-50MG, IM, Q4H, PRN NAUSEA,
                 (RJS).
               R=TIME TO RENEW

     IV-S:
     3/15 180.   IV LINE-FOLLOW PRESENT IV W FREAMINE 4.25% IN 25%/D,
                 1000ML W, SODIUM 30MEQ (AS CHLORIDE), POTASS 30MEQ (AS
                 CHLORIDE), POTASS 10MEQ (AS PHOSPHATE), CALCIUM 5MEQ (AS
                 GLUCONATE), MAGNES 8MEQ (AS SULFATE), MVI CONC. 5ML, REG
                 INSULIN 10U, X1BTL, 125ML/HR (31/125GTT), (HJK).
     3/15 181.   IV LINE-, ALTERNATE W FREAMINE 4.25% IN 25%/D,1000ML W,
                 SODIUM 30MEQ (AS CHLORIDE), POTASS 30MEQ (AS CHLORIDE),
                 POTASS 10MEQ (AS PHOSPHATE), CALCIUM 5MEQ (AS
                 GLUCONATE), MAGNES 8MEQ (AS SULFATE), REG INSULIN 10U,
                 X1BTL, 125ML/HR (31/125GTT)....OTHER MISC--(INSULIN IN Q
                 BOTTLE AND MVI IN Q OTHER BOTTLE), (HJK).

     TESTS AND SERVICES:
     3/10 115.   UNIT TESTS: URINE FOR GLUCOSE & ACETONE (DOUBLE
                 VOIDING), QID--IF SUGAR GREATER THAN 2% CALL MD. FOR
                 INSULIN ORDER., (HJK).
     3/10 138.   UNIT TESTS SPECIFIC GRAVITY, QID
     4/18 309.   (IN PROCESS) SMA-18 (PREP #1), TOM'RO, (04/19), (HJK).
     4/18 310.   (IN PROCESS) CBC, TOM'RO, (04/19), (HJK).

     PATIENT STATUS:
     3/6   36.   POSITIONING: ELEVATE FT OF BED-- 15 DEG X 15 MIN Q8H
                 TILL FULLY AMB., (HJK).
     3/6   37.   ACTIVITY, AMBULATE AS TOL, (HJK).
     3/6   42.   POSITIONING: ELEVATE HD OF BED 30DEG, (HJK).
     3/11 142.   VITAL SIGNS, QID, (HJK).
     3/10 117.   WEIGH PATIENT DAILY, (HJK).
     3/10 134.   *IV DRUGS ARE TO BE GIVEN THRU CVP-HYPERAL'N LINE WHEN
                 PERIPHERAL LINE IS DC'D., (HJK).
     4/18 312.   DIET: FULL LIQUID, (HJK).

                                   LAST PAGE
-*-
```

FIGURE 7.3B. Technician Medical Information System (TMIS) printed report. Sample order report. © 1985, an unpublished work by TECHNION DATA SYSTEMS CORP. All names are fictional.

a user group has been formed, and changes have been made to both the Duke implementation and the IBM support systems.

PCS has been called an application enabling package. It comes with the design of an HIS and a set of tools that enables the user to implement part or all of the initial HIS or to implement an alternative, compatible HIS. It is built using a standard DBMS and teleprocessing system. Thus, unlike TMIS, the PCS implementation is built on general-purpose software. The price it pays for this, however, is lowered responsiveness for equivalent equipment resources. Where TMIS provides a highly specialized package that can be modified for specific users, PCS is a very general development environment for producing HIS components. (The tools that constitute PCS are not specifically "medically oriented;" they can be used for any information application.) Thus one may view PCS as prototype Fourth Generation Language that supports the user, i.e., hospital, in the definition and implementation of its HIS.

The functions supported by each PCS implementation vary. Some are limited to the ADT function, others are focused on a single ancillary service such as radiology, whereas some provide a comprehensive HIS capability. The reports produced and user interfaces installed will vary from institution to institution. Few reports are as comprehensive as those shown in Fig. 7.3. Of course, this is a design decision and not a technical limitation. Light pens also are used with this sytem. Fig. 7.4 illustrates the processing flow for ordering a chest x-ray from the patient screen.[5] As in the case of all light pen or touch screen designs, one must go through a series of menus to initiate the process. An alternative design method, the use of commands, allows a direct branching to the desired activity. However, commands require more of an understanding of how to use the system and thus normally are reserved primarily for ancillary systems.

7.3.3. The HELP System

The two systems previously described were each designed to transfer and organize data. The PCS generally is operated by the nursing staff; physicians frequently use TMIS to process orders. Both manage information in Machlup's sense of "telling." They do not augment the data that are there; they simply present it. Of course, the orderly presentation of information aids in its use and has a beneficial effect on patient care. The next two systems to be presented, however, go beyond the passive display of information. Each applies medical knowledge to guide the decision-making process. In this sense they differ both historically and philosophically from the other systems.

The HELP system can be traced back to the early work of Warner and his association at the Latter Day Saints Hospital in Salt Lake City, Utah, in the late 1950s and early 1960s. Their goal was to make the computer a useful tool in the practice of medicine. They began with the processing of analog signals from patients, progressed to programs for the automated integration of these data, and finally came to the point where it was recognized that the integration of the output of each of the individual systems could be of greater importance than any of the individual systems by itself. Consequently, in 1970 the programs were modified to use a common database system. In 1975 the development of a language and system for processing medical decisions began. (This is discussed in Chapter 9.) By 1978 terminals had been placed in every nursing division and all the intensive care wards; surgical suites and clinical laboratories also had been instrumented for data acquisition and reporting.

```
aaaaaaaaaaaaaaaaaaaaaaaaaaaaaaaaaaaaaaaaaaaaaaaaaaaaaaaaaaaaaaaaaaaaaaaaaaaaaaaaaaTOP
                                                                09/28/77  0613
  PRE  4703-01   BAKER,ALBERT H

                        THESE PROCEDURES ARE DONE BY RADIOLOGY
                            --SELECT THE TEST DESIRED--
--------------------------------------------------------------------------------
    CALCANEOUS AND FOOT,RIGHT               CARDIOGRAM, CARBON DIOXIDE
                                                 DR.TO SCHEDULE
    CALCANEOUS,BOTH                         CEPHALOPELVIMETRY
                                                 SCHEDULE
    CALCANEOUS,LEFT                         CERVICAL AIR MYELOGRAM
                                                 SCHEDULE
    CALCANEOUS,RIGHT                        CHEMOPALLIDECTOMY,STEREO.STUDY

    CARDIAC FILMS SERIES                  ► CHEST, PA AND LATERAL

    CARDIAC FLUOROSCOPY                     CHEST-----PORTABLE--
         SCHEDULE
    CARDIAC FLUOROSCOPY AND FILMS           CHEST, SPECIAL VIEWS
         SCHEDULE
--------------------------------------------------------------------------------
                            PAGE BACK              PAGE FORWARD         RETURN
  RAD07
aaaaaaaaaaaaaaaaaaaaaaaaaaaaaaaaaaaaaaaaaaaaaaaaaaaaaaaaaaaaaaaaaaaaaaaaaaaaaaaaaaBOT
```

A

```
aaaaaaaaaaaaaaaaaaaaaaaaaaaaaaaaaaaaaaaaaaaaaaaaaaaaaaaaaaaaaaaaaaaaaaaaaaaaaaaaaaTOP
                                                                09/28/77  0613
  PRE  4703-01   BAKER,ALBERT H

                    --SELECT THE ALPHABET LISTING TO FIND THE
                      RADIOLOGY PROCEDURE YOU WANT TO ORDER--
--------------------------------------------------------------------------------
    ABD - ACE      CHE - COP      HEE - HIP      PAT - PUL      THI - TOM

    ACE - ANK      CRA - DUO      HIP - INT      PYE - RIB      TOM - TOM

    ANK - ARM      ELB - FAC      INT - KUB      RIB - SHO      ULT - VEN

    ARM - BAG      FAC - FOO      KUB - LAR      SHO - SIN      VEN - ZYG

    BAR - BON      FOO - FOR      LAR - MAM      SIN - SPI      * PORTABLE *

    BON - CAL      FOR - HAN      MAN - NEC      SPI - SPI      ABD - KUB

  ► CAL - CHE      HAN - HEE      NEC - PAT      SPI - THI      NAS - WRI

--------------------------------------------------------------------------------
                                                                   RETURN
  RADALPH
aaaaaaaaaaaaaaaaaaaaaaaaaaaaaaaaaaaaaaaaaaaaaaaaaaaaaaaaaaaaaaaaaaaaaaaaaaaaaaaaaaBOT
```

B

```
aaaaaaaaaaaaaaaaaaaaaaaaaaaaaaaaaaaaaaaaaaaaaaaaaaaaaaaaaaaaaaaaaaaaaaaaaaaaaaaaaaTOP
                                                                09/28/77  0613
  PRE  4703-01   BAKER,ALBERT H


                          SELECT THE CATEGORY OF ORDER
--------------------------------------------------------------------------------
                 CARE & TREATMENT                 HEART STATION

                 LAB                              RESP. THERAPY

               ► RADIOLOGY                        PHYSICAL THERAPY

                 DIETARY                          EEG

                 NUCLEAR MEDICINE                 ECT

                 CENTRAL PROC.SERVICE

  ..............................................................................
--------------------------------------------------------------------------------
                      MASTER                   CENSUS                  FUNCTION
  NORD11
aaaaaaaaaaaaaaaaaaaaaaaaaaaaaaaaaaaaaaaaaaaaaaaaaaaaaaaaaaaaaaaaaaaaaaaaaaaaaaaaaaBOT
```

C

FIGURE 7.4A-C. Patient Care System (PCS) processing flow example. A: The chest x-ray order process begins by selecting RADIOLOGY. B: The index to radiologic procedures is processed and a choice is made. C: Finally, the specific examination is selected.

```
@@@@@@@@@@@@@@@@@@@@@@@@@@@@@@@@@@@@@@@@@@@@@@@@@@@@@@@@@@@@@@@@@@@@@@@@@@@@@@@@@@@@@TOP
                                                                   09/28/77  0613
   PRE  4703-01  BAKER,ALBERT H                  CHEST

                             VALID FREQUENCIES FOR RADIOLOGY
                                 SELECT THE APPROPRIATE
-----------------------------------------------------------------------------------
                  ► ONCE                                           Q24H

                                           DAILY

                    QAM                                            ON CALL

                                           EARLY AM

                    STAT                                           DOWNTIME



-----------------------------------------------------------------------------------
                                                                    DELETE ORDER
 RADFREQ
@@@@@@@@@@@@@@@@@@@@@@@@@@@@@@@@@@@@@@@@@@@@@@@@@@@@@@@@@@@@@@@@@@@@@@@@@@@@@@@@@@@@@BOT
```

D

```
@@@@@@@@@@@@@@@@@@@@@@@@@@@@@@@@@@@@@@@@@@@@@@@@@@@@@@@@@@@@@@@@@@@@@@@@@@@@@@@@@@@@@@@@@@TOP
                                                                         09/28/77  0613
   PRE  4703-01  BAKER,ALBERT H                        CHEST

                                KEY IN CLINICAL IMPRESSION
-------------------------------------------------------------------------------------------

                       ► CHEST PAIN                               *
                                                                  *
                                                                  *
                                                                  *
                                                                  *
                                                                  *

                                               NOW PRESS ENTER KEY ◄

-------------------------------------------------------------------------------------------
                                                                        DELETE ORDER
 RAD
@@@@@@@@@@@@@@@@@@@@@@@@@@@@@@@@@@@@@@@@@@@@@@@@@@@@@@@@@@@@@@@@@@@@@@@@@@@@@@@@@@@@@@@@@@BOT
```

E

```
@@@@@@@@@@@@@@@@@@@@@@@@@@@@@@@@@@@@@@@@@@@@@@@@@@@@@@@@@@@@@@@@@@@@@@@@@@@@@@@@@@@@@@@@@@TOP
                                                                         09/28/77  0613
   PRE  4703-01  BAKER,ALBERT H

                      PLEASE REVIEW THE ORDER, AT THIS POINT YOU MAY
                             CHANGE ONLY THE DETECTABLE ITEMS
-------------------------------------------------------------------------------------------
               ORDER
     CHEST                                  FREQUENCY      BGN DT       BGN TM
                                            ONCE            0928         0700
        CLINICAL IMPRESSION
     CHEST PAIN                                 DUR        END DT       END TM
     ..............................             024        09-29         0700
     ..............................
     ..............................             ORDERING PERSON
     ..............................             DR. JONES
     ..............................
                                                DOWNTIME #          TRANSP
                                                ........             AF

-------------------------------------------------------------------------------------------
 XREVIEW                                        DELETE ORDER            ► ACCEPT
@@@@@@@@@@@@@@@@@@@@@@@@@@@@@@@@@@@@@@@@@@@@@@@@@@@@@@@@@@@@@@@@@@@@@@@@@@@@@@@@@@@@@@@@@@BOT
```

F

FIGURE 7.4D-F. Patient Care System (PCS) processing low example. D: The frequency is selected. E: The clinical impression is entered. F: The order is received and accepted.

Notice how the HELP system differs from TMIS and PCS. The last two systems were designed to meet the communication needs of the hospital. HELP, on the other hand, began with the analysis of physiological data and grew out of the need to integrate the data for medical decision-making. HELP was designed to support the clinical functions of the ICUs; once it can do this and communicate with the ancillary services, it can also support virtually all the other clinical functions. Because there is a medical decision-making module, the system can be used for surveillance as well as decision-making. Consequently, HELP routinely tests all orders for drug-drug and drug-test interaction. All clinical data must be organized by patient, and the need to identify patients establishes the need for an ADT system. Given this set of tools, most of the administrative functions can be installed with only limited additional effort.

All of the functions of TMIS and PCS also are provided by HELP. The major difference is that HELP was designed to meet the following objectives:

- Support an ever-expanding medical database with automated tools for acquisition, storage, and review.
- Implement a system to process medical logic.
- Serve both the medical and administrative needs of the hospital.
- Accommodate effective research subsystems to facilitate clinical research on the large database naturally acquired by the system.

Had HELP begun by focusing on the administrative functions, it would not be able to meet these clinical objectives.

As a result of a grant to Latter Day Saints Hospital, Control Data Corporation has gained the right to market the system. In October 1983, implementation of the first commercial system began at the Arnot-Ogdon Memorial Hospital, Elmira, New York. The treasurer of Arnot-Ogdon views HELP as "a real cost-containment mechanism." "The system will pay for itself in less than a year," he was reported to have said, "because of its accurate tracking of each test performed on a patient. This will ensure correct billing for all of a patient's tests." Thus, it would seem that to an administrator HELP is just like any other HIS. However, to a physician in the ICU, the best feature of HELP is that "it gives [doctors] an important second opinion."[6] How it does this is explained in Chapter 9.

7.3.4. PROMIS System

The fourth HIS differs from those previously presented in that its principal focus is the automation of a medical record system. Recall that the TMIS was designed to support the communication needs of the hospital. The design approach is primarily one of process control: it routes information for processing by the hospital units. In the case of the nursing station, the data are sorted and displayed in the form of plans and results. Within the pharmacy, the same data are interpreted as drug profiles, medication lists, work documents, and inventory actions. The goal of the system implementors is to identify the information needs of the various users, organize the data to meet these needs, and provide tools for the users to complete the processing cycle or provide feedback to the system. The second HIS, PCS, represents an alternative environment for performing the same functions.

HELP was designed to support medical decision-making. Although a discussion of the decision-making techniques has been delayed until Chapter 9, it was shown that HELP also contains the basic HIS communication functions. Here, the communications are required—not for process control functions—but to collect and exchange the data used by the decision making algorithms. In the case of the Problem-Oriented Medical Information System (PROMIS), the objective is to produce a system that will improve the delivery of care through the automation of the medical record.

In the late 1960s Weed developed the concept of the problem-oriented medical record. One objective was to interject the same disciplines into patient care and training that one used in research. By this criterion, clinical records should

- Be in a form that is easily audited and reviewed.
- Provide evidence of completeness and accuracy.
- Demonstrate sound analytical thinking coupled with good clinical judgment.

The method to achieve these ends was the use of a problem list with all diagnostic and therapeutic plans explicitly related to an item in the list, i.e., a Problem-Oriented Medical Record or POMR. Whereas the first POMR was a handwritten record, the computer offered a potential means for overcoming some of the deficiencies of manual record systems: lack of coordination of care, excessive reliance on memory, inability to access the logic of delivered care, and the difficulty of gaining feedback from the experience in treating individuals and patient populations.

The goal of PROMIS was to implement a health care delivery system around this view of the medical record's role. It differs from the previous systems in that it begins with a specific philosophy and imposes this philosophy upon all users of the system. Fig. 7.5 illustrates how the medical record and medical action are linked in PROMIS. The process begins with the establishment of a database (I) which results from a history, physical examination, and initial studies. Once the database has been established, it is organized into a problem list (II). The problems on the list are used to formulate plans (III) which results in more information (IV). The problem list (II) and the plans (III) may be changed in response to this follow up (IV). This basic flow is reflected in the PROMIS Master Frame (Fig. 7.6).

PROMIS operates using a touch screen. Medical knowledge is structured as a hierarchy of screens, and the user (i.e., physician) touches the screen to make selections, retrieve information, and branch through the knowledge base. Fig. 7.7 illustrates the flow for entering a symptom. In Fig. 7.7A the patient has been identified and it has been established that symptoms for depression are being entered. In the upper right corner "Relieved by" is in bold letters and below are the available choices. The lower half of the screen has standard fields for entering text, requesting instructions, and paging forward or back. (The number in the upper left is the frame number used only for system development.) In Fig. 7.7A

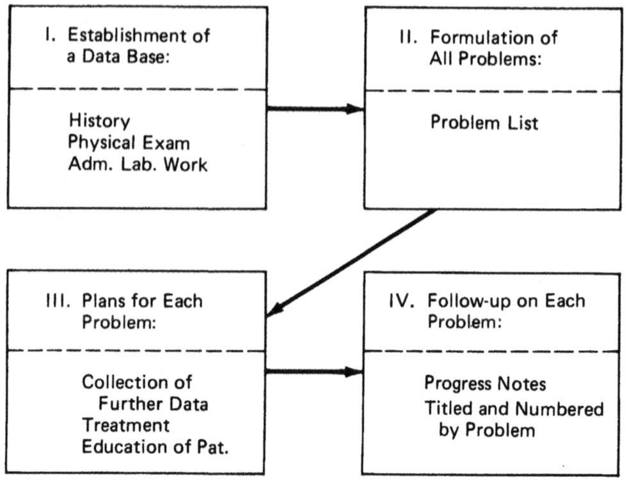

FIGURE 7.5. The Problem-Oriented Medical Information System (PROMIS) four logical phases of medical action.

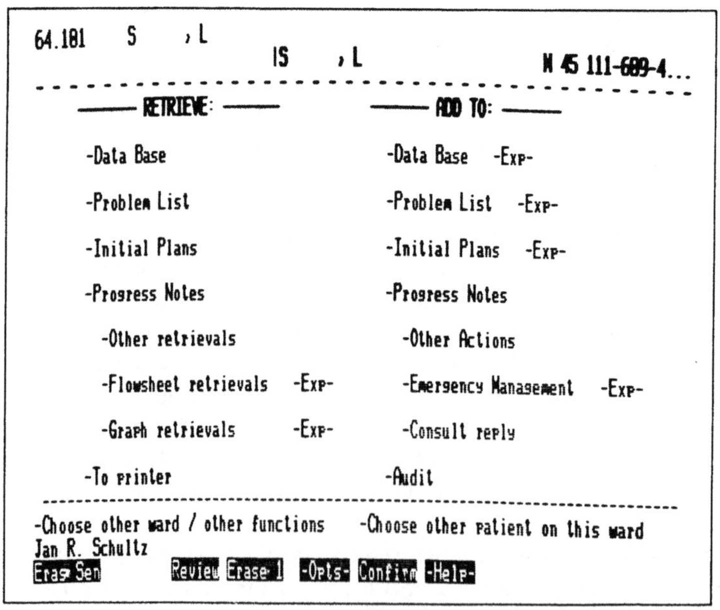

FIGURE 7.6. Problem-Oriented Medical Information System (PROMIS) master frame.

"counselling" is touched and it appears above the line in Fig. 7.7B. Here "antidepressants" is touched and in the next screen "solitude" is touched. Finally, in Fig. 7.7D the full patient illness record is displayed.

PROMIS maintains a completely automated medical record. It structures its contents through the method of entry, and every action is related to a problem. Because the knowledge has been organized, it is possible to audit clinical logic. Since the record is automated, one can access the data in many forms and formats. For example, there are flowsheets that display results and problems. The developers can integrate references to the literature to justify and explain actions; the screens can be modified for clinical specialties. However, the primary objective of PROMIS is the construction of a complete and well-organized medical record. It does this by managing the branching of screens in response to the user's input. Unlike HELP and some of the systems to be discussed in Chapter 8, it cannot initiate actions based on patient specific data.

Of the four systems presented, PROMIS clearly had the most sophisticated user interface. Yet, no major hospital is now using PROMIS. There are two reasons for this. First, the organization and structuring of knowledge is an expensive and difficult task. The methods for doing so are changing. (See Chapter 9 and the HKB example in Chapter 2. Weed has left the PROMIS Project to develop a microcomputer-based system that allows a physician to couple knowledge with the actions he or she takes.) Even more important, however, is the second reason. Where most HISs operate in a "cafeteria mode" in which the user may take only what he wants with no penalty for selecting, Weed's implementation of PROMIS required that all physicians use the system to write their records and specify their orders. Although a study indicated that it took no longer to enter information using PROMIS than it did using a manual POMR, the PROMIS users perceived that it did. This reflected a view that they were working for the system rather than vice versa.

During this same study, the investigator found that the overall yield of PROMIS was only slightly greater than that of the manual POMR, and he suggested that significant improvements would be necessary to motivate the users for whom it was designed. He concluded:

> The system also should be modified so that it is less demanding of user effort. Users have identified a number of areas that could enhance potential for physician support. Most important of these is simplification of data entry and retrieval.
>
> The PROMIS developers believe that the essential need for effective application is effective leadership. Dependence upon leadership to achieve user compliance, however, is unrealistic. Given the nature of human behavior, it is more likely that general acceptance and utilization of PROMIS will be determined, not by coercion, but by the attractiveness of the system to prospective users.
>
> The PROMIS developers seem to have defined as their major goal the design and implementation of computer software, which if used diligently, may provide an unequivocal record of patient care activities. It assumes dedicated and methodological use (of both input and output) by primary care providers. Thus, the major emphasis has been on technical components, with much less investment of time and energy in the design of user education programs and the assessment of user satisfaction with the system.

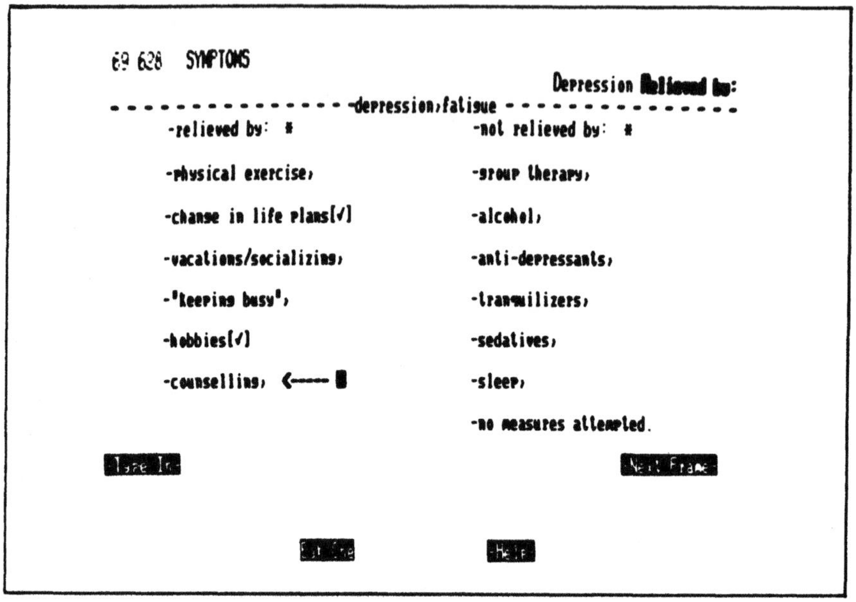

A

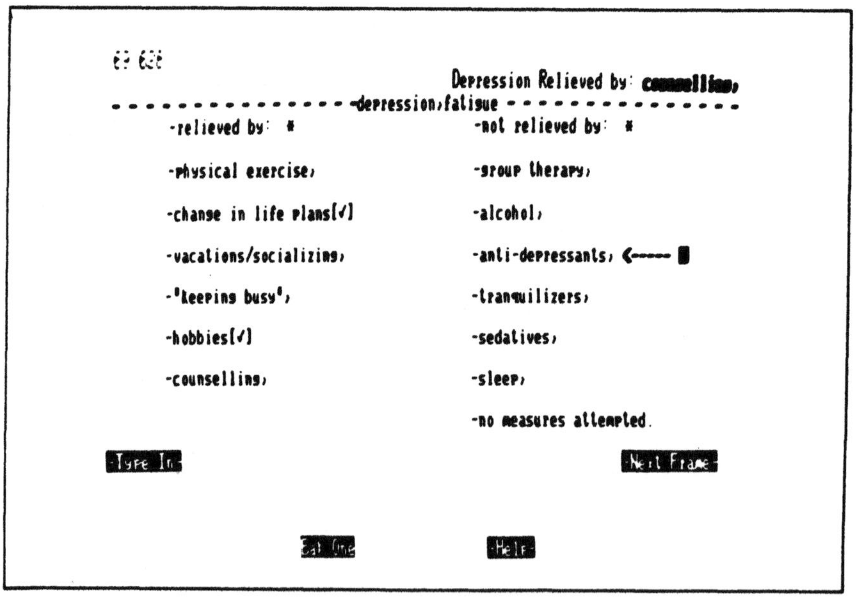

B

FIGURE 7.7A-B. Sample illustration of Problem-Oriented Medical Information System (PROMIS) use.

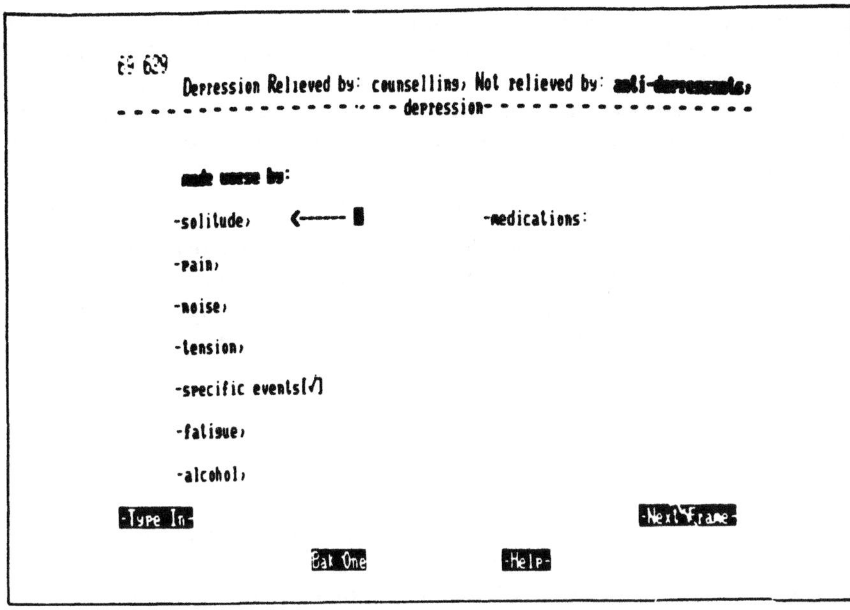

C

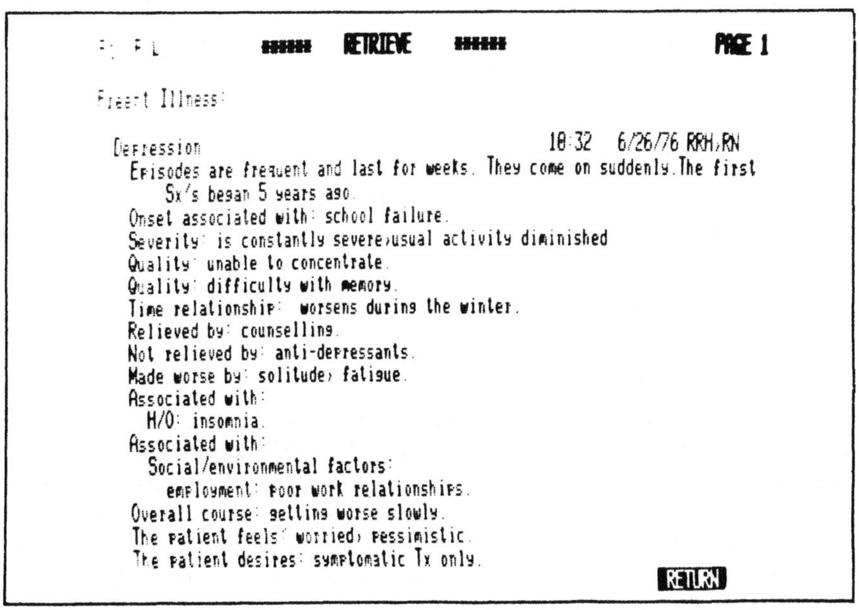

D

FIGURE 7.7C-D. Sample illustration of Problem-Oriented Medical Information System (PROMIS) use.

PROMIS is said to have greater potential than any other existing computerized medical information system. If so, this potential may remain largely unrealized until the PROMIS developers address themselves to the design of a serious strategy of user inducement. Paramount in such a strategy is (1) the identification of services desired by physicians, and (2) the provision of such services at relatively low personal cost of energy, time, or inconvenience to the physician.[7]

These comments are not restricted to the PROMIS experience; they are valid for all clinical information *and* knowledge-based systems. Moreover, it should be noted that a commercial version of PROMIS is now being marketed that is far more permissive: data need not be linked to problems, synonyms are allowed, etc. The conclusion, therefore, is that a well-designed system is a necessary, but not sufficient, requirement for success.

7.4. Evaluation

In Chapter 2 the general benefits of clinical information systems were outlined. This section shall examine the benefits of the HIS in further detail. It considers the effect of an HIS on operations within the institution, the user attitudes to the system, and the impact on costs. The role of the HIS medical record in decision-making will be postponed until Chapter 8 so that it may be considered with other types of clinical information systems.

7.4.1. Effect on Operations

The HIS is designed as a communication system. Thus one would expect three immediate benefits:

- Faster response times through the electronic transmission of messages
- Improved access to medical information (discussed in more detail in Chapter 8)
- Reductions in errors.

All have been documented. For example, the fact that reports are available for distribution as soon as they have been processed implies more timely service.

The ability to reduce errors comes from two sources. First, the computer provides a rigid, disciplined interface for describing actions. It will not accept an invalid test name and will not process incomplete orders. (Of course, this unforgiving nature of computers is also a source of user frustration.) Secondly, the computer has the ability to scan the data it processes and routinely apply logic to test for given conditions.

In the mid-1970s Simborg implemented several HIS components and evaluated their performance.† In a ward management system that processed orders, he

†Studies from the 1970s are cited to make the point that much of the material presented in this section has been known for quite some time.

compared an automated and unautomated unit and found that automation produced a reduction in transcription errors (1.7% for the automated unit as compared to 7.3% for the control). He also recorded a lower rate for failure to exactly carry out an order (5.8% versus 14.7%). The comparison of an automated unit dose and unautomated bulk distribution pharmacy system showed similar results. Errors of commission in the manual system were 4.6 times more frequent. Although the technology used for these early systems has rendered them obsolete, they represent some of the earliest demonstrations of the ability of the HIS to reduce errors.

When a comprehensive HIS is installed, there are more opportunities to coordinate data from multiple sources to apply logic and reduce errors. This has best been demonstrated at the Latter Day Saints Hospital where HELP is installed. In a 1976 report it was shown that—of over 13,000 patients monitored—(a) 5% of the patients' pharmacy orders indicated some form of drug-drug interaction and initiated an alert, and (b) 77% of these alerts resulted in changes in the orders. A more recent study at Latter Day Saints (1981-1982) found that 1.8% of the patients generated a pharmacy alert that was considered life-threatening, and that there was a 94% physician compliance to the life-threatening alerts. (As will be discussed in Chapter 8, the prevention of life threatening alerts does not seem to be a goal that can be achieved by additional education).

Another obvious benefit of the HIS is that it reduces clerical work. Once information is entered into the system it is available for other uses. It is no longer as necessary to copy information onto multiple forms or sort and rearrange data. In almost every instance, the installation of an HIS results in a reduction in the time nursing staff spend on clerical tasks. This is translated into more time available for patient care activities, a reduction in the number of nurses, or both. In some cases, the HIS is installed to alleviate a nursing shortage or to improve the working environment. In these cases, there may be no modification in the staffing pattern. In fact, in situations where there were vacancies, nurse staffing actually may increase; the HIS provides a better professional environment which facilitates recruitment.

7.4.3. User Attitudes

User attitudes will vary according to how the system is perceived to support the user. An early study of the TMIS installed at El Camino reported:[8]

- *Nursing acceptance*. Nursing acceptance of MIS, always high, continued to improve with time and experience until July 1974, when 92% of the nurses favored the system. Nurses perceived MIS as benefiting them in many ways, including a major reduction in clerical tasks, greater availability of patient data, improved legibility, and improved patient care planning.
- *Ancillary department acceptance*. Admitting, Pharmacy, Radiology, Laboratory, and other affected departments generally have shown good acceptance of MIS. This approval is due primarily to improved timeliness,

completeness, accuracy, and availability of information, and to reductions in clerical work.

- *Physician acceptance*. Physicians have increasingly accepted MIS until by August 1974, 61% of physicians who expressed a positive or negative opinion voted to retain and extend the system. Actual acceptance is even higher, since physicians who are major users of the hospital generally are also major users of the system.

Acceptance by the nursing staff and ancillary departments is generally high for all HISs. The success of the system, of course, depends on their cooperation. Since every HIS must be adapted to the hospital, it is essential that nursing and the ancillary departments play a key role in the modification of and user training for the HIS. Physician acceptance, on the other hand, is more variable. The computer is seen as one of many tools to help in patient care. Where the HIS provides an easy to learn, useful function, it will be accepted. Where it suggests a restrictive environment (e.g., the PROMIS evaluation) or where it infringes on the physician's domain (e.g., medical decision-making) it may be rejected. Wherever the computer demonstrates improved techniques for diagnosis or therapy, it is quickly accepted, e.g., CAT and radiation therapy planning. However, when a computer system demonstrates only an impressive potential capability, the physician correctly will view it as a research concept not yet ready for integration into clinical application.

At the present time most hospitals use their computers for administrative purposes, and only some 10% use them for clinical purposes. In most of the latter cases, the physicians are not required to interact with the system. The applications used most often by physicians are reporting of results and location of patients. There have been studies that trace how the use of the HIS moves from the older, influential physicians

to younger physicians through patient referrals and consultations. These physicians appear to follow the early adapter, in introducing computers in their practice only when they are convinced of the efficacy and utility of their use. (From Anderson JG, Jay SJ., The Diffusion of Computer Applications in Medical Settings, *Medical Informatics* 9, 3/4, p. 252, 1984. Reprinted with permission of Taylor and Francis Ltd., London.)

Thus, it would seem that physician acceptance is affected most by a naturally conservative approach coupled with a demand for significant and reliable improvement.

7.4.3. Impact on Costs

Drazen recently reviewed ten automated HIS (AHIS) cost studies and reported the following conclusions.[9]

- Few rigorous studies have been conducted of cost impacts of implementation of automated hospital information systems.
- Most of the work done in this area in the past has involved predicting cost

impacts. Somewhat overstated cost savings (largely the result of unrealistic labor savings and inclusion of revenue impacts) and understated system costs may have produced unrealistic estimates of the net cost impacts of AHIS.

- Little work has been done on validating the results of predictive methodologies. Therefore, there is very little documentation of actual impacts of an AHIS on the productivity of hospital staff or on overall changes to guide the conduct of cost assessments.
- Through improvements in information flow, an AHIS offers benefits to the quality of service delivery, and these are usually major motivations for a hospital to implement a system. More work needs to be done exploring the cost implications of improvements in the quality of service delivery, such as improved turnaround time for test results reporting and decreased loss of information.
- Revenue recovery from charge capture is not a measure of changes in the costs of operating a hospital and, therefore, should not be counted among the cost impacts.
- Cost studies have been conducted for different hospital settings and system configurations. The specific methodologies employed are generally applicable, however, to any setting or system type. The purpose in undertaking the cost study determines the approach that is used.

As these conclusions suggest, most cost studies are prepared to justify a purchase and are never evaluated. The reason for this is that the evaluation of an operational system is both difficult and expensive. For example, consider the experience of the El Camino HIS evaluation. Work began in the early 1970s, the data were collected in the mid-1970s, and the last report was issued in 1980. Clearly, over this period of time there were many changes in the El Camino Hospital, the national health care system, and computer technology. The conclusions of the final report were:

> The results indicate that the system improved productivity in the medical care departments and caused an overall reduction in patient length-of-stay. From a total hospital cost perspective, however, the results were not definitive. Under the assumption that support department cost increases that were found were not directly caused by TMIS, the system was estimated to be approximately 60 percent self-supporting in 1975.[10]

Read another way, this means that 40% of the system's operational cost produced the benefits cited in the first sentence. Of course, with increased experience and lowered equipment costs, there is no reason to believe that a modern HIS cannot be more fully self-supporting in the mid 1980s.

It is interesting to examine how the El Camino cost analysis was performed. Because of their contract with Technicon, El Camino Hospital conducted its own internal cost evaluation of the system. They computed the cost of TMIS operation and identified the cost savings derived from TMIS. To their disappointment, the saving was only 25% of what was required to break even. The benefits were limited to changes in work flow, e.g., form processing changes and keypunch service elimination. Consequently, they developed a second model that identified all the possible cost savings that might be associated with the system, for example, translating 8 hours of reduction in nursing time into the elimination of the need for one full-time nurse. It was discovered that this potential savings model produced approximately 50% of the amount needed to make the system cost-effective.

This was still not acceptable. Then, in the words of Gall, who led the analysis effort, they rediscovered the fact that the health care industry is a dynamic industry. Thus, one should look at cost containment trends and identify the role of the HIS in achieving savings over time. A comparison with other Northern California hospitals was conducted. It was shown that, after TMIS was installed, the rate of cost growth was lower for El Camino than it was for comparable hospitals. Fig. 7.8a illustrates how TMIS reduced the length of stay and Fig. 7.8b shows how the rate of increase in per diem charges was controlled during the period 1971-1974. With this interhospital trend comparison model, the cost of the system was fully justified.

How can the El Camino studies be applied to today's environment? First, the changes in methods used for hospital reimbursement may alter the evaluation criteria. For example, prospective payment based on a fixed payment by diagnosis may make reductions in length of stay more important than reductions in labor; the economic benefits of higher quality care may establish new evaluation criteria. Second, note that many of the changes attributed to TMIS were the result of system-independent management decisions. As shown in Fig. 7.8, El Camino's performance was always better than that of its neighboring hospitals. Good management without an HIS could maintain this lead; for some of the neighboring hospitals, an HIS without management changes could not produce the same benefit. Finally, recognize that many of the potential HIS savings are never realized. In part this is due to management's unwillingness to do so. In Gall's opinion:

> The major reason most computerized information systems are not cost effective is because most of the effort goes toward designing and implementing the technical aspects of the system and very little effort goes toward realizing the potential savings that might be associated with that system.[11]

However, it must be recognized that in many cases the potential savings cannot be realized. Eliminating the need for one full time equivalent (FTE) of a nurse when there is understaffing only relieves the understaffing; it does not change costs. Moreover, one FTE saving that is defined by combining small tasks over many units and shifts can never be achieved.

To conclude this discussion of HIS costs, we point out that the El Camino studies established that 95% of the savings came from reductions in labor; in the case of nursing, there was a 5% reduction in costs. Yet, no matter how the numbers are analyzed, the HIS does not seem to save money. It invests in a computer system to improve productivity, patient care, and the working environment. Preliminary cost studies project anticipated cost savings. Many of these cost savings are never realized. This lack of realization results from unrealistic

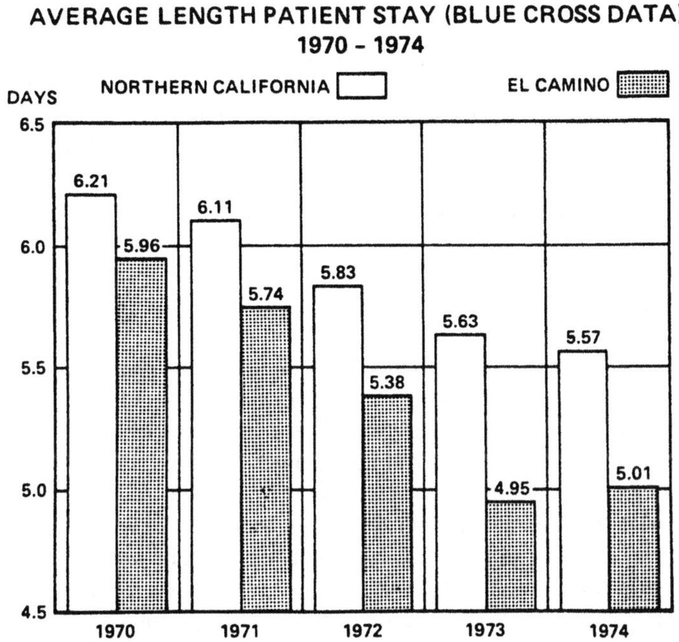

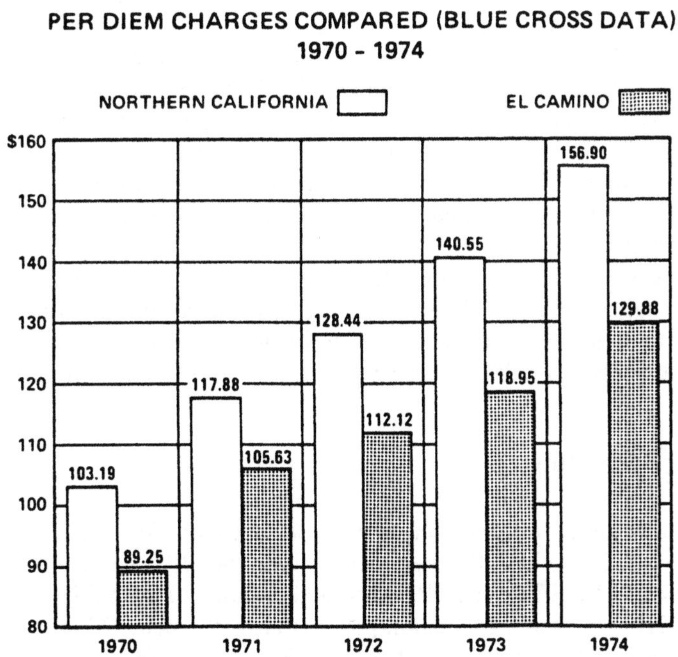

FIGURE 7.8. Some El Camino Hospital comparisons.

projections and limited management effort to achieve savings. Nevertheless, the conclusion seems to be that, although hospitals are labor-intensive, the HIS cannot significantly reduce the dependence on that labor. This should be an obvious conclusion. After all, most of a hospital's labor is directed to patient care functions. That support cannot be replaced by computers. However, it can be made easier, more productive, and effective. That is the proper role of the HIS, a role that it performs well and at little (if any) cost.

7.5. Concluding Remarks

This chapter reviewed the HIS. Two HIS models were discussed. The first implements a hospital-wide communication network to speed and monitor the flow of information within the institution. The second type of HIS adds tools to this model for medical decision-making and medical care. At the present time there are few examples of this second category of system; however, they represent a great potential for improvement in the delivery of care.

Methods for implementing an HIS were considered. The communication application is well understood and requires no knowledge of medical computing to implement. Two technologies are available: a single teleprocessing system or a network of independent but interfaced systems. The former is easier to implement and manage; the latter is more modular and easier to update with new features. It is probable that many of the newer medical decision support tools will be installed as distributed units in a network.

While the technology of an HIS is relatively independent of the medical application, the installation and use of the HIS is intractably associated with the health care environment that it must support. The design of user interfaces and system functions requires special knowledge that is gained only by experience with this application. The nursing and ancillary service departments will be the principal users of the system, and they must play a key role in the design and/or installation process.

Finally, we note that, although there have been cost studies, there is little evidence to suggest that the HIS saves money or enhances profitability. It does improve productivity and has the potential to improve care, control cost growth, and support management. These latter benefits justify the investment in an HIS.

For Further Reading

The book of readings *Information Systems for Patient Care* (BI Blum, ed, Springer-Verlag, 1984) has 10 papers dealing with the HIS. There are surveys, descriptions of PCS, HELP and PROMIS, and chapters on planning and installation of an HIS. Drazen's evaluation paper is also included. Other sources of information include DAB Lindberg, *The Growth of Medical Information Systems in the United States*, Lexington Books, 1979, as well as some of the references cited in Chapter 2. Finally, although somewhat out of date, MF Collen (ed), *Hospital Computer Systems*, John Wiley, 1974, contains much useful material. Of particular interest is RH Richart's chapter on evaluation.

For persons interested in specific systems, the American Hospital Association has a Hospital Technology Series that describes systems. The nonprofit organization, Medsy, also produces comparative systems reports. Two Federal Government activities provide additional sources of information. The Department of Defense has a TRIMIS program. Because most of their systems are procured, there is a good deal of useful requirements and evaluation literature now in the public domain. The Veterans Administration is also implementing some HIS components using MUMPS; these systems also should be in the public domain when completed.

References

1. Jydstrup, R. A. and M. J. Gross, Cost of Information Handling in Hospitals, *Health Services Research*, Winter, 1966, pp 235-271.
2. *Ibid*, p 260.
3. Johns, R. J. and B. I. Blum, The Use of Clinical Information Systems to Control Costs as Well as to Improve Care, *Trans. Am. Clinical and Climatological Assn*, 90, 1973, pp 140-152.
4. Lindberg, D.A.B., *The Growth of Medical Information Systems in the United States*, Lexington Books, 1979, p 10.
5. Patient Care Systems Terminal Operators Guide, IBM manual SH2000-1956-0, 1977, pp 41-43.
6. Warner, E., Expert System Helps Guide Hospital's Physicians Through Life and Death Decisions, *Computerworld*, July 9, 1984, pp 18-19.
7. Stratmann, W. E., A Demonstration of PROMIS, DHEW (PHS) 79-3247, September 1974, pp 7-8.
8. Demonstration and Evaluation of a Total Hospital Information System, DHEW (HRA) 77-3188, July 1977, p 32.
9. Drazen, E. and J. Metzger, Methods for Evaluating Costs of Automated Hospital Information Systems, DHHS (PHS) 81-3283, July 1981, p 37.
10. Coffey, R. M., How a Medical Information System Affects Hospital Costs: the El Camino Hospital Experience, DHEW (PHS) 80-3255, March 1980, Abstract.
11. Gall, J. E., Jr. Computerized Hospital Information Systems Cost Effectiveness—A Cast Study, J. van Egmond, P. F. deVries Robbe and A. H. Levy (eds), *Information Systems for Patient Care: Review, Analysis and Evaluation*, North-Holland, 1976, p 286.

8
Ambulatory Care Systems

8.1. Introduction

In the previous chapter, hospital information systems were discussed. The patients served by the HIS receive comprehensive treatment over a period of days or weeks. Each is suffering from an acute episode that requires some degree of continuous monitoring. The facility normally treats fewer than 500 patients at any one time and has a large staff to accommodate their needs. In addition to providing the care function, the hospital also supports a full range of hotel functions: food services, housekeeping, registration, etc. Thus, the hospital has a small number of patients, a great deal of information to manage for each patient, a large staff and overhead, and many ancillary functions to support. In this environment, it is not unrealistic to add \$5.00 or more per patient day for a computer system to help manage the patient's (and institution's) data.

In an ambulatory setting, however, the problem is quite different. Most of the care will be managed by the patient at home. The visit to (or encounter with) the provider is brief, the problems addressed are generally chronic or self-limiting but acute, and the support staff is small. Compared to a hospital, there are a large number of patients, but the amount of information to be managed for each patient is small; linkage between visits is essential for both medical and billing purposes but the costs for service are low. Moreover, there is no great demand for timely communication with other services, and where the need exists the patient can act as the courier. Thus, ambulatory care systems must be less expensive and not as complete as an HIS.

As in the case of the HIS, the ambulatory care system can be designed to support both the administrative and the patient care process. Naturally, when it does the latter, it also must do the former. Since an ambulatory care system does not focus on the communication functions, its primary impact on patient care is through the contents and availability of the medical record used by the providers and ancillary services. In what follows we shall present a model of the ambulatory care system, describe some representative systems, and evaluate our experience.

Because most of the benefits of these systems can be traced to the use of an automated medical record, the conclusions are equally valid for the HIS.

8.2. Automated Ambulatory Medical Record Systems

An automated Ambulatory Medical Record System (AAMRS) maintains a medical record and is designed to support patient care. A system typically has the following components:

- Medical record system
- Financial system
- Appointment system
- Management Reports
- System support, e.g., privacy and security

In the remainder of this chapter we shall consider only the medical record application.

Virtually all AAMRSs follow the flow shown in Fig. 8.1. If a patient is scheduled for an appointment, then the chart is prepared some time prior to the appointment. Preparation includes requesting radiographic films, medical records, or other materials. Many systems also include a computer printed encounter form. The AAMRS organizes the work flow so that when the patient arrives for the encounter, the materials have been assembled. All systems also must accommodate unscheduled patients. When they arrive, the encounter form is prepared and the medical records and films are retrieved. In either case, when the patient sees the provider, there is an encounter form and the necessary (or available) records. During and following the encounter, the form is updated. It then goes to a registrar where follow-up is scheduled. The completed form is used to update the database. Billing information, new appointments, and the updated medical record are produced from the updated database.

Different organizations will implement variations on this flow. A small practice may have sufficient control over the medical records to perform all retrieval on demand; in this case a standard data capture may be used or the preprinted encounter form may be produced on line. An emergency room system will see only unscheduled patients. A clinic in a large hospital may require interfaces with the hospital medical record department. There also may be a need to coordinate care with other clinics. Nevertheless, all AAMRSs support:

- Preparation for the encounter
- Recording key data from the encounter
- Updating the medical database
- Use of the medical database for medical, administrative, and financial applications.

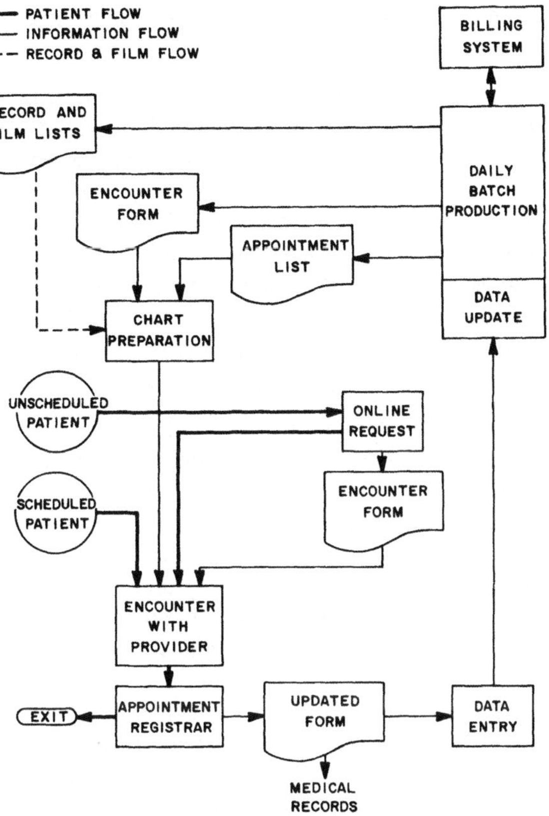

FIGURE 8.1. Typical Ambulatory Medical Record System (AAMRS) flow.

8.2.1. The Medical Record

The medical record plays a key role in today's medical practice. It is a medium for communication among providers, an informative source for follow-up, a resource for research, a legal record, and more. It is known that every record must identify the patient (except in research use where confidentiality requires suppressing the identification). There are many styles and forms for medical records; the problem-oriented medical record (POMR) is one example. All records contain some textual information (name and address) and some coded information (race and sex). The medical data may include text or codes for complaints, diagnosis, and therapies. Test results are incorporated into the record; they may be in the form of individual reports, flowsheets, or graphs. It is assumed that patient care is better when medical records are available than when they are not. However, the contents and structure of individual records are subject to personal preferences and local standards.

An automated medical record has several major advantages over the manual record:

- It is neither sequential nor physically constrained. That is, portions may be accessed directly or combined in alternative formats. Moreover, the record can be accessed from many different locations concurrently—it can always be found.
- It is consistent in format and always legible. Once a user is familiar with the system, data are easy to locate and read.
- It is expandable and easily integrated with other data sources. For example, laboratory data from another CIS can be incorporated into the basic record. Its contents can be processed as either text or numeric values.

The contents of an automated medical record will be defined by how it is used and the cost to collect and maintain the data. All systems code the diagnosis or complaint for reporting purposes. Such codes are useful for management reporting and effective in case finding and research, but they will be of little use in treating a specific patient. Textual information, the traditional form of the medical record, is most useful for conveying information to other providers; text is difficult to use in management and research. In some systems, the provider is offered a table of codes that can be augmented by text; in other cases, only text is entered and manual or automated coding follows; finally, some systems are limited to coded data.

User acceptance is linked to the form and contents of the medical record. If it is accessible and timely, if it contains the information desired, and if it is perceived to be easy to use, then the system will be accepted. Provider acceptance seems to be best when the provider was involved with the system design, participated in the installation decision, and received training in the use of the system.

Although the automated medical records have some clear advantages, there also can be frustrations. Access to the desired information may not be direct. Response time may be slow. (This is never a problem when viewing outputs in a book or paper.) Terminals may be limited in number or located inconveniently. Specification of the desired information may be confusing. (A system with very few options may be too constrained; one with many options can be too difficult to learn.) The printed text may seem more foreign than the provider's own handwriting. (This is especially common where the material recorded is used as a personal note intended for use by only the writer.) Finally, most users have been trained to find information by leafing through a paper record; it is a comfortable and natural approach. Most of these problems may be overcome through good design and training.

The automated medical record seldom eliminates the need for a paper record. It generally augments the paper chart. Yet, as we will see, there are many cases in which its availability reduces the need for the paper record. The most important attribute of the automated medical record, however, is that it is part of a larger system. This means that it can be expanded continuously and that it can be integrated with medical knowledge bases for prospective recommendations and retrospective analysis. In this way, the automated medical record has the potential to exceed the utility of the traditional record in both the AAMRS and the HIS.

8.2.2. The AAMRS in the United States

In 1975 Henley and Wiederhold conducted a state-of-the-art survey of the AAMRS. A literature search identified some 200 potential systems, many of which were no longer in operation. Seventeen operational systems (at 16 sites) were identified as useful for evaluating how such systems improve the use of the patient's medical record in different types of health care settings. It must be remembered that equipment costs were high (all systems had to be implemented using early 1970 technology), there was a limited experience base, and in some cases the expectations were unrealistic. It is not surprising, therefore, that one conclusion was that AAMRSs still required substantial development and evaluation.

Of the systems visited, five were outpatient clinics, four were health maintenance organizations (HMOs), four were university medical centers and there was one county health department, workman's insurance company, single-physician general practice, and single-specialty group practice. The role of the AAMRS ranged from supporting a completely automated medical record to encoding some data for administrative reporting. Of these systems, only four were classified as financially self-sufficient and one of these systems was developed with extensive federal support. Most system users, however, stated that cost reduction or containment was a goal.

In 1981 there was a follow-up to this study. Table 8.1 illustrates the status of the systems today.[1] Note that three of the systems used in patient care were visited in the follow-up study. Two other systems—a system in a specialty clinic primarily used to interface with a research databank (ARAMIS) and a multisite system designed to provide administrative assistance to family practices and residency programs—were also included in the follow-up study. From these two studies, the following points seem clear.

- There are several major systems that have been in operation for 10 or more years. During that time they have grown in scope.
- Financial pressures have limited the scope of some of the early systems. That is, in the competition for health care dollars, the cost of some of their clinical functions could not be justified.
- Despite the improvements in technology, the growth in experience, and the lowered costs for equipment, the second study did not identify new systems that could be compared with the COSTAR, RMRS, or TMR systems of the earlier study.

Thus, it would seem, the number of AAMRSs available for new users is still relatively small. The problem is not that we do not understand what an AAMRS should do. Most of the functionality of today's systems has been operational for at least 10 years. The limited number of AAMRS seems to result from the incentive to place the administrative functions first; there is no shortage of billing

TABLE 8.1. Current status of systems visited in 1975 AAMRS study.

	Systems Used in Patient Care
COSTAR	Harvard Community Health Plan, Laboratory of Computer Science, Massachusetts General Hospital, Cambridge and Boston, Massachusetts. A fully automated medical record system.
	This system was visited for the follow-up study.
RMRS	Regenstrief Institute, Indiana University Medical Center, Indianapolis, Indiana. Hospital-based clinics. Development of a medical record supplement.
	This system was visited for the follow-up study.
TMR	Duke University Medical Center, Department of Community Health Services, Durham, North Carolina. Student health services and hospital-based clinics. A total medical record system was planned; only administrative services were operational in 1975.
	This system was visited for the follow-up study.
MUSC	Department of Family Practice, College of Medicine, Medical University of South Carolina, Charleston, South Carolina. Residency family practice clinics. A fully automated medical record system, used in training.
	The orientation of the system is to provide a clinical, administrative, and research tool for practicing physicians (SCAMP). Several new features have been added.
CC	Cardiovascular Clinic. Oklahoma City, Oklahoma. Private group practice. A fully automated medical record system. Still in Operation.
HIP	Casa de Amigos, Department of Community Medicine, Baylor College of Medicine, Houston, Texas. Community—neighborhood clinics. The Health Illness Profile (HIP) supplements the medical record.
	The system is still in existence, but at reduced level.
LA	County of Los Angeles, Department of Health Services, Los Angeles, California.
	A Patient identifiecation and record retrieval system serving hospital-based clinics in the County Medical Center.
	The County Medical Center system has increased the amount of medical information provided.
IHS	Indian Health Service, Tucson, Arizona. Clinics on the Papago Indian Reservation. The Patient Care Information System (PCIS) is a supplement to the medical record.
	The system is now in a microfiche rather than an on-line mode.
	System Used for Research
ARAMIS	Division of Immunology, Stanford University Medical Center, Time-Oriented Data Bank (TOD), American Rheumatism Association Medical Information System (ARAMIS).
	ARAMIS remains operational; the number of remote sites has increased; development work continues.

and appointment systems. Thus, most users have a narrow choice between selecting among a very few systems or building (or modifying) a system to meet their needs. As Table 8.2 illustrates, the use of the AAMRS is still associated with a research environment.[2]

It is one thesis of this book that the AAMRS technology is mature even if the

TABLE 8.1. Current status of systems visited in 1975 AAMRS study—*cont'd.*

	Systems Used Primarily for Administrative Functions
MSIS	Multi-State Information System, Rockland State Hospital, Orangeburg, New York. Mental health services hospital and community-based clinics. the system collected primarily administrative data used to prepare required reports to supporting agencies. The system is now 100% user supported. Hardware and service improvements have been made.
DHD	Appalachi II District Health Department, Greenville, South Carolina, Public health clinics: program orientation. The system continues to be primarily administatively oriented, but is collecting medical data.
ELACYC	County of Los Angeles, Department of Health Services, Los Angeles, California. A Patient identification and record retrieval system serving hospital-based clinics in the County Medical Center and another system serving the East Los Angeles Child and Youth Clinic. The County Medical Center system has increased the amount of medical information provided. The ELACYC system has not changed significantly.
AUTOMED	Medical Data Systems Corporation, Olmstead Falls, Ohio. A private for-profit service bureau. Primarily financial services for solo practitioners and small groups. Some medical data in the record; amount depended upon individual user. This system is still in full operation.
ITC	Insurance Technology Corporation, Berkeley, California. An information system used in processing Workman's Compensation claims. The site visited in 1975 has been discontinued. Other sites remain operational.
	Systems No Longer in Operation
BELLEVUE	Pediatric Outpatient Clinic, Bellvue Hospital, New York City. Hospital-based clinic and emergency services. A supplement to the medical record, and medical record pulling service. The computer project serving the Pediatric Outpatient Clinic was terminated in 1976.
BUMED	The BUMED Computer Project, U.S. Naval Air Station Dispensary, Brunswick, Maine. Military dependents health services. A fully automated medical record. The project was cancelled at Brunswick in 1976.
YALE	Section of Medical Computer Sciences, Yale University School of Medicine, New Haven, Connecticut. A medical record information system for an HMO group practice with a goal to have the total medical record automated; minimally operational at time of visit. The system is no longer in existence.

marketplace has few offerings. An informed user community, less expensive equipment, and new development tools should all combine to produce a new generation of practical systems. In the following section several AAMRSs are described. There are few ideas presented that have not been in practical application for a decade.

TABLE 8.2. Follow-up study description of the characterisitics of a market for the larger AAMRS.

A group practice with four or more providers
A need for automated financial and administrative services. Practices have justified automated administrative services where there is:
a need for practice management data
evidence of lost charges, or
a problem with cash flow.
The potential to improve medical care by the acquisition of automated medical data services. The greatest potential for improved care from the use of medical services exists where there is:
A need for record availability, legibility, and common organization
A need for data organization and report formatting
A desire to improve quality of care or to improve procedures for quality of care assurance review
A setting where there is a desire to use the database for research
Research needs resulting from either the institutional setting or individual physician motivation.

8.3. Some Ambulatory Care Systems

In this section we shall describe some AAMRSs. We begin with a rather complete description of one system—COSTAR. We do this for several reasons. First, by illustrating how one system operates, we can show how the data are integrated for patient care, administration, and research. Secondly, COSTAR is a good example: it has a completely computer-stored medical record, it is available in the public domain, and many users have experience with it. Having presented one AAMRS as a complete system, we then present other systems as examples of other ways in which an AAMRS can be implemented.

8.3.1. The COSTAR System

The COmputer STored Ambulatory Record (COSTAR) was originally developed in the late 1960s by Barnett and his colleagues in the Laboratory of Computer Science (Massachusetts General Hospital) in collaboration with the Harvard Community Health Plan (HCHP). HCHP is a prepaid group practice in the metropolitan Boston area. In mid-1970 it handled 550 daily visits from a membership of 37,500. The fourth version of the system, COSTAR 4, has been integrated into HCHP operations since 1976. It is completely operated by the HCHP staff and is supported from the HCHP budget.

In 1978 a revision to that system, COSTAR 5 (or COSTAR V), was made available. The goal of COSTAR 5 was to expand the system for use by other ambulatory practices. This involved the removal of characteristics specifically designed for HCHP and the addition of new functions such as billing. Since the host language, MUMPS, was also undergoing standardization and revision at the time, it was decided to reprogram COSTAR as a highly modular system that could be adapted to practices smaller than HCHP. Once COSTAR 5 was available,

TABLE 8.3. Types of organizations using COSTAR (1982).

Organization type	Number of installations	Percentage
Hospital clinics/departments	18	25
Small group practices	16	22
Solo practitioners	8	11
Public health departments	7	9
Community clinics	7	9
Large group practices	5	7
Other clinics	4	6
Organizational health clinics	3	4
Research units	2	3
Unknown or other	3	4
Total	73	100

From Fiddleman, R.H., Proliferation of COSTAR—A Status Report, in B. I. Blum (ed) *Information Systems for Patient Care,* Springer-Verlag, 1984, p. 303. (Copyright 1982, by The Institute of Electrical and Electronics Engineers, Inc. Reprinted with permission from *The Sixth Annual Symposium on Computer Applications in Medical Care,* Washington, D.C., October 30-November 2, 1982.)

there was a need to distribute and evaluate its use in other practices. Since no major vendor elected to market the product, the National Center for Health Service Research chose to encourage commercial firms to act as COSTAR vendors by supporting some of their installation and programming services. The result would be a public domain version of COSTAR 5, many enhanced proprietary versions of COSTAR, and a large number of commercial agents experienced in the installation and modification of COSTAR systems. By mid-1982 there were 54 sites in operation and an additional 19 sites planned to install the system. Table 8.3 breaks down the organizations by type.[3]

Sixty-five percent of the sites were supported by a commercial vendor. Thus, the dissemination strategy seemed to be working. One disappointing fact was that 14 of the 54 sites did not use the medical records component of COSTAR, and—of those that did—it was difficult to determine how complete or extensive the medical record was. Put another way, there was evidence that the users perceived their most immediate need as the accounts receivable module. However, as has been noted frequently, when one has a clinical information system one can use the administration functions without using the clinical tools. On the other hand, where one has an administrative system, it is very difficult to add clinical tools onto it. Consequently, even though much of the current COSTAR deployment is administratively oriented, each system has the facilities to support clinical functions. One can anticipate that these tools will be adapted as the users become more familiar with the system.

In what follows we shall describe the COSTAR system. Most of the discussion will relate to version 5. However, many of the examples will be taken from earlier versions. We do this to emphasize the fact that there is a great deal of operational experience with AAMRSs.

The central objective of COSTAR has always been to facilitate patient care by improving the availability, accessibility, timeliness of retrieval, legibility, and organization of medical information. To support this function in a practice setting requires that the system also provide a billing system; tools for day-to-day operations; budgeting and planning; and support to the administrative and ancillary services. Finally, the design goals require that the system provide user-specified inquiry and quality assurance monitoring.

COSTAR 5 consists of six modules:

- *Security and Integrity Module*. This provides for identifying and logging in/out terminals and users for the purpose of preventing unauthorized access. It also provides routines to monitor system performance and prevent data loss. All COSTAR implementations require this module.
- *Registration Module*. This allows for the entry, service, and modification of the patient registration data—identification, demographic, insurance, and administrative information. It also is a required module.
- *Scheduling Module*. This supports an appointment system. It is an optional module.
- *Medical Record Module*. This processes the medical data by accepting inputs from encounter forms and providing access to the complete medical and administrative database. This optional module provides a large variety of facilities for recording, manipulating, organizing, and displaying data.
- *Billing and Accounts Receivable Module*. This uses the data captured during the registration and encounter form processing to prepare bills and, at practice option, to support other financial processing. It is an optional module.
- *Management Reporting Module*. This prepares preprogrammed standardized reports and also includes tools for searching and query. It too is optional.

Of the six modules, two perform control system functions (security and registration) and the remaining four may be implemented at the discretion of the practice. Two of these modules impact care: the Medical Record Module (for patient specific data) and the Management Reporting Module (for data about aggregates of patients or providers.) The following discussion will be limited to these last two.

COSTAR 5 uses a blank encounter form that is filled in manually by the registrar. If the patient is new to the practice, a separate registration session collects the necessary data; for returning patients the registration data need only be verified for accuracy. Unlike many of the AAMRS to be discussed below, the COSTAR encounter form—shown in Fig. 8.2—contains no preprinted information about the patient. This is possible because the full medical record is available on line (or preprinted if this is a scheduled visit). The examples shown in Figs. 8.2(A, B) illustrate the form used by the HCHP Medical Clinic in the mid-1970s.[4] The front of the form is primarily used to collect administrative information, the back of the form records the medical data. There are fields for entering the vital signs and checking problems. The list of problems was designed for internal medicine; other specialties use encounter forms with different lists. Problems may be classified as major (M), minor (a check), status/post (S/P), and so on. Short comments may be written after the code, added on the bottom of the form, or processed separately as a dictated note. (The last option is not encouraged and therefore seldom used.) In this case, it can be seen that the note for this visit would include:

Hematuria (Major problem). No previous hx prior 1 wk. In process of evaluation.
Initial Health Assessment—Generally healthy P.E. WNL
Obesity—Would like to lose at least 10#
S/P Appendectomy—1957

The problem codes are used for data entry and internal linkage. A set of codes has been defined for HCHP and COSTAR, but individual practices are free to modify the code dictionaries to meet their individual needs.

Once data are entered, they may be retrieved in the form of an encounter report that contains all data recorded for a single encounter, a case summary that includes current problems in a short format, a status report that contains a more complete medical record, or a variety of special flow sheets. As in the case of the HIS, not all installations use all possible outputs. Figure 8.3 contains a sample encounter report from the COSTAR 5 Functional Specifications, and Fig. 8.4 presents a case summary in the format currently used by the Primary Care Unit of the Massachusetts General Hospital Ambulatory Care Division. (Not shown in the summary figure are the sections that display current medications, physical examination findings, recent laboratory results, and planned dispositions.) A flowsheet designed for hypertensive patients is illustrated in Fig. 8.5. It presents laboratory values and therapies in both code and text. Other flowsheets are available for prenatal care, routine pediatrics, and other special patient populations. The flowsheets may be generalized to list out specified data by date, or they may be highly structured and specialized. For example, the routine pediatrics flowsheet lists length and weight by age and indicates the percentile ranking for each entry; it also displays the patient's immunization history.

Processing of COSTAR data follows the flow presented in the general model described in the previous section. A printed summary and an encounter form are available to the provider. Notes from the encounter are recorded on the forms and then entered into the database. This information is then used in subsequent medical records, for processing bills, and for administrative and management functions such as quality assurance, examination of the patient population characteristics, review of resource utilization, etc.

The Management Reporting Module may be used to produce standardized, preformatted reports such as:

- Distribution of patient population by age and sex
- Utilization rates by patient and provider
- Distribution of encounters by clinic or service
- Provider activity
- Problems addressed most frequently.

Since COSTAR is written in Standard MUMPS, it is relatively easy to add additional, practice-specific reports.

4) SITE
A___ MH-PH
B___ CAMBRIDGE
C_✓_ KENMORE
D___ KEN. TRIAGE
E___ CHMC
F___ PBBH
G___ BLI
H___ BI
J___ HOUSE CALL
K___ OTHER___________

5) TYPE
A_✓_ SCHEDULED
B___ WALK-IN
C___ TELEPHONE
D___ CANCELLED
E___ DNK
F___ CALL-IN
G___ IN-PATIENT
H___ EW
I___ NON-ENCOUNTER
J___ GROUP

NAME: Record, Sample Enr
UNIT: Ø7-39-Ø7 I
DATE: 4/4/75 DOB:
PROV #1: Plotkin
PROV #2: Imbernino
(if seen)

ABOVE MUST BE COMPLETE FOR INPUT

6) Hospital or EW Visit Approved: ___Yes ___No

************ THIS INFORMATION FOR FIRST VISIT/PRIMARY PROVIDER ONLY ************

7) PRIMARY MD Plotkin 8) PRIMARY RN Imbernino

9) RACE: A_X_ CAUCASIAN B___ BLACK C___ SPANISH SPKG D___ OTHER_______

10) MAR.STATUS: A___ SINGLE B_X_ MARRIED C___ WIDOWED D___ SEPARATED E___ DIVORCED

11) # OF CHILDREN Ø 12) PT. OCCUPATION Staff acct. - Boston based consulting Firm

PERSONAL BACKGROUND OF PATIENT - Only for primary providers
(To change, rewrite entire section; max. three lines. Do not repeat above data.)

Pt is a fairly active person, generally healthy and feeling well.
More physically active in summer - tennis, swimming. Commutes from
southern New Hampshire during summer

************ TO BE COMPLETED FOLLOWING EACH VISIT ************

40) DISPOSITION

Future appt w/ ______________________ in
(provider's full name)

A___ DAYS B___ WEEKS C___ MONTHS D___ PRN

E___ PT to call MD G___ PT to call RN
F___ MD to call PT H___ RN to call PT
I___ Other ______________________

REFERRALS

42) INTERNAL HCHP CONSULTATION

Consultation w/ Urology # L993
(enter specialty and provider's last name, if specified)

Consultation w/ ______________________
(enter specialty and provider's last name, if specified)

(IF A CONSULTATION NOTE IS NECESSARY, INCLUDE REASON FOR CONSULT IN ROUTINE DICTATION)

43) REFERRAL TO OUTSIDE AGENCY - NON-HOSPITAL

____
(enter full name & address of physician and/or agency)

DOCUMENTS TO BE FORWARDED: ______________________

44) HOSPITAL ARRANGEMENTS (make a choice in each column)

A___ BETH ISRAEL
B___ PBBH
C___ BOSTON HOSPITAL FOR WOMEN
D___ CHMC
F___ UNAFFILIATED

1.___ EMERGENCY WARD
2.___ URGENT ADMISSION
3.___ SCHEDULED ADMISSION

Date of Admission (if known) ___________

45) SUPPORTIVE SERVICES

A___ HOMEMAKER C___ HOMECARE
B___ VNA D___ TRANSPORTATION

46) DICTATION ___________ 47) REVIEW OF CHART ___________

48) FOLLOW-UP IMPORTANT ___________

FIGURE 8.2A. Harvard Community Health (HCHP) COSTAR encounter form. Front of internal medicine form. (From Policy Implications of Medical Information Systems, Office of Technology Assessment, 1977, p. 28.)

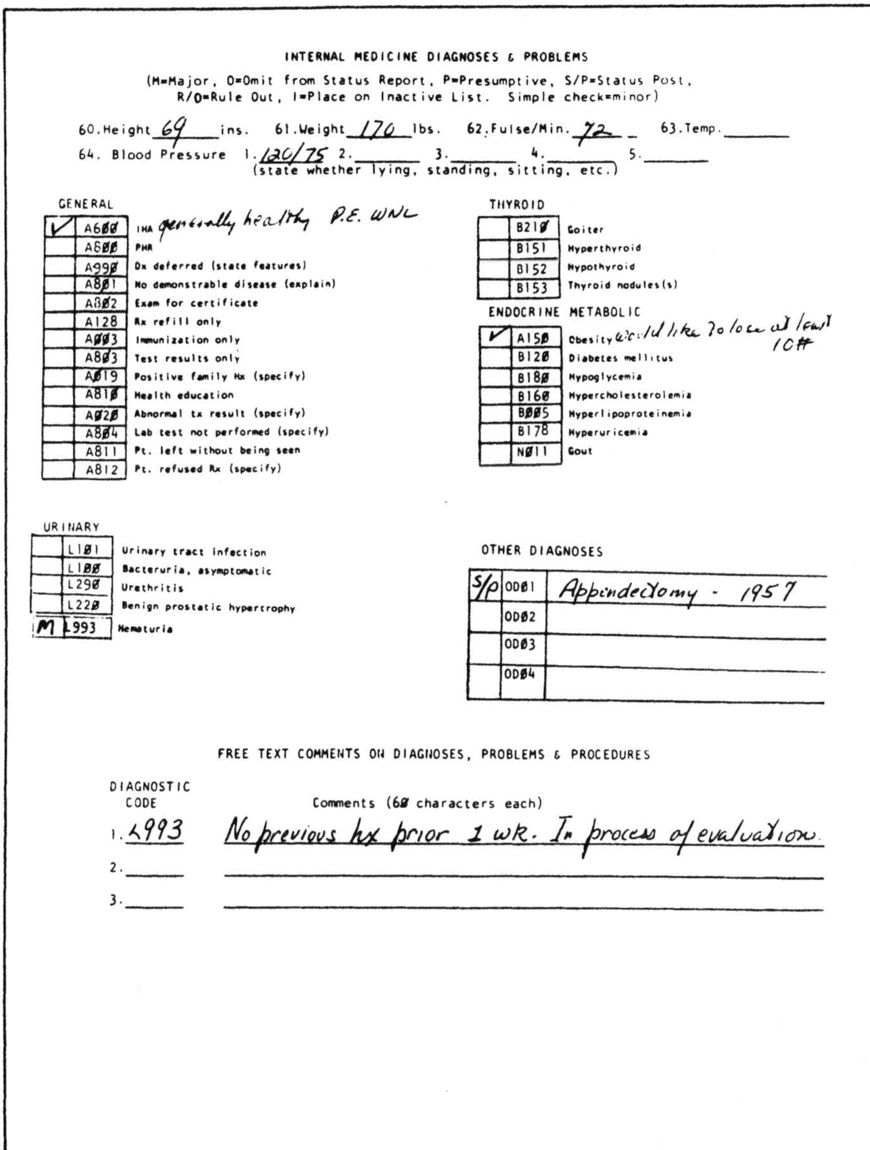

INTERNAL MEDICINE DIAGNOSES & PROBLEMS

(M=Major, O=Omit from Status Report, P=Presumptive, S/P=Status Post, R/O=Rule Out, I=Place on Inactive List. Simple check=minor)

60. Height 69 ins. 61. Weight 170 lbs. 62. Pulse/Min. 72 63. Temp. ______

64. Blood Pressure 1. 120/75 2. ______ 3. ______ 4. ______ 5. ______
(state whether lying, standing, sitting, etc.)

GENERAL

✓	A6ØØ	IHA generally healthy P.E. WNL
	A6ØØ	PHR
	A99Ø	Dx deferred (state features)
	A8Ø1	No demonstrable disease (explain)
	A8Ø2	Exam for certificate
	A128	Rx refill only
	AØØ3	Immunization only
	A8Ø3	Test results only
	AØ19	Positive family Hx (specify)
	A81Ø	Health education
	AØ2Ø	Abnormal tx result (specify)
	A8Ø4	Lab test not performed (specify)
	A811	Pt. left without being seen
	A812	Pt. refused Rx (specify)

THYROID

	B21Ø	Goiter
	B151	Hyperthyroid
	B152	Hypothyroid
	B153	Thyroid nodules (s)

ENDOCRINE METABOLIC

✓	A15Ø	Obesity would like to lose at least 10#
	B12Ø	Diabetes mellitus
	B18Ø	Hypoglycemia
	B16Ø	Hypercholesterolemia
	BØØ5	Hyperlipoproteinemia
	B178	Hyperuricemia
	NØ11	Gout

URINARY

	L1Ø1	Urinary tract infection
	L1ØØ	Bacteruria, asymptomatic
	L29Ø	Urethritis
	L22Ø	Benign prostatic hypertrophy
M	L993	Hematuria

OTHER DIAGNOSES

S/P	ODØ1	Appendectomy - 1957
	ODØ2	
	ODØ3	
	ODØ4	

FREE TEXT COMMENTS ON DIAGNOSES, PROBLEMS & PROCEDURES

DIAGNOSTIC CODE	Comments (6Ø characters each)
1. L993	No previous hx prior 1 wk. In process of evaluation.
2. ______	
3. ______	

FIGURE 8.2B. Harvard Community Health (HCHP) COSTAR encounter form. Back of internal medicine form. (From Policy Implications of Medical Information Systems, Office of Technology Assessment, 1977, p. 29.)

```
4782J          JOHN Q. ADAMS      M      76                   27 JAN 77

+++++++++++++++++++ OBJECTIVE DATA +++++++++++++++++++

MJKG4     BP                160/95 LYING
                            165/90 STANDING
MJKH7     PULSE             76
MJKL8     HEIGHT            69
MJKM3     WEIGHT            125

+++++++++++++++++++ DIAGNOSES/PROBLEMS +++++++++++++++++++

HDFC4 M HYPERTENSION, ESSENTIAL
          CONTINUE EXERCISE PROGRAM, GOOD COMPLIANCE WITH TREATMENT.

VDRR1   NEUROTIC DEPRESSION
          CHEWS FINGER-NAILS, OCCASIONAL RAPID-FIRE SNEEZING, SELDOM
          LASTING LONGER THAN TEN DAYS AT A TIME.

VCLM2   TOBACCO ADDICTION    HAS GIVEN UP FIGHTING AND IS SWITCHING.

GGKE2 > ABRASION     ICICLE FELL ON NOSE

+++++++++++++++++++ THERAPIES +++++++++++++++++++

TRSG3   DIET    - NO ADDED SALT

DFER9   CHLOROTHIAZIDE
          50 MG PO QD [11/12/76]
          (100 TAB, REFILL X3) [10/5/76]

PSCJ8 > REASSURANCE

+++++++++++++++++++ PROCEDURES +++++++++++++++++++

WSDR2 > APPLY DRESSING
          MAY HAVE SMALL SCAR ON NOSE

SPRS4   APPENDECTOMY [S/P:  1920]
          HAS SCAR IN RLQ -CLAIMS IS BIRTH-MARK

WAES3 * EKG    OCCASIONAL PVC, NON-SPECIFIC ST CHANGES

+++++++++++++++++ TESTS +++++++++++++++++++

WAUF6   CHOLESTEROL                 225
WASQ7 * URINALYSIS     FEW RBC AND CASTS IN SEDIMENT, 2+ PROTEIN
YJKL7   FBS                         95

 .    .    .    .    .    .    .    .    .    .    .    .    .    .
PODUNK MEDICAL CENTER ::  SCHEDULED :  LONG OFFICE VISIT
  RETURN VISIT - 6 MONTHS                          JOHN WARREN, M.D.
```

FIGURE 8.3. Sample COSTAR encounter report. (From COSTAR Functional Specifications, Version 5.3. MGH 4/15/1977.)

Although the Management Reports Module provides most of the outputs used for the standard reporting cycles, there also are occasional requirements for information that cannot be produced by the module. To satisfy this need, COSTAR supports a Medical Query Language (MQL) for ad hoc searches of the database. Most searches are used to identify groups of patients. The syntax of the search language is quite simple. A common form is:

```
WHEN <conditions> LIST <outputs>
```

For example:

```
WHEN SEX = MALE AND AGE > 40
LIST NAME,UNIT NUMBER,PRIMARY MD
```

```
                              CASE SUMMARY
PRIMARY PROV: JONES,WILLIAM J                      UN: DEMO-017
IMA-8                                              TEST,CASE
LAST VISIT: 5/18/83
ADDR: 121 LONGVIEW RD                              (M) 55 YRS  (4/22/28)
      APT 345                                      PH: 756-1111
      DORCHESTER,MA 02124                          OTHER PH: 793-9999 WK

DATE:________________ PROVIDER:__________________ SITE:______________
VISIT TYPE: [ ]NEW PT [ ]SCHED RTN [ ]UNSCHED RTN [ ]MED REFILL [ ]NO SHOW

REASON FOR VISIT:______________________________


HEALTH MAINTENANCE
  INFLUENZA VACCINE                                              9/10/82
  RECTAL GUAIAC    NEGATIVE                                       5/1/81

  CHECK & PROVIDE RESULTS IF DONE:

  GUAIAC:_____________________

  PNEUMOVAX:__________________

  FLU VACCINE:________________


ALLERGIES/SENSITIVITIES                              DATE FIRST ENTERED
* PENICILLIN ALLERGY                                             10/3/81
        AS CHILD, DETAILS VAGUE

MAJOR PROBLEMS
  ASTHMA                                                         10/3/81
        MINIMAL UPPER RESP INFECTION LAT WEEK; SOME DEGREE OF
        WHEEZING.                                              [3/18/83]

  HYPERTENSION                                                   10/3/81
        CONTINUES TO HAVE ELEVATED BP. NO HEADACHES. SEEMS TO BE
        CONCERNED ABOUT STARTING MEDICATION .  WILL KEEP CAREFUL
        NOTE OF EYE GROUNDS, MAY BE A THIRD HEART SOUND - CAN'T... [3/17/83]

  OBESITY                                                        10/3/81
        SIGNED UP WEIGHT-WATCHERS                                [3/8/83]

  ----------------------------------------------------------------------
  ----------------------------------------------------------------------
  ----------------------------------------------------------------------
  ----------------------------------------------------------------------
  ----------------------------------------------------------------------

OTHER PROBLEMS
  FOOT INJURY                                                     3/8/83
        STEPPED ON NAIL. SM PUNCT R FOOT -CLEAN.
  UPPER RESPIRATORY INFECTION                                    1/29/82
         1 WK COUGH, SOB, NO FEVER. USED OLD T.C.               [1/12/83]


STATUSES:  M/MAJOR     I/INACT     H/HO     R/RO     Y/SP     P/PRESUM
                  D/DO NOT DISPLAY      S/SHORT TERM PROBLEM
```

FIGURE 8.4. COSTAR case summary. (From Barnett, G.O., The Application of Computer-Based Medical-Record Systems in Ambulatory Practice, *NEJ Med*, 310: 1643-1650, 1984. Reprinted by permission.)

HYPERTENSION

TEST, MARY (F) 60 YRS UN: DEMO-031

DATE	WGT	BLOOD PRESSURE	BUN	CREA	URIC ACID	K+	MEDICATIONS
9/30/80		*160/110	*26	*1.7	8.2	3.7	HYDROCHLOROTHIAZIDE QAM 100MG PO CLONIDINE .4MG PO BID HYDRALAZINE 25MG PO BID
10/28/80	149	*154/96					
1/7/81	151	140/90					HYDRALAZINE 25MG PO 1 TAB BID QTY 100 X 1 YR REFILLS
2/17/81	147	*172/100					HYDRALAZINE 50MG PO BID
4/29/81	146	120/80					CLONIDINE 0.2MG 2 TABS BID QTY 200 X 1YR REFILLS
7/27/81	143	*140/100					
9/2/81	145	120/80	*28	*1.7	8.0	3.6	HYDROCHLOROTHIAZIDE 50MG BID CLONIDINE [DISC] [I] HYDRALAZINE [DISC] [I] METHYLDOPA (ALDOMET) 500MG BID
11/23/81	153	*180/100					HYDROCHLOROTHIAZIDE 50MG BID QTY 100 X 1YR REFILLS METHYLDOPA (ALDOMET) 500MG BID QTY 100 X 1YR REFILLS

FIGURE 8.5. COSTAR Hypertension Flow Chart. (From Barnett, G.O., The Application of Computer-Based Medical-Record Systems in Ambulatory Practice, *NEJ Med* 310: 1643-1650, 1984. Reprinted by permission.)

This search retrieves data from a two-dimensional space: patients and their attributes (SEX and AGE). Medical databases, however, are three dimensional. Time is always an important factor and all clinical data are normally identified by three index terms: the patient, the item, and the date. Note that there is a distinction between "the current diagnosis" and "the diagnosis at the time of a specific visit;" the value of the white blood cell count is meaningless without a time context. Thus, any medical query language must provide tools to manage this time context. The next example shows how MQL expresses the query to identify all male patients over 40 years of age with a diagnosis of hypertension noted by Dr. Smith during the last year:

```
WHEN SEX = MALE AND AGE OVER 40
  AND CODE = HYPERTENSION AND
  PROVIDER = SMITH AND DATE AFTER
  TODAY -1 YEAR
LIST NAME
```

A more complex time-dependent search might be for patients (a) with congestive heart failure, (b) who are on digitalis, digitoxin, or digoxin, (c) who are also on chlorothiazide, and (d) who have had a serum potassium value of < 3.0 recorded at least 1 month after an instance where chlorothiazide was noted as an active medication. Note that the four items may have been recorded at different dates and that a time relationship between only the last two is required. MQL uses a subcontext number appended to variable name to distinguish among the four times. The search thus becomes:

```
WHEN PATIENT
WHEN CODE1 = CONGESTIVE HEART FAILURE
WHEN CODE2 = DIGITALIS
  OR = DIGITOXIN
  OR = DIGOXIN
WHEN CODE3 = CHLOROTHIAZIDE
  AND STATUS3 IS NOT INACTIVE
        WHEN CODE4 = SERUM POTASSIUM AND VALUE4<3.0
WHEN DATE4 IS AFTER DATE3+1 MONTH
LIST NAME
NEXT PATIENT
```

From this brief discussion it can be seen that MQL provides a powerful tool to query the COSTAR database. The basic rules are limited in number and a user—with a knowledge of the attributes (e.g., CODE,PROVIDER,SEX) and values (HYPERTENSION,SMITH,MALE)—can present powerful queries with little effort. Unfortunately, the descriptive simplicity can result in valid queries that do not produce what is desired. For example, AGE is defined to be the patient's current age (TODAY–DATE OF BIRTH). A query for all patients age 5 years or younger diagnosed as having a specific disease at the date of their visit should not use AGE < 5 as a predicate. (AGE <5 means patients who are currently under 5 independent of their age at the time of the visit.) Naturally, this problem of incorrect queries is not limited to MQL. All query languages face the dilemma of choosing between ease of use and explicitness to avoid conceptual ambiguity.

This concludes the brief overview of COSTAR. We began showing how data could be captured and stored to produce a completely automated medical record. Records may be printed and discarded; the source is always available in the computer. The flow—print materials for encounter, record new data during and after encounter, and update automated files—was described. Finally, we noted that, although the primary objective was to maintain timely and accurate data about individual patients, the result was a large database that could be used for routine reporting or ad hoc queries. In the following subsections, several other AAMRSs will be described. They differ only in the needs of their users and the objectives and styles of their developers. However, there are more similarities to the COSTAR model than there are differences.

8.3.2. The Regenstrief Medical Record System

The Regenstrief Medical Record System (RMRS) presents an example of an AAMRS that has been in operational use for over 10 years in a teaching hospital. It differs from COSTAR in that (a) it does not relace the paper record but (b) it adds a reminder system. As McDonald put it:

> Physicians err. Government agencies and medical societies have attempted to reduce such errors with educational and motivational (Professional Standards Review Organizations) programs, with little success. We have argued that informational overload is responsible for many medical errors and have used a computerized reminder system to reduce such errors.[5]

To provide an information-rich environment to support the encounter, RMRS prepares three documents in anticipation of each visit:[6]

- *Patient Encounter Form.* This is a document on two part paper that (a) reports key data about the patient and (b) serves as an input document to update the database. It also contains the progress note which is filed in the paper medical record.
- *Flowsheet Summary.* This is in a standard flow sheet format. It contains time-ordered patient data stored in the clinical database; the specific contents may be modified for different practices.
- *Quality Assurance Report.* This is a set of reminders that are printed as the result of comparing the patient's data against a set of rules written by a physician.

A sample Encounter Form is shown in Fig. 8.6. This type of form is used by most AAMRSs. Since only a portion of the patient data will be retained in the AAMR, a paper record also is required. The appointment system is used to print out the encounter form. This form may supplement (or serve as a temporary surrogate for) the paper record. The progress note is written on the form. After the encounter, the top sheet is filed with the paper medical record, and the copy is routed for data entry. (Since COSTAR has a fully automated record, the record is printed prior to a visit and the encounter form is used only as a data entry form.)

Although the flow of the RMRS encounter forms is typical for most AAMRSs, its contents are not. The form is divided into four sections. In the upper left there is a place to record clinical observations. Some data are collected for all patients (e.g., WEIGHT) whereas others are collected for only specific patients. In this case, the patient is known to be using digoxin and so PND and edema were added as additional observations to be made. (Unfortunately, the two shades

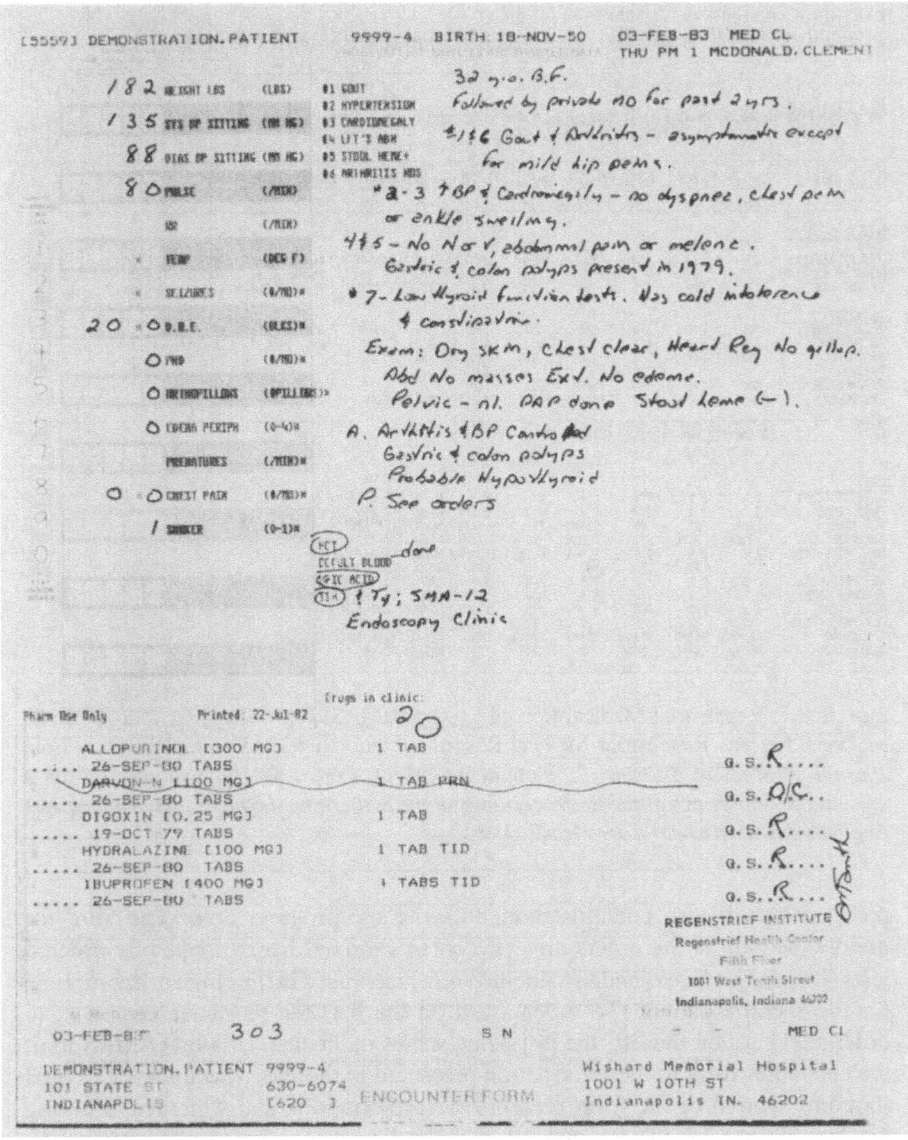

FIGURE 8.6. Regenstrief Medical Record System (RMRS) Encounter Form. (From C. McDonald et al., Regenstrief Medical Record System. Reprinted with permission from *Journal of Medical Systems,* 7, Plenum Publishing Corp., © 1983; modified from a version previously published in *Proceedings of the Sixth Annual Symposium on Computer Applications in Medical Care,* IEEE, 1982.)

of salmon on the form record as two shades of gray in Fig. 8.6, and some of the printing is obscured.) These data will be added to the data collected from other sources (e.g., clinical laboratory results) and displayed in the flowsheet.

The second section of the form, the upper right hand corner, contains the

BIRTHDAY 06-DEC-09 [5559]

WISHARD MEMORIAL HOSPITAL ¦DEMONSTRATION.PATIENT #9999-4

DX & COMPLAINTS

DX & COMPLAINT 10-AUG-79 HYPERTENSION, CARDIOMEGALY, LFT'S ABN, STOOL HEME+, ARTHRITIS NOS
13-OCT-78 GOUT, HYPERTENSION, CARDIOMEGALY

CLINIC DATA	26-SEP -80	16-MAY -80	19-OCT -79	07-SEP -79	10-AUG -79	22-JUN -79	16-MAR -79	13-OCT -78	18-AUG -78	10-MAR -78		
VITALS												
PULSE	72	82	80	68	72	.	.	80	.	85	/MIN	(60-100)
SYS BP SITTING	136	160	130	138	134	180*H	150	140	180*H	140	MM HG	(100-160)
DIAS BP SITTIN	90	84	72	84	80	110*H	84	90	100*H	80	MM HG	(60-90)
WEIGHT LBS	196	196	195	200	200	200	201*H	198	206*H	210*H	LBS	(50-200)
TREATMENTS												
ALLOPURINOL	300	300	300	300	300	300	300	300	300	300	MG	
COLCHICINE	D/C	1.3	0.6	0.6	0.6	1.3	0.6	1.3	1.3	1.3	MG	
DARVON-N	300	300	30	30	30	30	30	.	.	.	MG	
DIGOXIN	.	.	0.250	.	.	0.500	.	.	.	0.500	MG	
HYDRALAZINE	100	100	100	100	100	100	75	75	75	75	MG	
IBUPROFEN	1600	1600	1600	1600	1600	1600	1600	1600	1600	1600	MG	

SMA12	16-MAR -79	18-AUG -78	16-SEP -77	10-SEP -76	16-JUL -76	23-MAY -75		
SMA12								
CALCIUM (SMA)	9.4	9.8	9.8	9.8	9.4	9.7	MG/DL	(8.4-10.6)
PHOS (SMA)	3.2	3.1	3.7	2.7	2.9	5.2*H	MG/DL	(2.5-4.8)
GLU (SMA)	60*L	90	85	113*H	100	138*H	MG/DL	(70-110)
BUN (SMA)	24*H	27*H	21	29*H	22	26*H	MG/DL	(7-22)
URIC ACID (SMA	5.1	5.4	5.5	9.4*H	8.2*H	>12.0*H	MG/DL	(2.6-7.1)
CHOL (SMA)	173	190	183	187	200	175	MG/DL	(120-280)
TOT PROT (SMA)	7.8	8.1	7.9	7.9	7.8	8.0	G/DL	(6.4-8.2)
ALBUMIN (SMA)	4.2	4.1	4.2	4.2	4.0	3.7*L	G/DL	(3.8-4.8)
BILI (SMA)	0.4	0.5	0.5	0.6	0.5	1.3*H	MG/DL	(0.0-1.0)
ALK PHOS (SMA)	90	75	82	92	77	86	UNITS	(25-115)
LDH (SMA)	286*H	215*H	300*H	250*H	220*H	178	UNITS	(100-190)
SGOT (SMA)	47*H	46*H	54*H	39	26	38	UNITS	(8-40)

FIGURE 8.7. Regenstrief Medical Record System (RMRS) Flow Sheet Section. (From C. McDonald et al., Regenstrief Medical Record System. Reprinted with permission from *Journal of Medical Systems,* 7, Plenum Publishing Corp., © 1983; modified from a version previously published in *Proceedings of the Sixth Annual Symposium on Computer Applications in Medical Care,* IEEE, 1982.)

problem list. It also contains room to write the progress note. The third (or middle) section is the orders area. It contains a fixed list of frequently ordered tests. It may also be expanded to include other tests used in the clinic or appropriate for the specific patient. To order a test on the list, the physician circles it; to order a test not on the list, the physician writes in the test. (Many AAMRS limit the encounter form to the information presented in these two sections.) The final (bottom) section of the form presents the prescriptions that were active during the last clinic visit. These may be reordered or discontinued; the sig may be changed to modify the prescription; or new prescriptions may be written in.

The specific contents of a patient's encounter form are defined by the computer system at the time of printing. By referencing physicians' written protocols, the RMRS determines what parameters are to be displayed in the clinical observation section, what orders are to be presented in the order section, and even what diagnoses should be added to the diagnostic list.

A portion of a flowsheet is shown in Fig. 8.7. Data are organized in blocks that are decomposed into groups (e.g., VITALS) of individual parameters. The selection of blocks may vary with the practice or the status of an individual patient. Many systems that support flowsheets provide similar capabilities. The

```
SURVEILLANCE REPORT   DEMONSTRATION PATIENT   9999-4   BORN 18-NOV-50

Please record weight, PND, exercise tolerance, etc. in space allocated on
Encounter Form to document effect of change (-0.25) on 19-OCT-79) of
digitalis dose.

All women should have at least 2 annual CERVICAL PAP tests on record.
It has been more than a year since this patient's first test which was
done on 16-MAY-80.

Consider use of TSH to distinguish primary from secondary hypothyroidism
and/or to interpret borderline low T4 INDEX of 2.5 on 16-MAR-79.
```

FIGURE 8.8. Regenstrief Medical Record System (RMRS) Quality Assurance Report. (From C. McDonald et al., Regenstrief Medical Record System. Reprinted with permission from *Journal of Medical Systems,* 7, Plenum Publishing Corp., © 1983; modified from a version previously published in *Proceedings of the Sixth Annual Symposium on Computer Applications in Medical Care,* IEEE, 1982.

obvious advantage of the flowsheet is that it presents time-oriented data in a two-dimensional display. One can look for changes and trends rather than consider a parameter as a single number.

The ability to produce a flow sheet implies that the clinical data are available in the patient's database. In many cases these data are stored as panels in a format to facilitate display. (This is common in the HIS where results reporting is performed by treating the test result as a text string, e.g., the CBC result is processed as two lines of comments.) Where access is available to the values of the individual data elements, these data can be used to establish patient-specific recommendations. These recommendations—the quality assurance reports—are the third documents printed by RMRS for each encounter (Fig. 8.8). These reports are a variation of the alerts produced by HELP. In the case of HELP, the patient parameters are scanned against a set of physician defined interactions that will initiate an alert. With RMRS, the patient data are matched against physician defined interactions which produce a reminder. In the sample shown, the first message reminds the provider why data not previously supplied are necessary for the evaluation of this patient. The remaining two messages make recommendations for the current encounter. This Surveillance Report is used as a reminder and is discarded after the encounter. As we shall see in the following section, the provision of such reports strongly influences physician behavior.

For each encounter, RMRS produces documents that include both standard outputs and information tailored to the needs of a specific patient. To support this processing RMRS used a locally developed database system (RDB) and a query language for the medical records (CARE). As in the case of the COSTAR MQL, one may use CARE to produce reports from searches. The meaning of the following statement should be obvious:

```
REPORT PATIENT'S NAME AND ADDRESS IF
SEX = "M" AND (TODAY-BIRTHDATE/365) GT 40.
```

Yet CARE was defined to do considerably more than retrieve data from a clinical database; it was developed to describe the rules of practice (i.e., protocols) so that the computer could process these rules automatically (i.e., quality assurance).

In this sense, it is a schema for capturing medical knowledge. In Chapter 9 we shall see how HELP and some expert systems perform similar functions, and in Chapter 10 we shall detail how protocol-directed care is managed by OCIS. In what follows we briefly describe how CARE records queries for surveillance purposes.

One general form of a CARE statement is

```
IF <parameter> <condition> THEN <action>
```

where parameter is a term in a dictionary and condition is generally a verb. For example, to take an action if a potassium value has been recorded for a patient, one might write:

```
IF "K" EXISTS THEN <action>
```

Because CARE was designed to be used by physicians, it attempts to produce understandable statements. One way of doing this is to allow several verbs for the same condition. In the last example, IS, ARE, WAS, WERE, EXIST, and OCCURRED have the same meaning as EXISTS; the most appropriate sounding verb was used. For the purposes of surveillance, most of the actions will specify the text to be printed on the report. For example:

```
IF "AGE" WAS GT 65 AND TODAY IS AFTER 9/15 & BEFORE 12/31
THEN consider the use of flu vaccine
```

As was mentioned when discussing MQL, the complexity of medical query languages results from the need to establish time relationships among complicated sets of conditions. CARE has conditional verbs to establish time relationships and uses a DEFINE verb to reduce complexity. (MQL has a similar facility.) For example, the statements that would produce the quality assurance message that there is no documentation within the record of a measure of T4 index following the last change in levothyroxin dosage might be written:

```
DEFINE "THYROXIN CHANGE" AS LAST CHANGE [NE 0] OF
  "LEVOTHYROXIN" EXISTS
IF "THYROXIN LAST" WAS GT 0 AND NO "T4 INDEX" WAS
  AFTER "THYROXIN CHANGE"
  THEN SAVE
```

CARE can also be used to perform computations. To find the average serum SGOT level in the first year following the start of therapy, as might be of interest in a drug toxicity study, one could define a query similar to the following:

```
DEFINE "INH START" AS FIRST "INH" EXISTS
IF AVERAGE OF "SGOT" [AFTER "INH START" & BEFORE "INH
  START" + 1 YEAR] EXISTS
  THEN SAVE AS "INH.SGOT"
```

The result would be a record for each patient who had a serum SGOT level within the first year of INH treatment. The record would contain the average value of the SGOT during that year stored in a field called "INH.SGOT."

The language also accommodates verbs such as CHANGE, %CHANGE, INTERVAL and functions such as SIN, COS, LOG, and EXP. Finally, it allows the nesting of statements in a block structure to manage more complex queries and conditions.

RMRS currently manages a database of 60,000 patient records. The Quality Assurance (Surveillance) Reports are based on a knowledge base of over 1,400 rules written in CARE. The system has been in operational use since 1974, and the first evaluation of the effect of the Surveillance Reports on physician behavior was published in 1976. It also has been successfully installed at a second site, in Wilford Hall Medical Center in San Antonio, Texas. Thus, RMRS illustrates one very practical way in which a patient database can be used to support the process and improve the quality of care.

8.3.3. The Medical Record

The third AAMRS to be briefly described is The Medical Record (TMR) developed by Hammond and Stead. This system, like the previous two, was reviewed in both the initial and follow-up AAMRS studies. The system was developed for use by the Duke University Department of Community Health Sciences; it also has been transported to other institutions and is available as a commercial product. The system version that has received the most study is that of the Durham Veterans Administration Hospital Renal Dialysis Unit and Nephrology Clinic.

TMR provides tools for supporting the medical, administrative and financial needs of the organization. Although its goal is to replace the manual medical record, most implementations simply supplement it with an AAMR. The system produces well-formatted data in the form of encounter forms and flow sheets. The pharmacy subsystems can do things such as generate lists of patients whose medicines will expire on a given date, prepare prescriptions giving dosage choices, and calculate the day the prescription will run out. There are reports that can be used for both health and financial review. In general, the design is modular and comprehensive; users are expected to select from existing facilities. Naturally, special reports can be created to meet specialized needs. Fig. 8.9 contains a portion of the pre-encounter form used in the Nephrology Clinic.[7] It is supplemented by text notes and a flow sheet. The report in Fig. 8.10 illustrates how the coded data stored in the TMR database can be combined with occasional text modifications to produce a natural language output.

8.3.4. Cardiovascular Clinic System

The TMR previously presented is a general system that—in the example shown—has been installed in a specialty clinic. In this section we simply identify a system designed for a private specialty practice. It is unique among AAMRSs in that it

```
THE NEPHROLOGY SERVICE                                  * BROWN
Category: HOME HEMO/                              RV    *  CHARLES F.
 Primary MD: WILLIAM STEAD     4-100              WWS * 12 SHULTZ BLVD.
 Occupation:                                            *  PATTFORD, GH.   21456
   Employer:                                            *002-123-1234
                                                        *  Birthdate: 11/23/32
                                                        * 999-99-9977
Appointment: 14:30 - WILLIAM STEAD                      *
                                                        *  48 yo wh div male
10/12/81 10:07                                          ***************************

  ONSET   RESOLVED SEEN CODE        ALL PROBLEMS
04/23/70 04/24/70  __    189 APPENDECTOMY
01/23/72 ________  __      6 GLOMERULONEPHRITIS-MEMB
05/02/76 06/05/77  __    164   NEPHROTIC SYNDROME
02/15/81 ________  __     18   RENAL FAILURE (CHRONIC)
02/15/81 ________  __      1     HYPERTENSION-DIASTOLIC
02/15/81 ________  __    125     ANEMIA
02/15/81 ________  __    132     ACIDOSIS (METABOLIC)
06/25/81 ________  __    169     DIALYSIS THERAPY

________ ________  __  ____  ______________________________________

________ ________  __  ____  ______________________________________

  SUBJ/PHY      DATE      LAST VALUE                       TODAY'S VALUE
PRURITIS    09/10/81            MLD        MLD; MOD; SEV; N
NAUSEA      09/10/81              N        YN ____________________________
PAIN FLK                                   RT; LT; BILAT; N
WT          09/10/81           74 KG       #  ____________________________
WT DRY      09/10/81           74 KG       #  ____________________________
TEMP                              C        #  ____________________________
PULSE SIT                         MIN      #  ____________________________
BP SIT      09/10/81       140/90 MM       #/# ___________________________
ART NAR     09/10/81            MOD        MLD; MOD, SEV; N
EDEMA PED   09/10/81              0        0-4 ___________________________
RFLEX AKR   09/10/81              2        0-4 ___________________________
VIB LE      03/25/81             NL        INC; DEC; NL
KARNOF      03/25/81             95 %      #  ____________________________
__________ ________________________ :  __________ ______________
__________ ________________________ :  __________ ______________

---------------------------CURRENT THERAPIES--------------------------
        THERAPY                               DISP  RF    START      END
BASALJEL 620 MG C                              360   1  06/25/81  11/09/81  S R C
        3 QID /C MEALS & SNACK
CALCITRIOL .25 MCG C                            30   2  05/02/81  12/09/81  S R C
        1 QAM
TABRON 1  T                                     60   2  06/25/81  12/09/81  S R C
        1 BID
FLUOXYMESTERONE 10 MG T                         90   2  06/25/81  12/09/81  S R C
        3 QAM
TRIMEPRAZINE TARTRATE 2.5 MG T                  30   2  09/10/81  12/09/81  S R C
        1 Q6H PRN ITCHING
DIOCTYL NA SULFOSUCCINATE 100 MG C             120   2  02/15/81  12/09/81  S R C
        2 PO BID
```

FIGURE 8.9. The Medical Record (TMR) Preencounter Form. (From Stead WW, Hammond WE, Straub MJ. *J Med Syst* 7,2:103–109, 1983. Reprinted with permission from Plenum Press.)

was developed and supported by the practice, has been in operational use since the early 1970s, and provides a complete medical record designed for the practice's special patient population. A sample patient profile and hypertension flow sheet are shown in Figs. 8.11(A, B).[8] Note that these forms were in operational use almost a decade ago.

8.3.5. ARAMIS

The American Rheumatism Association Medical Information System (ARAMIS), as its name implies, was also designed for a specialized patient population.

THORACIC SURGERY SERVICE
DUKE UNIVERSITY MEDICAL CENTER

BROWN, CHARLIE
R99999
RANKIN, JS
SURGERY
06/22/84

OPERATIVE NOTE - CORONARY ARTERY BYPASS GRAFTING

NAME: BROWN, CHARLIE DATE OF SURGERY: 06/22/84
HX#: R99999 SSN: 000-00-0000
DIAGNOSIS: Coronary artery disease
PROCEDURE: CABG X 6
SURGEON: J. SCOTT RANKIN, M.D. ASSISTANT: WILLIAM L HOLMAN, M.D.
ANESTHESIOLOGIST: PAOLO FLEZZANI, M.D.

CLINICAL HISTORY:

The patient was a 53 year old male with ischemic heart disease. The patient had 3 vessel disease. Indication for operation was unstable angina. At surgery, he was NYHA Class IV. Ejection fraction was 54%. The patient was taken to surgery directly from the CCU. The operation was performed as a re-do procedure.

OPERATIVE PROCEDURE:

While monitoring the electrocardiogram and arterial blood pressure, the patient was anesthetized with Fentanyl and Halothane, positioned, prepared, and draped as a sterile field. A median sternotomy was performed, and the grafts were dissected from both legs. The pre-bypass period was characterized by arrhythmias. Heparin was administered, and the venae cavae were cannulated for arterial inflow and venous return. Cardiopulmonary bypass was begun at 10:17, and right superior pulmonary vein decompression was used. Coronary dissection was performed. The left ventricle was inspected and found to have a single scar. The aortic cross-clamp was applied after 101 minutes on the pump, and Plegisol cardioplegia was administered. Inflow temperature during cross-clamp was 20 degrees C., and the minimum esophageal temperature was 16 degrees C. Topical cooling was accomplished with pericardial lavage. Minimum myocardial temperature was 7 degrees C. The following grafts were completed:

	PD	RCPL1	LAD PROX	DIAG1	OD 1	CMA 1
ORDER OF GRAFTS	4	5	1	6	2	3
PROBE SIZE (MM)	1.2	1.5	1	1.5	1.54	1.5
ARTERY (GRAFT) QUALITY	fair	good	poor	good	fair	fair
ENDARTERECTOMY	no	no	no	no	no	no
BALLOON DILATATION	no	no	no	no	no	no
SUTURE MATERIAL	7/0 pr	7/0 pr	7/0 pr	7/0 pr	7/0 pr	7/0 pr
TECHNIQUE OF SUTURING	run	run	run	run	run	run
VEIN QUALITY	good	good	good	mamm	good	good

The optional diagonal 1 and circumflex marginal artery 1 arteries were bypassed with a sequential graft. The posterior descending and right coronary posterolateral 1 arteries were bypassed with a sequential graft. The total volume of cardioplegia administered was 2100 ml. After rewarming was begun, the aorta was unclamped. Clamp time was 111 minutes. One defibrillation was required. 3 proximal anastamoses were performed during the re-perfusion period. Both atrial and ventricular pacing wires were placed. After adequate rewarming, the ventricular vent was removed, and cardiopulmonary bypass was

FIGURE 8.10. Sample text report from The Medi al Record (TMR) database. (From Hammond W.E., personal correspondence. Reprinted with permission.)

```
                    CARDIOVASCULAR CLINIC PATIENT MEDICAL INFORMATION
                                      JUN 28, 1976

NONAME, JOHN    (N00000)                              ROBBINS
123 NW 45                                             SEX: M
TEST CITY, OKLA   73112                               BIRTH DATE: DEC 31, 1924
PHONE: 999-9999                                       STATUS: BYO
------------------------------------------------------------------------------
THE FOLLOWING INFORMATION WAS LAST REVIEWED DURING THE PATIENT'S
VISIT ON SEP 2, 1975.
------------------------------------------------------------------------------
                               PROBLEMS AND MEDICATIONS

PROBLEMS
   DUODENAL ULCER (UGI)                          12/27/74    1968
   HYPERCHOLESTEROLEMIA                          12/27/74
   FEMORAL POPLITEAL DISEASE                     12/27/74
   MYOCARDIAL INFARCTION                         12/27/74    ACUTE
   DRUG ALLERGY                                  12/27/74    PENICILLIN
   HYPERTENSION                                  12/27/74
   VENTRICULAR FIBRILLATION                      01/09/75
   ANGINA PECTORIS                               01/09/75    MILD
                                                 03/14/75    NONE - 1 MO
   SELECTIVE CORONARY ARTERIOGRAM                02/06/75    LAD ST. 90%, RC OCCL
   RENAL ARTERIOGRAM                             02/06/75    NORMAL
   HYPERTENSION PROTOCOL                         12/04/75

MEDICATIONS
   ISORDIL                    5 MG QID                        01/09/75
   PRONESTYL                  500 MG QID                      01/09/75
   DIUCARDIN                  50 MG BID                       02/13/75
   INDERAL                    40 MG QID                       03/14/75
   ZAROXOLYN                  5 MG QD                         11/12/75
   DYAZIDE                    1  BID                          12/04/75

------------------------------------------------------------------------------
                                   PRESENT ILLNESS

LAST PRESENT ILLNESS (03-14-75): SO FAR NO MORE ANGINA PECTORIS.  TOLERATING
     MEDICATION WELL BUT BP CONTROL STILL NOT ADEQUATE.  ELECTED TO
     INCREASE INDERAL.

------------------------------------------------------------------------------
                               HISTORICAL RISK FACTORS
                                    INFARCTION
            EXP ALIVE HYP CVA <39 40-50 >50 HD  DM  CAB CAC MAL
MOTHER      63         1   1
FATHER      78                        1         1
BROTHER(S)       3                    1
SISTER(S)

MARITAL STATUS: MARRIED                      SOCIO-ECON. TYPE: MIDDLE
WORK TYPE: SEDENTARY                         EXERCISE PROGRAM: NONE
HOME: LIVES WITH OTHERS                      DISABILITY RATING: 4D

END OF REPORT
```

FIGURE 8.11A. Output from cardiovascular clinic system. (From Rodnick J. The use of automated ambulatory medical records. *J. Fam Pract* 5(2), 1977. Copyright 1977, Appleton-Century-Crofts. Reprinted with permission.)

Unlike the AAMRSs considered previously, ARAMIS maintains a national database that is used primarily for research. It is one of the first systems to implement a time-oriented databank (TOD, Fries and Wiederhold) and was included in the 1975 AAMRS study. Because the goal of ARAMIS is research, data are collected at each encounter, recorded on forms, and sent to the national center for processing. This flow cannot support the printing of encounter forms or provide

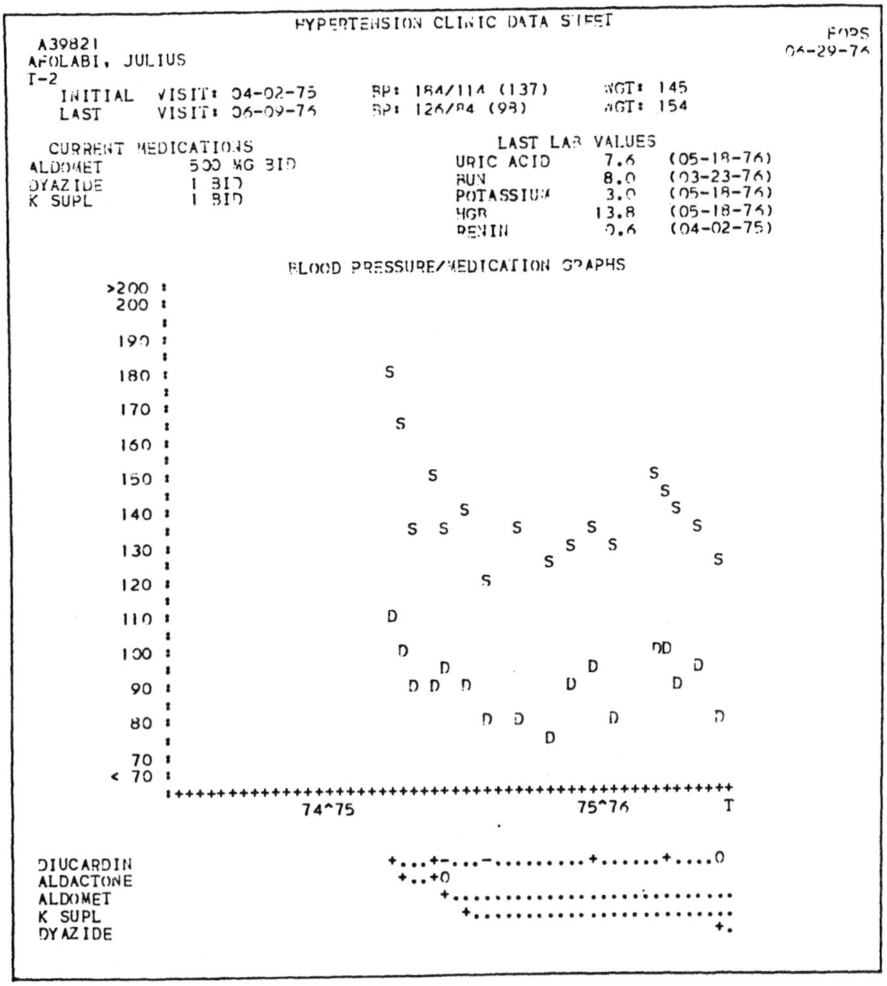

FIGURE 8.11B. Output from cardiovascular clinic system. (From Rodnick J. The use of automated ambulatory medical records. *J. Fam Pract* 5(2), 1977. Copyright 1977, Appleton-Century-Crofts. Reprinted with permission.)

timely access to a patient's data. However, the availability of a large database allows one to analyze how a group of patients responds to therapy. For example,[9] the output in Fig. 8.12 shows the outcomes for a group of 40 patients who were identified as having the same diagnosis (RA), sex, age group, and Wintrobe sedimentation rate as the patient Jane Doe.* This report can also be formatted as a natural language report similar to that shown in Figure 8.10.

*HELP provides an extension of this capability, see Chapter 9.

OUTPUT FROM LD:AUTOSET

Jane Doe
Medical Record Number: 654321
Date: SEP 8, 1976
Referring Physician: A. Harlow
Ward or Clinic: ARAMIS

Stanford University Hospital
Stanford, California 94305
COMPUTER PROGNOSTIC ANALYSIS

40 patients have been selected with the following criteria:

Diagnosis: RA	Patient value	Range used for selection			
Sex	0	0	to	0	(code)
Age of pt. to date	45.0	25:0	to	68:0	(years)
Wintrobe Sedimentation Rate	20:0	3:00	to	38:0	(mm/hr)

CLINICAL FINDINGS

Age (mean) 45.4 years
Sex: 0 male, 40 female

Arthritis (% of patients)	100.0	%	
Symmetry of Arthritis (% of patients)	72.5	%	
PIP Involved (% of patients)	82.5	%	
Wrists Involved (% of patients)	77.5	%	
Knees Involved (% of patients)	65.0	%	
Subcutaneous Nodules (% of patients)	20.0	%	
Dry eyes (% of patients)	12.5	%	
Hematocrit (mean)	41.1	%	(+/- 5.23)
White blood count (mean)	8.35	x1000/cumm	(+/- 3.42)
Sedimentation rate (mean)	22.4	mm/hr	(+/- 9.54)
Grip strength (mean)	232	mmHg	(+/- 149)
FANA: % patients	27.5	%	mean titer 1:94
Latex Fixation: % patients	57.5	%	mean titer 1:638

THERAPY

Drug	# Pts.	Mean Dose	Associated Therapy	Subsequent Therapy
Aspirin	22	17.0 tabs/day	Plaq(2)Indo(2)	Pred(1)Buta(2)Indo(1)
Prednisone	14	12.1 mgm/day	ASA(11)Plaq(2)Indo(1)	Indo(3)ASA(2)Plaq(2)*

Other Therapy (6):
Indomethacin(3),OH-Chlor(2),Pred + Aza(1)

OUTCOME

Per cent of patients experiencing each event.

End Event

ASPIRIN GROUP	1	2	4	6	8	10	12	14	16	18
Death (cumulative %)	0	0	0	0	0	0	0	0	0	0
Arthritis, exacerbated (%)	27	27	43	43	43	43	43	43	43	43
Arthritis, remission (%)	0	0	0	0	0	0	0	0	0	0
MCP joint improvement (%)	14	19	19	19	19	19	19	19	19	19
Prednisone, increased (%)	0	0	0	0	0	0	0	0	0	0
Neuropathy, observed (%)	5	5	5	5	5	5	5	5	5	5
Patients followed (number)	22	15	10	6	5	4	4	3	2	2

(Months)

PREDNISONE GROUP	1	2	4	6	8	10	12	14	16	18
Death (cumulative %)	0	0	0	0	0	0	0	0	0	0
Arthritis, exacerbated (%)	7	7	7	7	7	7	7	7	7	7
Arthritis, remission (%)	7	7	7	7	7	7	7	7	7	7
MCP joint improvement (%)	7	15	26	26	26	26	26	26	26	26
Prednisone, increased (%)	7	7	7	7	7	7	7	7	7	7
Neuropathy, observed (%)	14	14	14	14	14	14	14	14	14	14
Patients followed (number)	14	10	9	6	6	6	4	4	2	1

FIGURE 8.12. Sample output from the American Rheumatism Association Medical Information System (ARAMIS) Summary Time-Oriented Record.

8.3.6. The SCAMP System

SCAMP was developed by Shapiro as a tool for practice management which also would allow primary care physicians to perform research. It is in use at five large family medical clinics and a private practice. The features of SCAMP that add to those that have been previously described are (a) the use of natural language and (b) the incorporation of medical knowledge.[10]

SCAMP allows the user to write queries in free text. For example:

HOW MANY VISITS WERE THERE IN THE CLINIC LAST YEAR?

The query

LIST MY PATIENTS WHO NEED FLU SHOTS.

assumes that the eligibility for the vaccine has been entered into the patient's record. The query then matches patient, eligibility, and immunization history to produce a response. This next question, however, requires more knowledge:

TELL ME THE NAMES OF PATIENTS WHO DEVELOPED ADVERSE DRUG REACTIONS WITHIN ONE MONTH AFTER TAKING ONE OF THE SHORT-ACTING ANTI-ANXIETY AGENTS.

In this case "adverse drug reactions" and "short-acting anti-anxiety agents" must be defined. SCAMP provides dictionaries of classes, subclasses, and supraclasses for problems, lab tests, and immunizations.

The system also allows the user to encode rules for surveillance or retrieval. Rule definition and editing are controlled by a menu driven program; emphasis is placed on a user-friendly interface. Here is a listing for a rule to ensure that the patient's blood pressure is recorded at least once a year.

THIS RULE WILL SELECT PATIENTS WHO:
(1) HAVE THE PROBLEM 'HYPERTENSION, UNCOMPLICATED': AND
(2) HAVE NOT HAD A BLOOD PRESSURE MEASUREMENT WITHIN 365 DAYS.
IF A PATIENT MEETS ALL OF THE ABOVE CONDITIONS, HIS APPOINTMENT WILL BE FLAGGED WITH THE MESSAGE 'CHECK BP: NO BP IN PAST YEAR.'

Next is a rule that establishes a time relationship between prescriptions, laboratory values, and problems in the record text. This might be used to produce a report.

THIS RULE WILL LOCATE THE PATIENTS WHO:
(1) RECEIVED CHLORTHALIDONE FOR TREATMENT OF 'HYPERTENSION': AND
(2) HAD A SERUM POTASSIUM LESS THAN 3.3 WITHIN 8 WEEKS AFTER AN RX FOR CHLORTHALIDONE: AND
(3) HAD THE CONCEPT 'HYPOKALEMIA' MENTIONED IN THEIR RECORD WITHIN 2 WEEKS BEFORE OR 2 WEEKS AFTER THE PRESENCE OF A POTASSIUM LESS THAN 3.3

It will be noted that these features of SCAMP are identical to functions available in RMRS; they differ only in their orientation to the users.

NAME: STOREONE.TEST CLINIC: RDC PART A
UNIT NUMBER: 85 72 81-0 BIRTHDATE: / /

DATE CLINIC PROVIDER			8-28-80 TO 10-02-80	10-23-80 RDC A363	11-13-80 RDC X000	12-24-80 TO 1-25-81	3-12-81 RDC A363	4-09-81 RDC A363	5-21-81 RDC A363	06-23-81 RDC
PROBLEMS/MANIFESTATIONS	**ONSET***	**UNITS***								
1. SYSTEM LUPUS ERYTH	1976	0-3			0		0		INACTIVE	
2. ARTHRALGIA 567	10/80	0-3 SCALE			2		1		0	
3. LUPUS PROFUNDUS RASH	10/80	0-3			3		1		0	
4. MESANGIAL PROLIF GN	10/80									
5. HIGH BLOOD PRESSURE	1977	MM HG		120/90	120/90		100/70		130/85	
6. BURSITIS		0-3			2		1		1	
7. OBESITY	REMOTE	LBS		210	209		192			
12. UPPER RESPIRATORY INF	5/21/81									
THERAPIES	**ROUTE***	**UNITS***								
1 PREDISONE	PO	MG			15 QOD		5 QD	5 QOD	0	
2 LASIX	PO	MG		80 BID	80 BID				80 BID	
3 INDOCIN	PO	MG		25 TID	25 TID				25 BID	
4 KENALOG	IM	MG		40 Q MONTH	40 Q MONTH					
5 PROPANOLOL	PO	MG		80 BID	80 BID				80 BID	
6 TNG	SL	1/150 GR	PRN			PRN				
LABORATORY		**UNITS***								
434 ANTI-DS DNA ANTIBODY		NG/25 MC	7.8		10.8	3.1	4.0	15.1	18.3	
473 COMPLMNT. TOT (CH50)		CH 50 U	36.5		35.2	34.0		37.8	36.8	
365 PROTEIN .UR						NEG	1+	1+	TR	
368 HEMOGLOBIN .UR						NEG	NEG	NEG	NEG	
369 WBCS .UR		/HPF				<2	2-5	2-5	2-5	
370 RBCS .UR		/HPF				<2	2-5	2-5	2-5	
902 POTASSIUM		MEQ/L	4.2			4.3				
BLANK SPACES										

FIGURE 8.13A. Sample Summary Time-Oriented Record (STOR) Record. Principal patient data.

8.3.7. Summary Time-Oriented Record

The Summary Time-Oriented Record (STOR, Simborg and Whiting-O'Keefe) is an interesting variation on the previous AAMRSs. In this case, the encounter form is presented as a time-oriented flow sheet. Most systems use flow sheets to display clinical data. (Examples were presented for COSTAR and RMRS.) STOR also presents the problems and medications summary in a time oriented format.[11] Fig. 8.13 displays a sample form that is generated prior to the encounter. Part A contains the principal patient data. The right-hand column is blank and provides a space for recording observations and data for the current encounter. Part B contains problems or therapies deemed inactive or of less importance by the physician. The assignment of data to part A or B is done by the provider after each encounter.

8.3.8. The Oncology Clinical Information System

Each of the systems presented was designed for ambulatory care. The Johns Hopkins Oncology Clinical Information System (OCIS, Blum and Lenhard) is

```
NAME: STOREONE,TEST              CLINIC: RDC                    PART B
UNIT NUMBER:  85 72 81-0         BIRTHDATE:  /  /

*************************************************************************************************
***PROBLEMS/MANIFESTATIONS*** **ONSET***   ***UNITS***   *LAST DATA** **************   **DATE**   PRVR CLIN
-------------------------------------------------------------------------------------------------
  8  ANGINA PECTORIS           1978         #TNG/WK       10                          1-25-81    X000 GM2
  9  ALLERGY: PENICILLIN       REMOTE                                                 8-28-80    X000 GM2
 10  HX ALCOHOLISM             REMOTE                                                11-13-80    X000 RDC
 11  S/P HYSTERECTOMY          1972                                                  11-13-80    X000 RDC
 13  SMOKER                                                                           5-21-81    A363 RDC

**************************** **********   ***********   ************ **************   ********   **** ****
***THERAPIES**************** **ROUTE***   ***UNITS***   *LAST DOSE** ***FREQ********   **DATE**   PRVR CLIN
-------------------------------------------------------------------------------------------------
  7  MOTRIM                    PO           MG            D/C                           3-12-81    A363 RDC

**************************** **********   ***********   ************ **************   ********   **** ****
***LABORATORY*************** **********   ***UNITS***   **RESULT**** **************   **DATE**   PRVR CLIN
-------------------------------------------------------------------------------------------------
442  ANTINUCLEAR ANTIBODY                  TITER         1:160                         3-12-81
368    HEMOGLOBIN      ,UR                               NEG                           6-22-81    A363 RDC

**************************** **********   ***********   ************ **************   ********   **** ****
***SUMMARY TYPE*************************REPORT***********************************   **DATE**   PRVR CLIN
-------------------------------------------------------------------------------------------------
  1  SUMMARY:                  MANY COMPLAINTS BUT NO OBJECTIVE EVIDENCE OF DISEASE   5-21-81    A363 RDC
  2                            EXCEPT HIGH ANTIDSDNA.
  4  ORDERS:                   D/C PREDNISONE.  CHECK SEROLOGIES.  RTC 6 WKS.          5-21-81    A363 RDC

  1  SUMMARY:                  ? ASEPTIC NECROSIS OF L SHOULDER.  NO OBVIOUS          4-09-81    A363 RDC
  2                            EVIDENCE OF LUPUS ACTIVITY, ALTHOUGH ELEVATED ESR IS
  3                            WORRISOME.  ? STEROID WITHDRAWAL SX.
  4  ORDERS:                   DECR PREDNISONE TO 5 QOD.  CHECK SEROLOGIES, UA, CBC.  4-09-81    A363 RDC

  1  SUMMARY:                  RECENTLY DISCHARGED FOR 2ND R THR.  WEAK P SURGERY     3-12-81    A363 RDC
  2                            AND HX OF ALOPECIA, BUT NO OTHER SYMPTOMS OF DISEASE
  3                            ACTIVITY.
  4  ORDERS:                   CONTINUE PREDNISONE 5 MG QD.  CHECK SEROLOGY.  RTC     3-12-81    A363 RDC
  5                            1 MONTH.
```

FIGURE 8.13B. Smaple Summary Time-Oriented Record (STOR) Record. Problems or therapies deemed inactive.

one of the few examples of a system that integrates both inpatient and outpatient care. OCIS was designed to support the needs of a comprehensive cancer center where treatment modalities encourage ambulatory care combined with inpatient admissions. The system prints plots and flow sheets of clinical data for use at each patient visit. Access to an abstract of the medical record plus a history of therapies at the center also are available. This system is discussed in further detail in Chapter 10.

8.3.9. Core Record System

This is the final AAMRS to be described. It differs from the other systems in two major respects. First, it was designed to act as a low-cost adjunct to the medical record for use in a large teaching hospital. Its primary purpose was to provide access to the essential *mini*mal medical *record* (i.e., minirecord) when the paper record was not available. Through use of this minirecord, a core AAMR would be available online. This core record would identify major problems and therapies, link visits among different sources of care, and provide access to this record in situations where a complete medical record was not available (e.g., emergency visits or follow-up to a clinic that locally maintains only notes from that clinic.) The second way in which the Core Record System (CORE, McColligan) differs from the previous systems is that it was designed to be independent of all other hospital systems. This independence is not a virtue; it was a requirement imposed by the limited funding available for its implementation.

CORE operates in the Johns Hopkins outpatient clinics.[12] In the Orthopedic clinic, the flow is essentially the same as that described in Section 3.1. There is an appointment system and preprinted encounter forms; the forms serve as a progress note, a data collection form, a charge capture device, and as instructions to the patient. (Forms are modified for special clinics; for example, the Orthopedic Clinic contains back-to-work information and instructions.) CORE is also used in the Emergency Department. Here all forms are printed on demand during the triage process. The printing of the form initiates a time stamp that is updated during the patient visit (e.g., registration, release, admission). Thus the system can also serve as a patient locator and management tool.

The encounter form is printed on a two-page form. The first page contains registration and clinic specific information. The second page contains a summary of previous OPD visits, and lists of allergies, problems and medications. Clinic specific data collection forms are also printed (see Fig. 8.14). Because the system was designed to be low in operational cost and independent of other hospital systems, the minirecord portion is limited to data readily entered by the provider. The problem lists uses free text. (Another system has the tools to convert this text to codes for use in longitudinal studies.) The medication summary is limited to identification of the drug; the computer-stored record does not include the sig. (Since verification of input data required an investment in labor that was not practical, the decision was made to enter only data in which a keypunch error would have little impact. Thus, misspelling of digoxin would be easily recognized; an error in the sig might not be so obvious.) Naturally, the laboratory results are not recorded. When one compares CORE to the systems previously described, it indeed is minimal. Nevertheless, it must be recognized that most patient registration systems and office practice systems have no access to other clinical data. The flow sheets and surveillance facilities all assume the availability of such data in nontextual (processible) format. Where the data cannot be accessed automatically, the cost of capture makes its entry impractical. Consequently, the systems described in Sections 8.3.1 through 8.3.8 represent total systems that may be effective only in larger facilities. However, institutions that have limited resources are able to implement minirecords (or problem lists) that augment the administrative database with some useful clinical data.

8.3.10. Office Practice Systems

Most office practice systems are designed to manage the administrative and financial operations of a practice. Few offer any clinical support; and where clinical data are entered, they tend to be used for management rather than patient care functions. Naturally, there are exceptions and several very impressive systems have been described in the literature. In general, most are similar to CORE in the data they collect. Some also provide flow sheets; because the users can

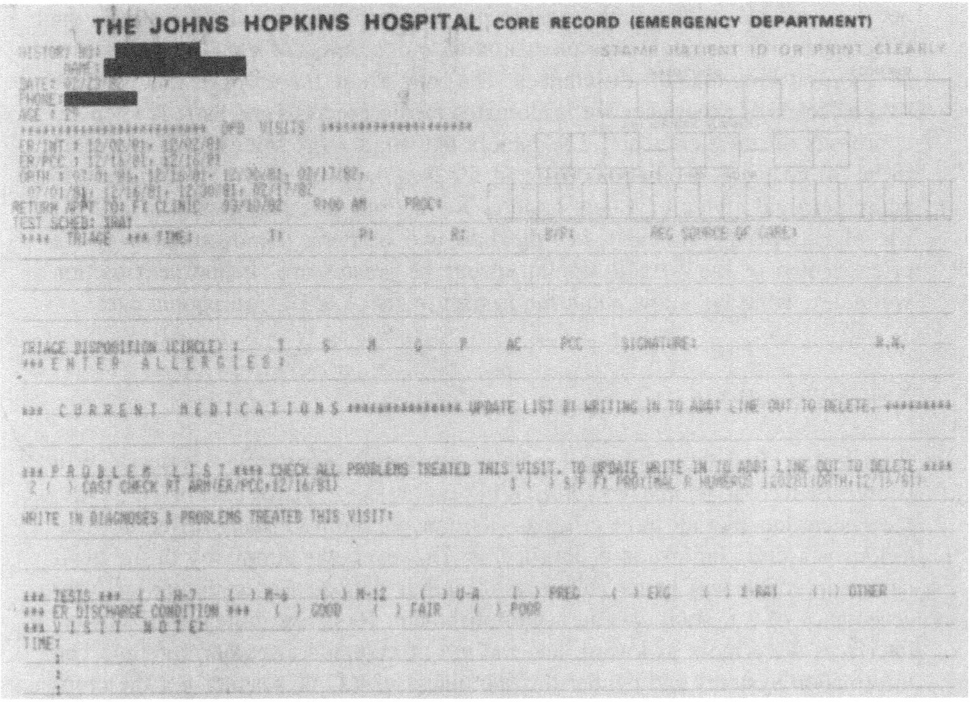
THE JOHNS HOPKINS HOSPITAL CORE RECORD (EMERGENCY DEPARTMENT)

HISTORY NO: [redacted] STAMP PATIENT ID OR PRINT CLEARLY

NAME: [redacted]

PHONE: [redacted]

*** TRIAGE *** TIME: T: P: R: B/P: REG SOURCE OF CARE:

TRIAGE DISPOSITION (CIRCLE): T S M G P AC PCC SIGNATURE: R.N.

*** E N T E R A L L E R G I E S :

*** C U R R E N T M E D I C A T I O N S *** UPDATE LIST BY WRITING IN TO ADD; LINE OUT TO DELETE.

*** P R O B L E M L I S T *** CHECK ALL PROBLEMS TREATED THIS VISIT. TO UPDATE WRITE IN TO ADD; LINE OUT TO DELETE ***

WRITE IN DIAGNOSES & PROBLEMS TREATED THIS VISIT:

*** TESTS *** ( ) H-7 ( ) H-6 ( ) H-12 ( ) U-A ( ) PREG ( ) EKG ( ) X-RAY ( ) OTHER

*** ER DISCHARGE CONDITION *** ( ) GOOD ( ) FAIR ( ) POOR

*** V I S I T N O T E:

TIME:

FIGURE 8.14. Portion of a CORE medical record.

provide quality control over the data entry process, most include the sig with the medication.

The availability of microcomputers has resulted in the production of many office practice systems designed for this equipment. All support registration and billing, management reporting, and appointment processing. Some allow the inclusion of problem lists and medications (as in the fashion of CORE). However, the level of detail recorded and the needs of the practice seldom make such systems useful tools in clinical situations. These data are best used in retrospective analysis, quality assurance, and follow-up.

8.3.11. Some Final Remarks

In this section many AAMRS examples were described. They vary in scope from maintaining a fully automated record to providing access to a minimal record when the chart is unavailable. Some systems provide routine surveillance, others ad hoc query support. Some are designed for specific patient populations, others are very general. Although there are many differences among these systems, the differences are in (a) style of implementation and (b) intent of use. The similarities are more striking than the differences. The conclusion, therefore, is that we have over a decade of experience with automated medical records and there is a general consensus on their contents. The factors that limit more widespread use seem to be (a) cost for installation, (b) cost for data capture, and (c) willingness to adapt personal styles to a new system. Reductions in equipment cost and the use of networking should lower the first two barriers; demonstrations of the effectiveness of the AAMR should encourage greater use. In the next section we review what we know about the impact of the AAMRS on patient care.

8.4. Evaluation

Barnett has cited three informal tests in evaluating information systems: Will people use it? Will people pay for it? Will people steal it? In the case of COSTAR, the system has met all three criteria—its transportation to many different institutions is a clear indication of its success. However, the simplicity of the evaluation approach was better suited to an earlier period. A decade earlier, user acceptance of a system was an accomplishment. Response times were slower, interfaces were more awkward, and the use of computers seemed foreign. The information systems had neither the usefulness of a CAT scanner nor the completeness of the traditional record. Most of these problems have ceased to be factors in the microcomputer era.

Once the system was accepted, there was the challenge of getting the user to pay for the service. COSTAR, RMRS, and TMR are among the systems that are paid for out of patient care revenues; the Cardiovascular Clinic System, OCIS, and CORE were exceptions in that both the development and operating costs came from internal sources. Today—with little research support for such activities—virtually all new installations are funded by the users. Finally, that leaves the question of "stealing," i.e., the export of products and ideas. Of the nine systems described, only two are actively being "marketed" (COSTAR and TMR) and another two are available for external use (RMRS and SCAMP). Considering that there is over a decade of experience with these systems, this is not much of an accomplishment. Perhaps the AAMRS will follow the path of the HIS. At first, the emphasis will be placed on the administrative functions and then—as it is recognized how the systems benefit patient care—the existing systems will be upgraded to (or replaced by) a more clinically oriented system.

How does the AAMRS assist in the delivery of care? One obvious way is by providing access to clinical information when the medical record is not available. The CORE record was designed for a large teaching hospital in which location of the paper record was not always easy. One short evaluation of an earlier version of the system found that 17% of the patients in a medical clinic had no charts available on the day prior to the visit and 10% had no charts available at the time of the visit. In contrast, 95% of all patients had a printed automated record in time for the encounter.[13] Similar results have been reported elsewhere.

Once the paper medical record has been located, will the desired information be found? The more complex the case, the greater the number of sources of care, the higher the probability that the desired information will not be found. Some facetiously refer to the paper medical record as a "write only memory." As we have seen from the AAMR examples, the computer-stored record is always available and easily organized to present the key information of current interest. One study was designed to see to what extent the full medical record was used. In this case, the providers were divided into two groups. The first group received a manually maintained flow sheet plus the complete record; the second group received only the flow sheet but were allowed to request the chart as well. At the end of each encounter, a physician reviewed all charts for overlooked clinical information. Fifty-nine percent of the study group physicians (flow sheet only) did not choose to receive the full record. Moreover, the study group was found not to differ from the control group with regard to the follow-up of clinical information as measured by the pre- and post-encounter chart reviews. The investigators concluded

> that a flow-sheet type of summary medical record can serve as the sole source of clinical information in a substantial number of outpatient follow-up encounters in a medical subspecialty clinic without deterioration in the communication of clinical information.[14] (From Whiting-O'Keefe QE, Simborg DW, Epstein WV. *Medical Care*, 1980.)

This was the origin of STOR.

The previous study suggests that a selected portion of the current medical record, when properly displayed, presents sufficient information for most outpatient follow-up visits. The differences in AAMR formats reflect different approaches to identifying and displaying the most useful information. Some systems always use a fixed format; others provide flexibility in selecting the encounter forms and record contents as a function of the clinic and patient. Nevertheless, in each case the presentation of data is relatively passive. It suppresses unnecessary detail and organizes the data to help the provider recognize trends or necessary actions. The recognition of the action is a responsibility of the provider, and—as we shall see—even the well-organized computer-printed record has too much information to be assimilated readily.

The description of RMRS pointed out that three forms are available for each encounter. The first two—the encounter form and flow sheet—are passive; all interpretation is performed by the provider. The third form—the Surveillance Report—is active; it makes recommendations and the provider is expected to react to them. We have seen in the discussion of HELP that alerts alter physician behavior; what can be said of surveillance reports? Fortunately, McDonald and his colleagues have conducted some careful studies of the impact of reminders on clinician behavior.

TABLE 8.4. Percent of times clinician responded to protocal action.

	Reminder	No reminder
Order recommended test	36%	11%
Change drug order	28%	13%

From McDonald CJ. *Ann Intern Med* 84: 162–167, 1976. Reprinted with permission.

The first of these studies was published in 1976.[15] Since RMRS maintained a complete database, it was possible to identify what actions were taken during an encounter, e.g., ordering a test, prescribing a medication. This provided an environment to determine if the actions of a clinician differed when reminders (i.e., surveillance reports) were presented. Over a period of 8 months, some 600 patient visits were assigned to a control and a study group. Only the study group received the reminders. However, for both groups the reminder suggestions and the encounter actions were recorded. The results are summarized in Table 8.4. Although it is clear that the protocol-created reminders were not accepted as appropriate for most of the cases, they did affect behavior. This was even more dramatically noted in the case of clinically significant changes in therapeutics, where the responses were 47% with and 4% without computer assistance.

In this evaluation, the patients were assigned to the study or control group; few patients saw the same provider in successive visits. McDonald next asked the questions, What if there was continuity of care and the clinicians were assigned to study and control groups: could the reminder system be used as a "training" tool to "perfect" the physicians' performance? A crossover study was designed with two groups of physicians.[16] One group spent 7 weeks with the reminders and then 9 weeks without them; the other group spent the first 7 weeks without reminders and the final 9 weeks with them. All groups using the reminders were asked to comment on them and indicate if they agreed or disagreed with the protocol or if there were insufficient data to determine if the protocol applied to the given patient. As shown in Table 8.5, response to events was greater when reminders were present.

It was expected that the reminders would alter behavior. However, there was no difference in the behavior of the two groups during the control period. That is, there was no residual change in performance (no training effect) for the group that initially used the reminders. Moreover, when one divided the physicians by level of training, one could find no significant overall effect on the results. There also were some interesting anecdotal results. For example, the reminders had "the greatest effect on a highly regarded second-year resident who responded to 71% of study events and 25% of control events. Interestingly enough, at the onset of this study the latter physician insisted that what was needed was education of bad physicians about what they did not know, not reminders to good physicians about what they knew."[16] Another example of the difference between perception and action was recorded when the physicians' comments on the reminders were analyzed.

TABLE 8.5. Results of McDonald's crossover study.

Reminder type	Control		Study	
	Events	Responses	Events	Responses
Suggest an observation	163	30	153	66
Suggest a test	165	37	119	72
Suggest a therapeutic change	57	17	55	28
Totals	385	84 (22%)	327	166 (51%)

From McDonald CJ. *Ann Intern Med* 84: 162–167, 1976. Reprinted with permission.

Excluding the suggestion with missing data, there is a 77% physician agreement with the protocol logic. Interestingly enough, the physician's words and actions were not always congruent. In some cases they agreed with a suggestion by their word and disagreed with it by action, and in some cases, vice versa. (From McDonald CJ, Protocol-based computer reminders, the quality of care and the nonperfectability of man, *N Eng J Med* (295): p.1354, 1976.)

Since this study, McDonald has conducted other tests and continues to find that the impact of reminders is independent of level of training, the availability of literature sources, or other factors. Thus, his 1976 conclusions seem to be true:

I believe that the results are most consistent with the initial hypothesis: that the amount of data presented to the physician per unit time is more than he can process without error. The computer augments the physician's capabilities and thereby reduces his error rate. The hypothesis is also relevant to the substantial rates of physician noncompliance with standards observed by Brook and Appel, Payne et al., and Sibley et al. (98 per cent, 60 per cent and 30 per cent noncompliance respectively.) It is very likely that the physicians in these studies were simply unable to detect all the multitudinous conditions specified by the standards used.[16]

Although the most complete analysis of the effect of protocol directed reminders in behavior was carried out using RMRS, the same results have been repeated in other environments. In one case, Barnett and his associates used COSTAR to identify patients with (a) a positive throat culture for ; hemolytic streptococci and (b) no record of appropriate antibiotic therapy within 4 days after the results were known. In such cases, a protocol generated reminder was sent to the physician. As a result of this activity, the number of records without a documented record of follow-up fell from about 8% of the cases to under 1%.[17] In many of the cases, the change was only in the documentation; the therapy actually had been started. However, there was also evidence that sore-throat patients showed significant improvement under the concurrent review system.

In the concurrent review cited, the system affected provider behavior. One reason for this is that it followed the normal flow of data: patient seen and test ordered; test result received and action taken. The encounter and the action taken occurred at different times; the action was related to the test result and not the encounter. Thus, a reminder of the test result could stimulate the action if it already had not been taken. Concurrent review proves to be less effective when it is not associated with the action to be taken. In the case of another COSTAR study, hypertensive patients were identified and a study and control group were selected. The study group received follow-up reports, but there was no perceptible difference in control of hypertension between the groups. Other studies in different situations—such as feedback about overutilization of laboratory tests—also suggest that the information tends to be effective ony when it is available at the time of the action. (Indeed, the reason McDonald had the users comment on the applicability of the reminders was to ensure that they were read. Even then, there were discrepancies between the agreement and the action.)

By way of summary, we note that the limitations of the human being place a ceiling on the quality of care that can be delivered. Given a large, unstructured, paper record, important information will not be found. Continuity of care relieves the reliance on the written record, but the human mind can recall and process only a small number of facts at any one time. The availability of a smaller, better organized record improves the identification of pertinent data. A computer-stored record facilitates access, restructuring, and coordination. A medical record database can be used to produce reminders, follow up, and quality assurance reviews. But the delivery of care is very complex. In some cases, one can identify life-threatening events correctly to alert providers. (Recall the 94% HELP compliance rate.) But in other situations, established protocols are not always appropriate. (Review the study columns in Table 8.5.) Information overload seems to limit the facts on which decisions are based. Reminders clearly help; too many reminders (or citations, or presentations of "knowledge") simply may result in another level of information overload.

Thus, we conclude this section on evaluation by noting that automated medical records (both in an inpatient and outpatient setting) are superior to the written record and that automated medical record systems provide tools to improve the quality of care. Most of the evidence to support these claims has been available for almost a decade. Yet the number of such systems is limited. Why? Cost seems to be the primary factor. Clinical systems have been traditionally reviewed in the context of cost benefit where quality of care was excluded from the equation. Registration and appointment systems are viewed as cost saving devices and purchased as such. (As in the case of the HIS, there is little evidence that the cost benefits are achieved. See p58). There is not yet a broad enough recognition of how automated medical record systems do improve care. However, where this benefit is acknowledged, one can expect a new demand—first in the larger institutions such as hospitals and HMOs, then in the smaller organizations and offices. Perhaps the changes in reimbursement mechanisms will accelerate further this move to new tools that help improve the quality of care.

8.5. Concluding Remarks

This and the previous chapters provided an overview of the CIS in patient care. The systems were classified by where they are used: hospitals and ambulatory care settings. However, most of the AAMRSs discussed are used in teaching hospital clinics. Many of the benefits of the HIS are derived from its ability to satisfy the communication needs of the institution. As we gain more experience with small computers and networks, one can see that it will not be long before there is a need to link private practices to the laboratories that provide their data and the hospitals that admit their patients. When this need matures, there will be less of a distinction between the two types of systems.

The primary focus of this chapter was the automated medical record. Many examples were shown. Such displays, however, can be misleading. There is a difference between a program to print an AAMR and an AAMRS. The latter requires a trained support staff, timely and accurate collection of data, and a continuous commitment by the users. In Chapter 7 we spoke of a 6- to 24-month installation period for an HIS. The installation of an AARMS is as complex a process. It cannot be installed as a new device to be used; and once installed it must be used to be effective. Like spinach on the cafeteria tray, it must be ingested before any benefit can be derived.

The author's philosophy has been so liberally exposed throughout these chapters that there is no need to attempt any review here. It will be noted that all of the systems presented in Chapters 7 and 8 were examples of information systems that anticipated the need for data to "tell" the clinician what is important. The clinician was also given tools to retrieve additional information as necessary. All decision-making is done by the clinician; the CIS simply reduces the "noise" in the information transfer. The next question is, can the information system (or automated system) play an even more active role in the clinical decision making process? That is the subject of the next chapter.

For Further Reading

The book of readings *Information Systems for Patient Care* (ed, B. I. Blum, Springer-Verlag, 1984) has 14 papers dealing with ambulatory care systems including chapters on COSTAR, RMRS, TMR, SCAMP, CORE, and several office practice systems. J. Zimmerman and A. Rector, *Computers for the Physician's Office*, Research Studies Press, 1978, provides an earlier overview of the subject. These references, those previously cited, and the notes provide a good set of initial readings.

There are several books designed to provide an introduction to computers and medical practice. H. D. Covvey and N. H. McAlister have produced a very readable two volume *Computers in the Practice of Medicine*, (Addison-Wesley, 1980). An AAMSI committee has sponsored B. B. Oberst and R. A. Reid (eds) *Computer Applications to Private Office Practice* (Springer-Verlag, 1984). Both are introductory in nature and contain little specific details about office practice systems. E. J. Neiburger, *Computers for Professional Practice* (Andent, Inc., Waukegan, IL, 1984) is a thorough introduction and "how to" softcover. Finally, there is a continuing series of articles on office practice systems in the journal *M. D. Computer.*

References

1. Kuhn, I. M., G. Wiederhold, et al, Automated Ambulatory Medical Record Systems in the U.S., Stanford Report CS-80-928, August 1982, and the summarized report in B. I. Blum (ed) *Information Systems for Patient Care*, Springer-Verlag, 1984, pp. 199-217.
2. *Ibid*, p. 5.
3. Fiddleman, R. H., Proliferation of COSTAR—A Status Report, in B. I. Blum (ed) *Information Systems for Patient Care*, Springer-Verlag, 1984, p. 303.
4. COSTAR figures can be found in Barnett, G. O., COSTAR, A Progress Report, MGH, no date, COSTAR Functional Specifications (Version 5.3), MGH, 4/15/1977, and Barnett, G. O., The Application of Computer-Based Medical-Record Systems in Ambulatory Practice, *NEJ Med.*, 310 1984. Search examples are taken from P. D. Beaman, N. S. Justice and G. O. Barnett, A Medical Information System and Data Language for Ambulatory Practices, *Computer* 12:11 1979.
5. McDonald, C. J., G. A. Wilson, and G. P. McCabe, Physician Response to Computer Reminders, JAMA 244 1980 p. 1579.
6. The CARE examples which follow have been taken from the chapter on RMRS in B. I. Blum (ed) *Information Systems for Patient Care*, Springer-Verlag, 1984, and the description of the CARE language, Appendix C in C. J. McDonald *Action-Oriented Decisions in Ambulatory Medicine*, Year Book Medical Publishers, 1981.
7. Taken from W. W. Stead, W. E. Hammond and M. J. Straube, A Chartless Record—Is It Adequate, *J. Med. Sys.*, (7,2) 1983, pp. 103-109.
8. Taken from J. E. Rodnick, The Use of Automated Ambulatory Medical Records, *J. Fam. Pract.* (5,2) 1977, pp. 253-264.
9. This example is taken from the ARAMIS users manual (V. Weiderhold, Stanford University, September 1976). The manual also illustrates the input sequence and an equivalent text report.
10. Examples are taken from the A. R. Shapiro, SCAMP System, in B. I. Blum (ed) *Information Systems for Patient Care*, Springer-Verlag, 1984.
11. Simborg, D. W. and Q. E. Whiting-O'Keefe, Summary Time Oriented Record—A Progress Report, SCAMC-5, 1981, pp. 100-104.
12. See E. E. McColligan, Care Record System, in B. I. Blum (ed) *Information Systems for Patient Care*, Springer-Verlag, 1984.
13. Blum, B. I. C. J. Johns, E. E. McColligan, C. R. Smith, D. M. Steinwachs, Low Cost Ambulatory Medical Information Systems, *J. Clin. Eng.* (4,4) 1979, 372-377.
14. Whiting-O'Keefe, D. W. Simborg and W. V. Epstein, A Controlled Experiment to Evaluate the Use of a Time-Oriented Summary Medical Record, *Medical Care*, (18,8) 1980 pp. 842-852.
15. McDonald, C. J., Use of a Computer to Detect and Respond to Clinical Events: Its Effect on Clinical Behavior, *Ann. Int. Med* (84) 1976 pp. 162-167.

16. McDonald, C. J. Protocol-Based Computer Reminders, The Quality of Care and the Non-Perfectability of Man, *N. E. J. Med.*, (295) 1976 pp. 1351-1355.
17. Barnett, G. O., R. N. Winicoff, J. L. Dorsey, et al, Quality assurance through automated monitoring and concurrent feedback using a computer-based medical information system, *Med. Care* 16, 1978, pp. 462-769.

9
Medical Decision Making

9.1. Introduction

Chapter 2 introduced the concepts of data, information, and knowledge-oriented systems. It was suggested that knowledge applications were an area of research and that the technology required to support the data and information applications existed and was well understood. This view is summarized in Table 9.1. It suggests that for data and information applications, advances will be made by identifying medical and health care problems and engineering the computer systems to implement solutions. The research will emphasize biomedicine and health care; implementation will be primarily an engineering activity. Knowledge-oriented applications, however, are still topics of active research. The paradigms vary from the rigorous application of mathematic principles to the use of artificial intelligence (AI) techniques. This diversity of approaches is not without emotion, hyperbole, or controversy. Yet, as will be shown, this emphasis on medical knowledge processing identifies a broad research area that addresses common problems using different methodologies. From this activity, a science of medical informatics should emerge.

It is important for the reader to recognize that we are now considering applications that are fundamentally different from all of those discussed earlier. The clinical use of computers may be viewed by the role they play in the health care process:

- *Mechanization.* Here the computer automates a process normally performed manually or by some other machine. Examples are the processing of bills, the management of a clinical laboratory, and the reporting of results in an HIS. In each case, the work flow has changed, but the ultimate user (e.g., physician) perceives no change except in media, accuracy, timeliness, etc.
- *Complementation.* In this case the computer augments a human user's performance by doing well-defined tasks that the user cannot do as well. Examples are maintenance of a legible, integrated medical record, computation of EKG metrics, and display of a CAT image. Here the user sees the system

TABLE 9.1. Scope of medical computing.

	1950s	1960s	1970s	1980s
Data applications	Research	Prototypes	Mature	Refinement
Information applications	Concepts	Research	Prototypes	Mature
Knowledge	Concepts	Concepts	Research	Prototypes

as a tool that augments his capabilities and improves his productivity or performance.

- *Collegial Assistance*. In this role the system acts more like an associate than a tool. The distinctions between the user and system role are less clear; the system assumes responsibility for functions that were traditionally in the user's domain. Examples are closed loop clinical systems that implement patient management judgments within previously determined limits, and medical decision-making systems. Because of their potential infringement on the users' responsibility, these applications receive little acceptance until they are perceived to be efficatious tools that complement the users' capabilities.

If one accepts this allocation of roles, then there is an inherent conflict. Medical decision-making systems are intended to improve on an imperfect—imperfectable in McDonald's view—human process. Limitations in success, difficulties in evaluation, and an entrenched social structure all inhibit change. Thus, in addition to the enormous technical challenges, there is also a need to present a comprehensible interface that instills confidence; that is, a technical solution is a necessary but not sufficient condition for the success of an application.

In what follows we shall first examine the medical decision-making process. Then we shall consider ways in which computers are being used to support this process. The techniques are divided into two groups: those that are not considered AI applications and those that are. A final section identifies the commonalities among the systems presented.

9.2. Medical Decision Making

In a seminal 1959 paper on medical decision making, Ledley and Lusted began:

> The purpose of this article is to analyze the complicated reasoning processes inherent in medical diagnosis. The importance of this problem has received recent emphasis by the increasing interest in the use of electronic computers as an aid to medical diagnostic processes. Before computers can be used effectively for such purposes, however, we need to know more about how the physician makes a medical diagnosis.
>
> If a physician is asked, "How do you make a medical diagnosis?" his explanation of the process might be as follows. "First, I obtain the case facts from the patient's history, physical examination, and laboratory tests. Second, I evaluate the relative importance of the different signs and symptoms. Some of the data may be of first-order importance and

other data of less importance. Third, to make a differential diagnosis I list all the diseases which the specific case can reasonably resemble. Then I exclude one disease after another from the list until it becomes apparent that the case can be fitted into a definite disease category, or that it may be one of several possible diseases, or else that its exact nature cannot be determined." This, obviously, is a greatly simplified explanation of the process of diagnosis, for the physician might also comment that after seeing a patient he often has a "feeling about the case."[1]

The authors then proceeded to show how the medical knowledge used in the process could be structured by use of symbolic logic. Consider a very simple example in which there are two symptoms S_1 and S_2 and two diseases D_1 and D_2. The possible logical combinations would be:

S_1 S_2 D_1 D_2 (or 1111)
S_1 $\bar{S}_2$ D_1 D_2 (or 1011 where $\bar{S}_2$ is not S_2)
$\bar{S}_1$ S_2 D_1 D_2 (or 0111)
etc.

After one removed all combinations that could not exist, one might have only the following three combinations which were consistent with experience:

S_1	S_2	D_1	D_2
1	1	1	1
1	1	1	0
0	1	0	1

Assuming that a patient did not present symptom S_1 but did present S_2, then—according to the logical database—disease D_2 was present. However, if the patient presented both S_1 and S_2, then there would be two possible diagnoses: only D_1 or both D_1 and D_2. In this case, the symbolic logic would not be sufficient to make a determination; one would need to know something of the relative occurrences in the patient population of $D_1 \bar{D}_2$ and $D_1 D_2$. Using Bayes' theorem (to be discussed in greater detail below) one could use this occurrence distribution to compute the conditional probability that $D_1 \bar{D}_2$was true given S_1 S_2 (written $P(D_1 \bar{D}_2|S_1 S_2)$).

Of course, decision-making does not end with diagnosis; decisions are required for therapy as well. Viewing therapy in the context of a decision tree, Ledley and Lusted projected the alternatives and possible outcomes and interventions. They then assigned subjective values at each decision point to determine the best (in the context of the values) path of action. This can be clarified by summarizing the illustration they used. A 5-week old infant has progressive difficulty in breathing. The physician decides (from the symptoms S_1, respiratory distress, S_2, several surface hemangiomas, and S_3, mediastinal mass on chest x-ray film) that one or more of three abnormalities are causing the respiratory distress:

D_1 A prominent thymus gland
D_2 A deep hemangioma in mediastinoum
D_3 A dermoid cyst.

The treatments available are x-ray therapy (T_1) or surgery (T_2). T_1 will be effective for D_1, may be effective for D_2 and will have no effect on D_3; it can be done quickly, with little discomfort, but cancer of the thyroid may develop later. On the other hand, surgery (T_2) will allow for the removal of the cyst (D_3) and will allow for a definite diagnosis. The dangers are a potential for hemorrage if D_2 plus normal surgical risk. What should the physician do?

With three symptoms and three possible diseases, there are $2^3 \times 2^3$ or 64 possible combinations. However, a single symptom complex has been identified, and medical knowledge can be used to reduce the number of possible disease complexes. In this example, the medical knowledge is:

- If a patient has D_1 and also D_2 or D_3 then he must have both symptoms S_1 and S_3
- If a patient does not have D_2 then he does not have symptom S_2.
- If a patient does not have D_1 but does have D_2 and D_3, then he has symptom S_3.

By logically applying the symptom values to this medical knowledge, it can be shown that only four disease complexes are possible:

$$
\begin{aligned}
D_1\ \overline{D}_2\ \overline{D}_3 &= C_1\\
\overline{D}_1\ D_2\ \overline{D}_3 &= C_2\\
\overline{D}_1\ \overline{D}_2\ D_3 &= C_4\\
\overline{D}_1\ D_2\ D_3 &= C_6
\end{aligned}
$$

Now the problem has been narrowed, and subjective values (on a scale from -10 to 10) can be assigned for each disease complex. The result of this exercise in value theory is the following table.

T	C_1	C_2	C_4	C_6
X-ray (T_1)	+3	−2	−3	−2
Surgery (T_2)	−2	+6	+10	+8

The choice of therapy would depend on relative occurrence of the conditions C_1 C_2 C_4 and C_6. That is, if the probabiity of condition C_1 occurring was very low, then X-ray therapy was not to be considered; however, if the combined probabilities of C_2 C_3 and C_4 were low, then surgery would not be appropriate.

The value of a therapy is computed as the sum of the products of the value and probability for each disease complex. The computational methods are straightforward, but how could one collect the data for deriving the probability distributions? The approach described by Ledley and Lusted was the use of notched-edge cards that indicate disease symptom complexes. (See Fig. 9.1.) Each time a patient was diagnosed, a card would be created.

To make a diagnosis, sort out those cards that correspond to the symptom complex presented by the patient. The disease complex part of these cards gives all possible disease complexes the patient can have. Separate these cards by the symptom complexes: the

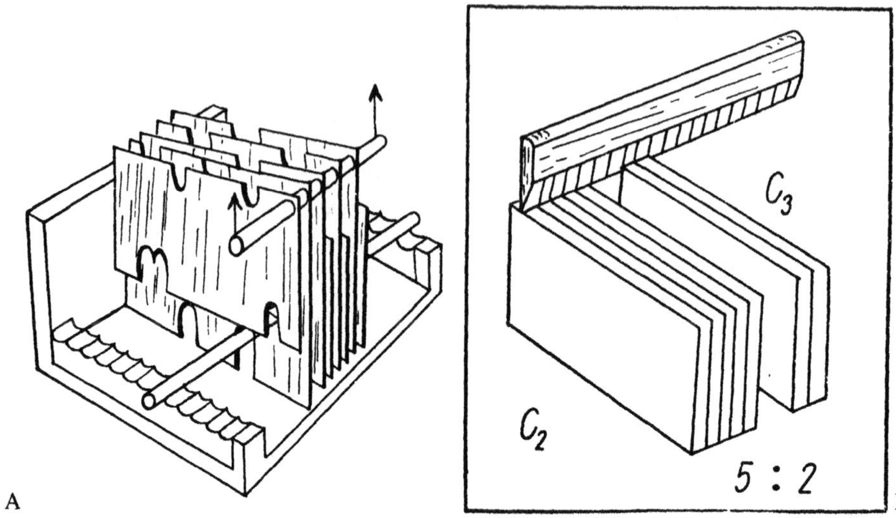

FIGURE 9.1. Notched-edged card illustrations. (From Ledley RS, Lusted LB, *Science* 130:9–20, July 1959. Copyright 1959 by the American Association for the Advancement of Science.)

thicknesses of the resulting separated decks will be proportional to the probability of the patient's having the respective disease complexes.[2] [See Fig. 9.1B]

The technology of notched-edge cards limited the size and scope of the database. It was suggested that computers could process much more complete sets of disease-symptom complexes. (They noted, however, that in a realistic application with 300 diseases and 400 symptoms—such as would occur within a medical specialty—some 10^{200} logical combinations would have to be considered.)

In 1961 Warner demonstrated the Bayesian statistical basis for medical diagnosis in congenital heart disease, and the concepts first presented in 1959 continue to remain active areas of research. As we shall see in the following sections, there are many examples in which mathematical techniques have proven to be very effective. (The HELP system is one example.) Nevertheless, there are also many workers in the field who disagree with this approach. In 1977 Feinstein made the following indictment.

Iatromathematical enthusiasts could make substantial contributions to clinical medicine if the efforts now being expended on Bayesian and decision-analytic fantasies were directed to the major challenges of algorithmically dissecting clinical judgement, based on the way the judgements are actually performed. Instead, however, the enthusiasts usually become infatuated with the mathematical processes and with the associated potential for computer manipulations, so that the basic clinical challenges become neglected or evaded.[3] (From Feinstein AR. *Am Soc Pharmacol Exp Ther* 21(4):495, 1977. Reprinted with permission of CV Mosby.)

Ledley and Lusted began their paper with a description of the cognitive process and showed how the process could be supplemented by logical analysis. Feinstein presented the view that, in many cases, the resulting analysis produced models that were inappropriate for the process and therefore of little value. Mathematical tools do not reflect how physicians actually make the decision; neither do they account for subjective factors, i.e., "feelings about the case."

The method of making a differential diagnosis, that presented in the initial quotation, involves decision-making with uncertainty. Not all the data are available; conditions vary with time; and there may be several diseases present that produce confusing combinations of symptoms. This analysis process has been studied extensively by Elstein and his colleagues. They have developed a four-stage hypothetico-deductive model for how physicians perform medical problem solving.[4] The stages are:

- *Cue acquisition.* This includes taking a history, performing a physical examination, reviewing test results, etc.
- *Hypothesis generation.* Retrieval from long-term memory of alternative hypotheses of the diagnosis.
- *Cue interpretation.* The data are now considered in the context of the hypothesis previously generated.
- *Hypothesis evaluation.* The data are weighted and combined to determine which hypotheses are supported or ruled out.

The process is iterative. It may result in a decision that more data are required (i.e., tests and procedures are to be ordered) or that a probable diagnosis (and recommended therapy) are suggested, or both.

In analyzing this model, the researchers found that the generation of early hypotheses has considerable natural force; medical students generated early hypotheses even when asked to withhold judgment. The number of hypotheses is usually around four or five and appears to have an upper bound of about six or seven. The generation of hypotheses was based more consistently on single salient cues rather than on combinations of cues; very few cues seemed to be used. Hypotheses selection is also biased by recent experience. (That is the source of the joke so common in medical schools: when one hears the sound of hoof beats, one immediately thinks of zebras.)

They also found that cue interpretation tended to use three measures: confirm, disconfirm, or noncontributory. The use of seven-point weighting schemes had no greater explanatory power. The accuracy of cue interpretation was related to the accuracy of diagnostic outcome, but it was independent of the thoroughness of cue acquisition. In fact, one researcher found "that greater thoroughness in the history and physical examination are associated with increased costs, but not with greater diagnostic accuracy."[5] The lack of thoroughness is not as important a cause of error in diagnosis as problems of integrating and combining information; however, it was shown that a conscious effort to employ useful heuristics does appear to help in decision-making.

Table 9.2 contains a list of heuristics prepared by Elstein and others for use in a course in clinical decision analysis.[6] Note how often probabilities are required

TABLE 9.2. Heuristics for medical problem-solving.

Generating a list of alternative hypotheses or actions:

a. *Multiple competing hypotheses*. Think of a number of diagnostic possibilities compatible with the chief complaint and preliminary findings. Avoid making snap diagnoses. Key on "good" symptom clusters; organ-system links are helpful. Nesting overcomes limits of working memory.

b. *Probability*. Consider the most common diagnoses first.

c. *Utility*. Consider seriously those diagnoses for which effective therapies are available and in which failure to treat would be a serious omission. Try to keep separate your estimates of the probability of a disease and the cost of not treating it.

Gathering data:

d. *Form a reasoned plan* for testing your hypotheses, one that reckons with probability and utility. Sequence laboratory tests to rule out first the most common diseases (probability), and next the diseases most needing treatment (utility).

Corollary 1: Diagnostic decisions should be realted to treatment alternatives. There is no reason to pursue a differential among diagnoses that will make no difference in the action to be taken, and your data gathering should reflect this.

Corollary 2: There should be a reason for every datum gathered. For example, if a test result does not change your opinion about any of your diagnostic hypotheses, ask yourself why the test was ordered and what range of values could have changed your mind.

e. *Branch and screen*. History-taking and the physical examination should be branching procedures. Develop adequate screening tactics to help make overly detailed examinations unnecessary. For example, if a patient denies changes in weight, the physician can omit going down the branch that realtes to certain endocrinopathies.

f. *Cost-benefit calculation*. Consider the harm tests might do and their cost. Balance these against the information to be gained.

g. *Precision*. Strive for the degree of reliability needed for the decision at hand. More is not necessary.

Aggregating data, evaluating hypotheses, and selecting a course of action:

h. *Disconfirmatory evidence*. Actively seek out and evaluate evidence that tends to rule out any hypotheses or action alternative as well as the evidence that tends to confirm it. Be aware of the tendency to discount or disregard evidence likely to disconfirm your favorite alternative.

i. *Multiple diagnoses*. Don't forget the possibility that a patient with multiple problems or complaints has more than one disease.

1. The joint probability of two common diagnoses may well be greater than one rarer diagnosis.
2. When failure to treat both hypothetical diagnoses might have disastrous results, and neither can be confirmed or ruled out, act as if both were established.

j. *Bayes' theorem*. Revise probabilities after collecting data.

1. In assessing the probability of a particular diagnosis, give special weight if it is common.
2. If the clinical findings are relatively more likely in diagnosis A than in diagnosis B, revise your opinion in favor of A.
3. If hard data are missing about how common a disease is, or about how likely particular symptoms are in it, make rough approximations, It is usually possible to weight each finding as at least tending to confirm, disconfirm, or not change one's prior belief.
4. If you rank order diagnoses on the basis of the predominance of findings of their support, weighted as described in (3), this ranking will correspond roughly to a probability scale.

TABLE 9.2. Heuristics for medical problem-solving—*cont'd.*

k. *Probability and utility should guide action.* When a course of action is finally selected, consider both the probability of the diagnoses for which this action is appropriate and the benefits/penalties that would accrue. Combine the two considerations to estimate expected value and choose so as to maximize expected value.

Corollary 1: Consider clustering diagnoses that would be treated identically. This nesting effectively reduces the number of alternatives to be evaluated.

Corollary 2: Among the benefits and penalties of medical action, consider quality of life and morbidity as well as mortality.

to determine a course of action. Note, too, how much knowledge and data are required to make these decisions. We know that physicians have difficulty in appraising or combining large quantities of complex probabilistic information. We also know that physicians seldom compute probabilities using Bayes' Theorem; they tend to rely on subjective approximations. Yet, probabilities can be very counter to intuition. For example, assume that a disease is found in 3% of the population and that there is a test that will identify correctly 95% of the people with the disease and incorrectly identify 10% (i.e., 10% are false-positives). What is the probability that a patient diagnosed as positive actually has the disease? The correct, but counterintuitive, answer is 22.7%.*

From this brief survey, the reader can sense that there will be two general approaches to medical decision-making. The first uses mathematical models and probabilities; that is, decisions are derived from empirical evidence. The second approach structures the knowledge used by the physician and relies on an inference mechanism to arrive at a decision; that is, deductive reasoning is applied. The former uses algorithmic and statistical techniques, the latter applies AI methods. The clinician, on the other hand, uses both approaches. His or her acceptance of facts is based on a prior statistical demonstration. Through experience, he or she is able to generate the correct hypotheses rapidly. Cue acquisition is supported by both explicit and subliminal processes so that not all cues can be available to a computer. Nevertheless, man is imperfectable. He finds it difficult to combine patterns of cues, his intuitive probability estimates are unreliable, and his short term memory is easily saturated. The goal is to produce tools that complement man's strengths and bridge over his limitations.

In the following two sections we shall consider these two approaches to medical-decision making. As we have just seen, the process is far too complicated to expect to have it "computerized." Still, clinicians need help, and there now are many applications that can supply reliable collegial advice. Unfortunately,

*The probability of a positive given the presence of the disease is .95; .227 is the probability of having the disease given the presence of a positive result. The fact that only 3% of the population has the disease lowers the second probability. This is discussed in further detail in the next section.

few are sufficiently transportable, robust, or friendly to be used routinely in a clinical setting.

9.3. Strongly Formalized Techniques

It is useful to separate the clinical decision making tools into those that are strongly formalized—i.e., those that use algorithmic methods or statistical pattern classification techniques—and those that rely on symbolic reasoning approaches—i.e., artificial intelligence. As in the case of the data, information, knowledge division, the organization is artificial and has been chosen simply to facilitate discussion. The reader should be aware, however, that some researchers perceive the division to be deeper than it actually is.

9.3.1. Algorithmic Methods

We begin by considering algorithmic methods. It has been shown that this is the method chosen for most of the embedded applications: ECG, CAT imaging, etc. An understanding of the process is modeled and then formalized as an algorithm. The algorithm is a sequence of processing steps that will terminate with the anticipated outcome; it is a representation of the knowledge of the process' behavior. When algorithms are used to manage the clinical decision process they are called protocols. The word protocol has various shades of meanings. In a clinical research setting, the protocol defines the process necessary to manage a patient and collect data to evaluate a hypothesis. In ambulatory care, it implies tools designed to guide non-physician providers.

The use of protocols in primary care settings was experimented with widely in the 1970s. The following is the abstract of a representative evaluation.

> A symptom-oriented protocol for acute pharyngitis was evaluated in a busy general medical clinic staffed by physicians and graduate and student physician's assistants. We observed significantly improved performance by all providers in collection of medical data, utilization of laboratory tests, and appropriate use of antibiotics after introduction of the protocol. Patient charges were less when the protocol was used, but these savings were offset partially by the cost of audit. Compliance with and acceptance of the protocol differed among the various health providers, with physicians demonstrating significantly lower levels than nonphysicians. Patient-care protocols provide an effective means of monitoring the process of medical care, detecting weakness in supportive clinic services, and affording educational feedback for all health providers.[7] (From Grimm RH et al. Reprinted by permission of *The New England Journal of Medicine* 292:507, 1975.)

In this case the protocol was a manual check list that referenced a chart maintained in the clinic.

The automation of clinical protocols also was experimented with in the 1970s, but the costs and response times limited their utility. However, the availability of Automated Ambulatory Medical Record Systems (AAMRS) with their monitoring and database facilities provided an environment for integrating protocols with the CIS. In fact, the Reigenstreif Medical Record System (RMRS) uses protocols to adapt the encounter form to the patient's diagnosis; it also produces protocol-directed reminders. It should be noted, however, that in both the above study and the RMRS evaluations there were significant deviations between protocol suggestions and physician actions. This would suggest that the primary care protocols are general guides rather than formal rules to be rigidly followed.

A different application of protocols was tested by Wirtschafter, Mesel, and colleagues in a cancer research environment. In this case, the objective was to make the experience of a cancer center available to community physicians through a consultant-extender system. In its first (mid-1970) application, a protocol form was prepared for each patient with Hodgkin's disease who was to be treated by a specific therapeutic regimen (i.e., protocol). The form indicated data to be collected with recommended therapies based on the patient's response. (For abnormal situations, the recommendation was, "IF YES, call Center.") The physician filled out the form with the data and actions taken and then mailed it to the Center. Here it was processed, and a new form was created and sent back in time for the next encounter. Later versions of the consultant-extender used computer processing of the data and generation of the forms.

The results achieved by the consultant-extender system were quite favorable. In a breast cancer study, the system was used by both the center and 75 physicians located throughout the state of Alabama. Compliance with the protocol was measured at 97%, and disease-free intervals of those patients treated in a prospective clinical trial were indistinguishable from a comparable group of patients treated in an academic setting. Another study showed that there was a 94% protocol compliance with extender supported physicians and only 64% from a group without the care protocols. Moreover, two measures of hematologic toxicity were associated more often with noncompliance. Thus, it would seem that physician acceptance of protocols is high in areas where relatively uncommon diseases are treated by new and potentially life-threatening means. Once the protocol is learned, the extender system is no longer required. However, where the therapy is subject to change—as it is in a research setting—the consultant-extender provides the only means to access current protocols. It also provides the beneficial effect of increasing the number of patients who can be included in the study analysis.

In some cases it is possible to identify a special area, define the medical decision-making process as an algorithm, and then implement the algorithm as an interactive program. Bleich was one of the first to demonstrate this approach successfully. He chose as his topic acid-base disorders, and, extracting his expert knowledge, he flowcharted the decision criteria and selections. A portion of the flow chart is shown in Fig. 9.2.[8] Note that the flow chart allows both "yes/no" and computational branching. The design allows the program to make recommendations even if data are missing; if crucial information simply is not available,

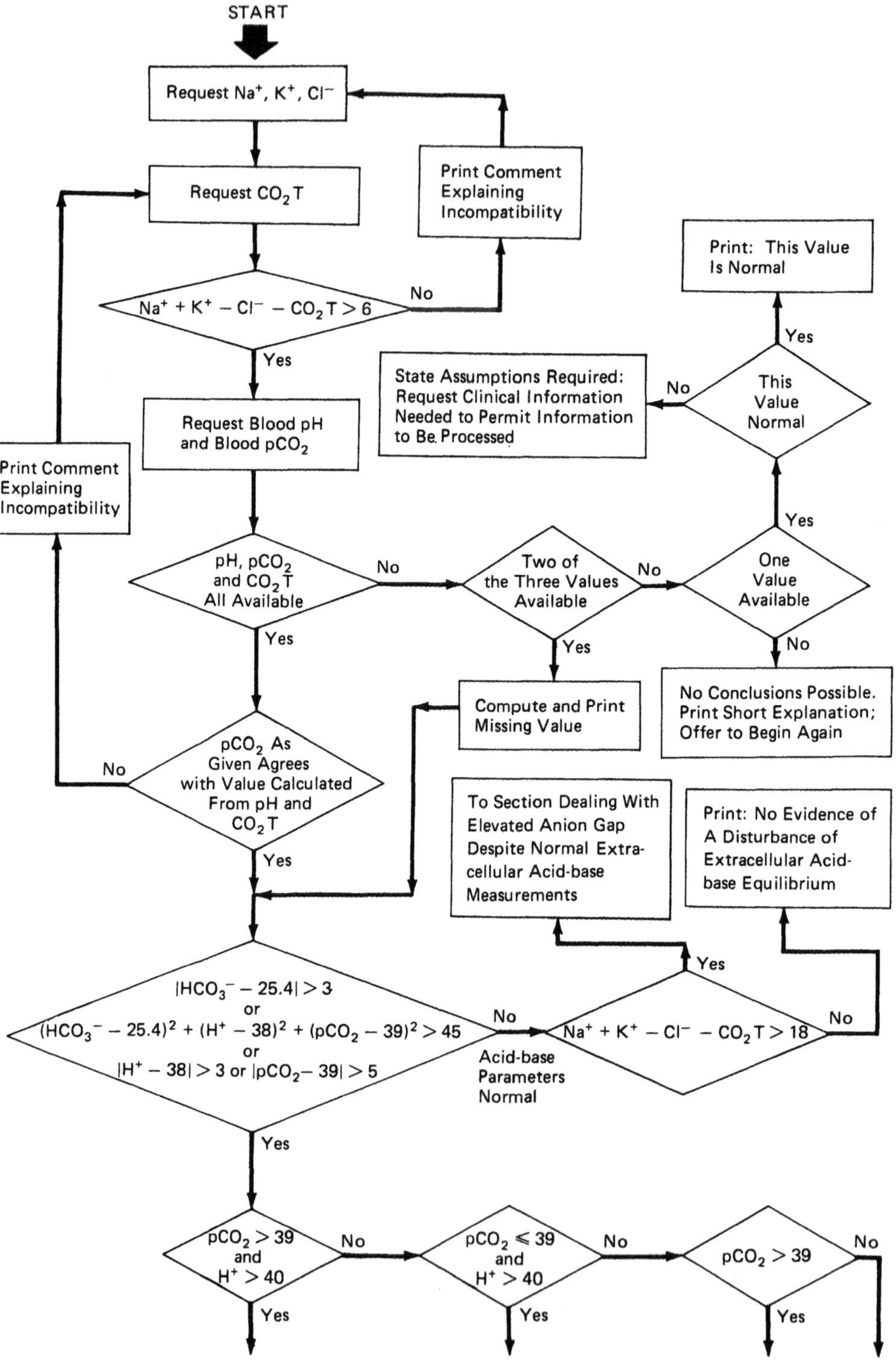
START
Request Na+, K+, Cl−
Request CO2T
Print Comment Explaining Incompatibility
Na+ + K+ − Cl− − CO2T > 6
No
Yes
Request Blood pH and Blood pCO2
Print Comment Explaining Incompatibility
pH, pCO2 and CO2T All Available
No
Yes
Two of the Three Values Available
No
Yes
One Value Available
Yes
No
This Value Normal
Yes
No
Print: This Value Is Normal
State Assumptions Required: Request Clinical Information Needed to Permit Information to Be Processed
No Conclusions Possible. Print Short Explanation; Offer to Begin Again
Compute and Print Missing Value
pCO2 As Given Agrees with Value Calculated From pH and CO2T
No
Yes
To Section Dealing With Elevated Anion Gap Despite Normal Extracellular Acid-base Measurements
Print: No Evidence of A Disturbance of Extracellular Acid-base Equilibrium
|HCO3− − 25.4| > 3 or (HCO3− − 25.4)2 + (H+ − 38)2 + (pCO2 − 39)2 > 45 or |H+ − 38| > 3 or |pCO2 − 39| > 5
No
Acid-base Parameters Normal
Na+ + K+ − Cl− − CO2T > 18
Yes
No
Yes
pCO2 > 39 and H+ > 40
No
Yes
pCO2 ≤ 39 and H+ > 40
No
Yes
pCO2 > 39
No
Yes

the program draws the most useful conclusion possible based on the data provided. The output is a text report that is designed to review the pathophysiology of the disorder and assist the physician in its management; key references are included.

The system was installed on a time-shared computer in 1969, and in the first year approximately 40 hospitals located in 10 states dialed up to process 1,500 consultations. The system was later extended to include electrolyte disorders, but it could not sustain its initial interest. In part, this was the result of its educational impact: after a few times physicians could anticipate its analysis. The decline in usage was also due to the limitation of the scope of the program. There was no feedback or follow-up; it was not designed to pursue specific etiologies or interrelationships among possible etiologies.

The limitations of algorithms are clear. They are representations of knowledge. Where the knowledge is not otherwise available—as in the case of nonphysician administered care or nonspecialist administration of chemotherapy—they provide useful guides. Where the knowledge is available, the provider may justifiably override the algorithm's direction. (Recall that not all physicians responded to RMRS's recommendations or to HELP's life-threatening alerts.) When the algorithm is implemented as a program, there are necessary limits on the scope and flexibility of the algorithm. All situations must be anticipated and explicitly programmed. Nevertheless, the algorithm can perform computations that the physician finds cumbersome. This has proven helpful in applications where access to pharmacokinetic models (such as for digitalis dosing) is necessary. However, it is an unrealistic approach for most clinical decision-making situations; there are too many variables and alternatives.

A variation of the algorithmic approach is the use of decision analysis. Again, the conceptual structure is a flow chart. In this case it is represented as a tree and the emphasis is on the branching logic. Figures 9.3 (A,B) contains a decision tree for diagnosis and treatment of urinary tract infection (UTI). All possible paths are identified and probabilities are associated with branch points. The probabilities may be derived from published results, analysis of local data, or subjective evaluations. Values may also be associated with the nodes, e.g., a cost in dollars, projected days with disease, and/or probability of death. Starting at the lowest node, one then multiplies these values by the probabilities to compute the "expected" values at the next highest node. By continuing in this manner until all decision nodes have values, one may then use the values as a guide to selecting alternatives under conditions of uncertainty (i.e., where data are missing). Similar techniques are used to allow patients to assign their own values to aid in the selection of the therapeutic approach that is best for them. Pauker, for example, has shown how patients can supply values (utilities) regarding survival

FIGURE 9.2. Portion of Bleich's acid-base flowchart. Reproduced from *The Journal of Clinical Investigation,* 1969, 48:1690, by copyright permission of The American Society for Clinical Investigation.)

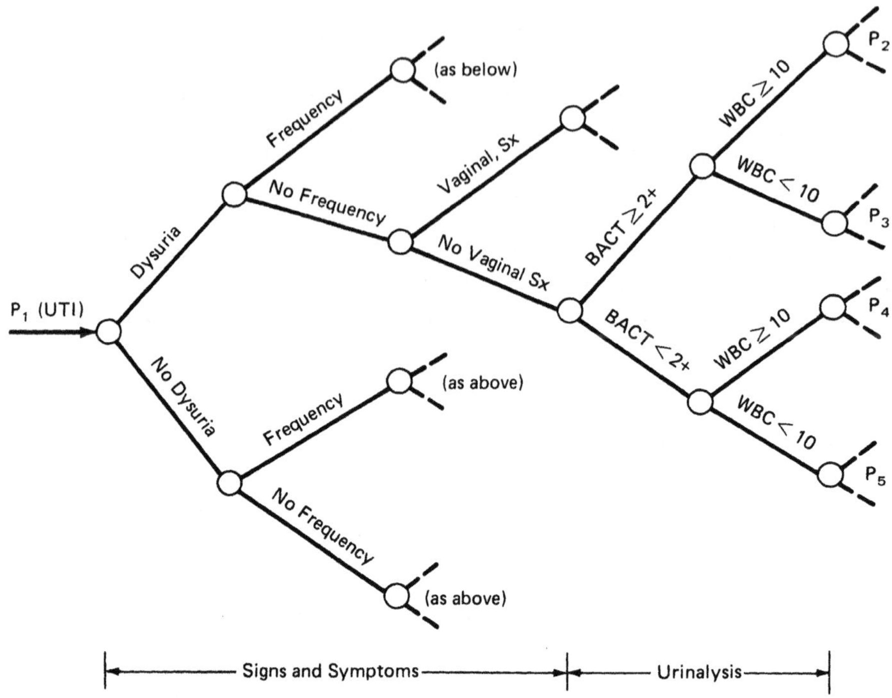

FIGURE 9.3A. UTI Decision Tree. (From Pass TM, Sherman H, Komaroff AL. Clinical Algorithms and Decision Analysis, *Fourth Illinois Conference* of *Medical Information Systems*, 1978, pp. 1-18. Reprinted with permission, AAMSI.)

and degree of disability which are then integrated into a decision tree for coronary bypass surgery. Nevertheless, it is important to recognize that the concept of decision analysis assumes the existence of an exhaustive decision table (or equivalent tree). In this sense, it is as restrictive as the algorithms previously discussed.

9.3.2. Bayesian Statistical Approaches

Throughout this chapter reference has been made to the use of probabilities in decision making. At each branch in Fig. 9.3 probabilities are given whose sum is 1. Of course, each of those outcome (O) probabilities assumes the existence of conditions (C) that lead to the node. Thus, the probability really is that of the outcome O given that the conditions C exist, written $P(O|C)$. In many cases, we know $P(C|O)$ and wish to find $P(O|C)$. To do this, we use Bayes' formula. By way of illustration, recal that in Section 9.2 we spoke of a test for a disease that is 95% accurate in identifying presence of the disease and produced a false-positive in 10% of the cases. The disease was found in 3% of the population. From this we have

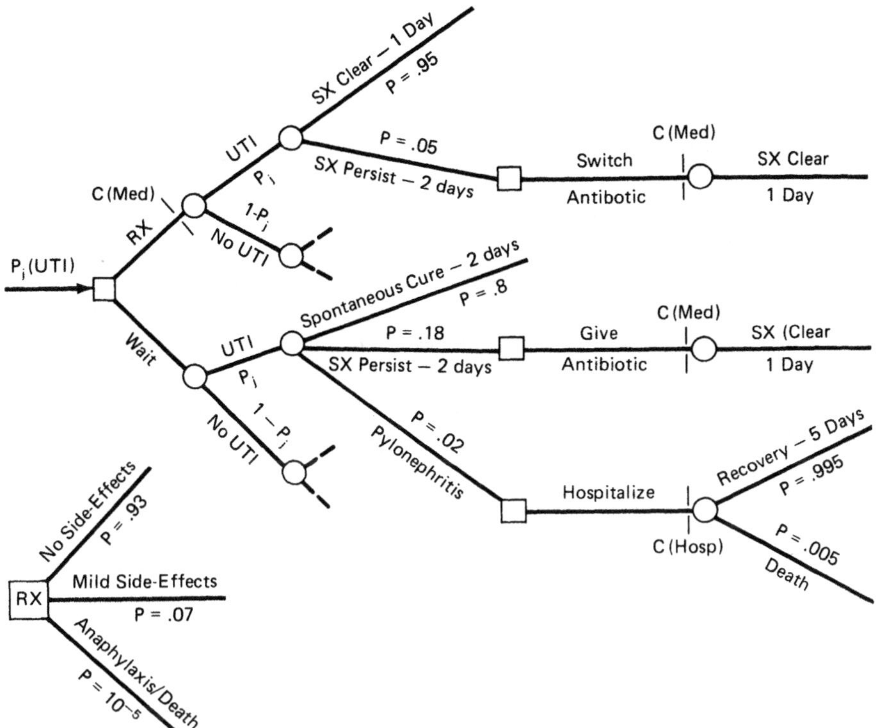

FIGURE 9.3B UTI Decision Tree. (From Pass TM, Sherman H, Komaroff AL. Clinical Algorithms and Decision Analysis, *Fourth Illinois Conference* of *Medical Information Systems,* 1978, pp. 1-18. Reprinted with permission, AAMSI.)

- Probability of the disease: $P(D) = .03$
- Probability of a positive test result on the condition that the disease is present: $P(T|D) = .95$
- Probability of a positive test result on the condition that the disease is not present: $P(T|\overline{D}) = .10$
- Probability of the disease given a positive test result: $P(D|T)$—to be computed.

Bayes' Theorem for this case states

$$P(D|T) = \frac{P(D) \cdot P(T|D)}{P(D) \cdot P(T|D) + P(\overline{D}) \cdot P(T|\overline{D})}$$

$$P(D|T) = \frac{(.03)\,(.95)}{(.03)\,(.95) + (.97)\,(.10)}$$

$$P(D|T) = .227$$

In a more general form for diagnosis D_i from the evidence E it becomes:

$$P(D_i|E = \frac{P(D_i) \cdot P\ (E|D_i)}{\sum_{j=1}^{n} P(D_j) \cdot P\ E|D_j)}$$

where $P(D_j)$ represent all of the *a priori* probabilities and the sum of these *a priori* probabilities is 1. This implies that the formula is valid only if the D_i are mutually exclusive and the D_i represent all possible selections.

In his book, *Computer-Assisted Medical Decision Making*, Warner shows how conditional probabilities can be used for making diagnostic decisions.[9] The example he uses is a pair of bags, A and B, each containing 1,000 marbles. The problem is one of selecting a marble from either bag A or B and presenting it to a judge. The judge must then determine from which bag the marble was taken. (The parallel with the diagnostic process is obvious.) Without prior knowledge, the probability that the marble came from bag A is 1,000/2,000 or .5. However, if there were some facts about the contents of the bags, then this information could be used in judging a single marble. Warner's example notes that some of the marbles were dirty and others rough with the following distribution:

	Dirty	Rough
Bag A	103	292
Bag B	810	651

Now, given a dirty marble (D), the probabilities can be computed

$$P(A|D) = .113$$
$$P(B|D) = .887$$

If it is rough and dirty, the conditional probability can be determined using P(A|D) from the previous computation

$$P(A|D,R) = \frac{P(A|D) \cdot P(R|A,D)}{P(A|D) \cdot P(R|A,D) + P(B|D) \cdot P(R|B,D)}$$

All the data are available to establish that

$$P(A|D,R) = .054$$

Therefore, when the judge is given a rough and dirty marble, he now has a 95% chance of making the correct decision.

Warner then extended the example to illustrate utility theory. Suppose the judge received a \$1,000 reward each time he correctly recognized a marble from bag A, and received a penalty of \$100 each time he was wrong; he also had a reward and penalty of \$100 and \$200 for bag B marbles. In tabular form:

	Source	**Bag**
Declared Source	**A**	**B**
A	1000	−200
B	−100	100

In this case we would adjust the selection threshold to ensure equal utility values for declaring either bag A or B, that is $U(A) = U(B)$. We then have the following formulas:

$$U(A) = 1000 \bullet P(A) + (-200) \bullet P(B)$$
$$U(B) = (-100) \bullet P(A) + 100 \bullet P(B)$$

substituting $P(B) = 1 - P(A)$ we find that a value of $P(A) = .21$ satisfies the above equations. Thus, a threshold (with no prior knowledge but taking the utility rewards into account) for making the decision that a marble came from bag A is .21 (and not .5). Put another way, one should select bag B only if one expects that the probabiity that the marble came from bag B to be .79 or higher. Naturally, the analysis is valid for $P(A|D)$, $P(A|D,R)$, etc.

Several things should be noted from this example. First, each additional attribute added information. With no attributes, the selection had a 50% chance of being correct. With the attribute dirty, the chance of a proper classification grew to 89% (for a dirty marble), and with two attributes it became 95% (for a rough dirty marble). Secondly, see how the complexity grows as attributes are added. With one attribute, we have four cases to consider:

$$\begin{matrix} AD & A\bar{D} \\ BD & B\bar{D} \end{matrix}$$

With two attributes there are eight cases.

$$\begin{matrix} ADR & AD\bar{R} & A\bar{D}R & A\overline{DR} \\ BDR & BD\bar{R} & B\bar{D}R & B\overline{DR} \end{matrix}$$

The number of cases is 2^n where n is the number of attributes. Also note how the computation allows the attributes to overlap, i.e., not be mutually exclusive. Given a database, the individual attribute distributions can be calculated by simple counting processes. Finally, recognize that the utility function value varies as the precision of the probabilities improves. These last points suggest that the computational complexity exceeds what can be reasonably expected of a physician, but the processing is ideally suited to a computer.

One often cited, early demonstration of the power of the Bayes' Theorem is the work of deDombal and his associates in the assessment of acute abdominal pain. Their first step was to collect data summarizing clinical and laboratory findings on 304 patients treated in the emergency room for acute abdominal pain. A computer program then used these attribute counts and distributions of diseases with acute abdominal pain as a symptom to compute an *a posterior* probability of the diagnosis. One then could specify the attribute values for patients with acute abdominal pain, and by use of the *a posterior* probabilities, determine the most likely diagnosis. In the initial 1971-1972 studies, the data were batched and used to confirm the physician's unaided diagnosis; subsequent use of the system made the results immediately available to the physician.

A comparison of the accuracy of the clinicians and computer system showed that the computer-aided system was 91.8% accurate, whereas that of the senior clinician to see each case was 79.6%. (A later study with 552 patients reported accuracies of 91.5% and 81.2% respectively.) The system also proved to be more reliable than the clinicians; surgeons performed 20-odd negative laparotomies whereas the computer recommended only six cases in which a laparotomies would have been negative. In the second study, where the results of the computer analysis were available to the physician after he made his initial decision, the proportion of appendices that perforated before operation fell from 36% to 4%, and the rate of negative laparotomy rate dropped sharply.

The system developed at Leeds University clearly showed that—with a narrow spectrum of diseases—computation using Bayesian statistics could produce better results than physicians. In a subsequent study (Leaper), they replaced the computed probabilities with expert estimates, and found that the system performed *less* well than the clinicians when expert (rather than computed) probabilities were used. This is consistent with the experience in cue processing and probability estimations which were discussed in the previous section. Thus, although Bayesian analysis offers no intuitive explanations, it does seem to provide reliable projections based on empirical evidence.

The Leeds system had access to only limited data restricted to patients with a single symptom. All data reflected the information available at the time of initial registration. It was noted that in only 45% of the cases was the admitting diagnosis identical to the final operation diagnosis, but the Leeds system chose not to use additional information to refine its predictions. What if a computer system were to have access to all current clinical data for all patients treated at the institution and was provided facilities to update and revise the probabilities as new data were processed? Clearly such a system would overcome some of the limitations imposed by the need to collect data and restrict the range of judgments (e.g., diagnosis, therapy). That system would also be able to provide the clinician with the objective data needed to make or evaluate his or her decisions; data that he or she understands and accepts as reliable but is unable to compute or estimate. HELP is such a system.

HELP was considered briefly as an HIS in Chapter 7. The present discussion will be limited to illustrating how it uses Bayesian statistics and its HIS database to assist in medical decision-making. We already have seen that the system reviews orders and prepares alerts when abnormal conditions are recognized. Conditions for these alerts are defined in HELP sectors. For example, Fig. 9.4 contains a HELP sector to be used whenever the conditions are satisfied which imply the printing of the message shown in line A. The sector causes testing for a relationship between the last reticulocyte count and the red blood cell count. If the sector is satisfied, then the alternative message is processed. The HELP sectors differ only in style from the AAMRS query languages presented in Chapter 8. Just like the RMRS CARE language, HELP sectors structure medical knowledge so that they can produce appropriate recommendations when matched against patient data. However, HELP also provides facilities that use Bayes' formula to compute *a posterior* probabilities. Thus, the quality of the information processed

```
SECTOR 5
HYPOCHROMIC MICROCYTIC ANEMIA—SUSPECT A HEMOGLOBINOPA-
THY. SUGGEST ORDER A HGB ELECTROPHORESIS
INHIBIT LOGIC = 6 7
*EVAL A AND (D GT 5000)
-----------------------------------------------------------------
A  (4) HYPOCHROMIC MICROCYTIC ANEMIA. SUGGEST ORDER RETI-
       CULOCYTE COUNT AND LOOK FOR BLEEDING
B      (A) RETICULOCYTE COUNT (×10)% LAST
C      (A) CBC, RED BLOOD COUNT (RBC ×100) MIL/M3 NEAR EVNT B
D      B*C
-----------------------------------------------------------------
```

FIGURE 9.4. Sample HELP sector. (From Warner H. *Computer-Assisted Medical Decision-Making*, 1979. Reproduced with permission, Academic Press.)

by HELP is far superior to the information available to a typical CIS: it contains both the raw data (e.g., laboratory results, diagnosis) and the calibrated data (i.e., interpretations of the raw data based on the medical knowledge in the HELP sectors). Moreover, HELP also provides for the integration of physician- or patient-supplied values in the decision-making process.

To illustrate how the Bayesian statistics are applied, consider a HELP sector designed to calculate the likelihood of pleural fluid in a patient (see Fig. 9.5). It is known that 10 out of 1,000 (1%) of the Latter Day Saints Hospital patients for whom a chest x-ray film is ordered have pleural fluid. That is the *a priori* probability that pleural fluid is present in this population. If one knows that it is a type 1, 2, 3, 7, or 56 x-ray procedure, then the *a priori* probabilities can be adjusted to a value from 7.9% to 52.4%. The computation of these probabilities is quite simple. Count the number of patients for whom chest x-rays were ordered and divide them into two categories: those with and without pleural fluid. Of course this probability has built into it the chest x-ray ordering patterns at Latter Day Saints, the patient mix at Latter Day Saints, the presence of pleural fluid at Latter Day Saints, etc.

Now we begin to structure the medical knowledge. There are different reasons for ordering a chest x-ray. One would expect the distributions to vary with these reasons. The key general reasons are pre-op, follow-up to known disease, and post-op. The specific reasons are chest pain, coronary artery disease, or suspected pleural effusion, pneumothorax, or pulmonary embolus. It would also help to know if the patient was ambulatory or if pleural fluid was reported in the last 2 days. Finally, the patient's age and albumin, hemoglobin, and calcium test results provide additional information about the likelihood of pleural fluid.

Part of a HELP sector designed to use this knowledge is contained in Fig. 9.5. Lines (items) in the sector are defined by letters A . . . Z, AA . . . . References to an item are by this identifier. Item A indicates that this sector should be executed each time a new chest x-ray exam is to be processed. B

		Pleural Fluid	Final Evaluation II
A		X-ray, chest, specific exam	
B		10	
C		If (A EQ 7) then B = 524	
D		If (A EQ 1) or (A EQ 2)) or (A EQ 3) then B = 150	
E		IF (A EQ 56) then B = 79	
F		Chest pain (reason)	
G	?	Pleural effusion (reason)	
H		Pre-op (general reason)	
I		Followup known disease (general reason)	
J		Chair (transportation)	
K		Post op (general reason)	
L		Walk (transportation)	
M	?	Pneumothorax (reason)	
N		Coronary artery disease (reason)	
O	?	Pulmonary embolus (reason)	
P		Pleural fluid reported in last 2 days	

		(Item)	(Prior prob.)	P(S/D)	P(S/D)
Q	Prob binary	F	B	.022	.070
R		G	Q	.193	.029
S		H	R	.009	.150
T		I	S	.210	.146
U		J	T	.546	.420
V		K	U	.395	.225
W		L	V	.004	.084
X		M	W	.059	.021
Y		N	X	.004	.030
Z		O	Y	.053	.018
AA		P	Z	.243	.036

BB	(A) SMA-12, Albmin GM%
CC	(A) CBC, Hemoglobin GM%
DD	(A) SMA-12, Calcium MG%
EE	(A) Age

		Item	(P)	Min	Max	(1)	(2)	(3)	(4)	(5)	(6)	(7)	(8)
FF	Prob dist	BB	AA	1.1	5.4	6/2	12/4	16/8	23/13	22/19	12/25	6/17	2/12
GG	Prob dist	CC	FF	4.7	18.0	5/2	14/7	18/9	23/11	18/19	13/23	6/16	2/14
HH	Prob dist	DD	GG	6.8	11.0	6/2	12/4	15/10	21/15	18/28	18/27	6/10	3/3
II	Prob dist	EE	HH	0	100	1/1	4/6	5/11	8/11	25/24	34/31	18/13	5/3

FIGURE 9.5. HELP sector logic for calculating likelihood of pleural fluid in a patient. Reprinted with permission from *Journal of Medical Systems*, 7, Plenum Publishing Corp., © 1983; modified from a version previously published in *Proceedings of the Sixth Annual Symposium on Computer Applications in Medical Care*, IEEE, 1982.

assigns the *a priori* probability as 10/1,000 and items C, D, and E adjust the probability for different test types. Items F through P identify the medical factors listed in the previous paragraph that can be evaluated in a binary (yes/no) fashion. Items Q through AA provide the *a priori* probabilities for each item in the previous list. For example, in item Q, the numbers .022 and .070 reflect the probabilities that, for an inpatient at Latter Day Saints with and without pleural fluid by x-ray, chest pain (F = yes) would be given as a reason for ordering the x-ray film. The value of item B is to be used as the prior probability in

Bayes' formula when item Q is executed. If the item is not true (F = no), then the prior probability is unchanged.

The value of item Q is used in the calculation of item R in the same way. In this manner, AA reflects the posterior probability of pleural fluid under the conditions B through P. Items BB through EE represent continuous functions. HELP breaks each into 8 discrete bins and computes the *a priori* probabilities for each bin. In this case, item FF indicates that the percent of patients with and without pleural fluid whose last albumin value was in the bin 1.1—1.5 GM% was 6% and 2%. In the bin 1.6—2.0 it was 13% and 4%, and so on. As in the case of items Q through AA, items BB through EE find the last value for the clinical parameter identified and items FF through II apply Bayes' formula to the last result. The final probability is found in II.

The format of the HELP sectors seems confusing and unfriendly at first. However, all the necessary information is presented in a clear fashion. There are over 2,000 such sectors that formalize medical knowledge, and researchers have access to system tools to define more specialized sectors. Printed outputs eliminate the housekeeping details of the HELP sectors. Fig. 9.6 illustrates a consultation report. Superficially, it resembles the types of report that one might reasonably expect to find from RMRS, SCAMP, or COSTAR. The major difference, of course, is that the HELP system uses medical knowledge to compute *a posterior* probabilities which it then uses in selecting comments. These probabilities are derived from seemingly obscure numbers, e.g., the probability that chest pain was given as a reason for ordering a chest x-ray at Latter Day Saints for patients with and without pleural fluid. Such numbers are easily counted when access to a comprehensive database is available.

DeDombal showed that Bayesian analysis could produce better results than clinicians. The HELP developers have shown that computers can manage the large amounts of data necessary to apply this technique in a general way. Further, HELP demonstrates that these functions can be integrated with an HIS. (Current technology places a limit on the number of HELP sectors that can be processed on demand in the clinical areas. Consequently, the Latter Day Saints researchers are now developing a microcomputer supported terminal/workstation for more complex decision-making support at the patient's bedside.) Nevertheless, there are limits to the use of Bayesian statistics. They reflect local experience and not universal truths. For example, the Latter Day Saints probabilities may not provide accurate recommendations for an Elmira, New York patient population. Neither will they "explain" why a recommendation was made. Nevertheless, HELP illustrates a practical realization of the concepts prophetically described by Ledley and Lusted in 1959. It is in routine clinical use and is undergoing commercial/marketplace evaluation. Moreover, the techniques employed are readily transferred to other CISs.

9.3.3. Other Analysis Techniques for Databases

The availability of a large clinical database presents many alternative approaches for processing data used in medical decision-making. Among the most common

```
       341086                  SEX - M              AGE 66
   DR. NELSON, R.R.            ROOM 4N80            ADMIT 11/4/78

ADMIT DX
   AORTIC VALVE, STENOSIS                          4      5      6

HISTORY FINDINGS:
   1      CHOLECYSTITIS                            *

MEDICATION REACTION:
   2      SUGGEST THAT PATIENT RECEIVE A
          POTASSIUM SUPPLEMENT AS THE
          PATIENTS HYPOKALEMMIA OF 3.0
          MEQ/L INCREASES THE RISK OF
          DIGITALIS TOXICITY                              *

COAGULATION FINDINGS:
   3      PROLONGED PTT. SUGGEST ORDER
          COAGULATION SCREENING PRO-
          FILE (PT AND PLATELET COUNT)             *

   4      COMMON PATHWAY FACTOR DEFI-
          CIENCY IS SUSPECTED. SUGGEST
          ORDER NORMAL PLASMA DISTRIBU-
          TION TESTS

PULMONARY FINDINGS:
   5      MILD RESTRICTIVE CHEST DISEASE
          ORDER LUNG VOLUME AND DLCO
          TESTS IF CLINICALLY INDICATED                          *

ECG FINDINGS:
   6      ATRIAL FIBRILLATION, MODERATE
          VENTRICULAR RATE                         *
```

FIGURE 9.6. Sample online display of HELP decision. (From Warner H. *Computer-Assisted Medical Decision-Making,* 1979. Reproduced with permission, Academic Press.)

tools are the standard statistical packages. These are available for mainframe, minicomputer, and microcomputer systems. Most support interactive analysis and can produce plots, multiway tables, and descriptive statistics. Although most systems are primarily used in a research setting, these packages can be loaded with clinical data to produce effective extensions of the ad hoc query capabilities normally included with an information system. Systems—such as CLINFO—that have been designed for clinical research have increased the clinician's sensitivity to the benefits of these tools. The emerging generation of microcomputer systems that can communicate with larger databases should increase interest in the application of such personalized, off-line decision support tools.

In addition to HIS databases, there are also databases designed to collect detailed data about a specific disease. The database may be restricted to a single institution or it may be part of a national databank. Where such data are available, well-structured and reliable, they may be used to measure prognostic indicators and compare responsees to various therapies for specific subgroups of patients. An example of a report from ARAMIS was presented in Chapter 8. In that instance a national arthritis databank was used to project the outcome for a given patient based on the experience with aspirin and prednisone therapy for similar patients. Rosati and his colleagues implemented a similar system that was limited to patients who have undergone coronary arteriography; their system produced reports called a prognostigram. In each of these two cases, the cost for processing the report is charged to the patient as if it were a laboratory study. Such systems illustrate the potential benefits from consulting (querying) a specialized database system to evaluate alternative therapies for individual patients.

Finally, databases may be used as a resource for statistical pattern recognition analysis. The approach is similar to the Bayesian analysis previously discussed in that an existing database is used to detect predictive factors. In the case of pattern recognition, a discriminant function is computed from a set of features. The features are properties that the researcher would expect to be related to the diagnosis or prognosis, and the discriminant represents the posterior probability as a function of the features and associated weights. That is:

$$P(D|X) = a_1x_i + a_2x_i + a_2x_2 + \cdots + a_nx_n$$

where a_i are weights and the x_i are the descriptive variables (i.e., features).

Pattern analysis is performed after a training set has been prepared. This contains the descriptive variables for the features that the investigator believes will define an effective discriminant function. The training set is processed using one of a dozen of mathematical techniques, and the discriminant function is produced. It must then be evaluated against individuals (both in and outside the training set) to validate its predictive utility. To illustrate, Faught and his associates defined the following discriminant function based on the data of 87 stroke patients.[10]

```
D =  8 * NUMBER OF TRANSIENT ISCHEMIC ATTACKS
  +  6 * NUMBER OF ARTERIES CATHETERIZED
  + 14 * PRESENCE(DIABETES MELLITUS)
  + 11 * PRESENCE(SEX = FEMALE).
```

They observed that when D was calculated to be more than 55 for one of their patients, that patient had a .77 probability of having a neurological complication from arteriography. When D was less than 55, there was only a .02 likelihood of a complication. Thus, a simple calculation can be used to provide a powerful predictor of risk that can be used by many different systems. In fact, the above discriminant function is shown in the syntax of KMS so that it can be integrated into an expert system (Reggia).

9.4. Artificial Intelligence in Medicine

In Chapter 2 the field of Artificial Intelligence (AI) was briefly addressed and one subfield—expert systems—was identified as being of particular interest to medicine. In fact, the term Artificial Intelligence in Medicine (AIM) is generally limited to the use of expert systems for clinical decision-making. There is no precise definition of AI. It is a branch of computer science that studies how to make computers do things that people currently perceive as requiring intelligence. Naturally such perceptions vary with time and experience. As we noted in Chapter 1, Turing introduced a test for computer intelligence. Place a terminal in a room with a test subject. In another room, connect the terminal to both a computer and a human tester. If the subject cannot tell from his dialogue whether he is interacting with the computer or the human tester, then the machine is said to be intelligent. (Of course, to exhibit intelligent behavior, the machine may have to introduce unnecessary delays, respond with false answers, etc.). He later made the following observation.

The extent to which we regard something as behaving in an intelligent manner is determined as much by our own state of mind and training as by the properties of the object under consideration. If we are able to explain and predict its behaviour or if there seems to be little underlying plan, we have little temptation to imagine intelligence. With the same object therefore it is possible that one man would consider it as intelligent and another would not; the second man would have found out the rules of its behaviour.[11] (From Turing AM. In: *Machine Inteligence* 5, 1970, p. 23. Reprinted with permission of Halstead Press.)

Therefore, it might be better to refer to AI techniques rather than AI since once a technique is understood it loses its quality of intelligent behavior. In fact, it will be shown that it is common to develop applications in an AI research environment and then implement them using more traditional programming languages.

Why use AI techniques? Szolovits suggests that they are a good engineering approach to capturing the best-understood source of existing expertise on medicine. He continues:

The choice to model the behavior of a computer expert in medicine on the expertise of human consultants is by no means logically necessary. If we could understand the functioning in health and in disease of the human body in sufficient depth to model the detailed disease processes which disturb health, then, at least in principle, we could perform diagnosis by fitting our model to the actually observable characteristics of the patient at hand. Further, we could try out possible therapies on the model to select the optimum one to use on the patient. Unfortunately, although biomedical research strives for such a depth of understanding, it has not been achieved in virtually *any* area of medical practice. The AIM methodology does not dogmatically reject the use of non-human modes of expertise in the computer. Indeed, accurate computations of probabilities and solutions of simple differential equations—tasks at which human experts are rather poor without special training—play a role in some of our programs. Nevertheless, most of what we know about the practice of medicine we know from interrogating the best human practitioners; therefore, the techniques we tend to build into our programs mimic those used by our clinician informants.

Relying on the knowledge of human experts to build expert computer programs is actually helpful for several additional reasons: First, the decisions and recommendations of a program can be explained to its users and evaluators in terms which are familiar to the experts. Second, because we hope to duplicate the expertise of human specialists, we can measure the extent to which our goal is achieved by a direct comparison of the program's behavior to that of the experts. Finally, within the collaborative group of computer scientists and physicians engaged in AIM research, basing the logic of the programs on human models supports each of the three somewhat disparate goals that the researchers may hold:

- To develop expert computer programs for clinical use . . . .
- To formalize medical expertise . . . .
- To test AI theories in a "real world" domain . . . .

(From Szolovits P. (ed) *Artificial Intelligence in Medicine*, 1983, pp. 3-4. Westview Press, Boulder, CO. Reprinted with permission.)

Researchers have an interest in AIM because the attributes of medical reasoning make it an ideal subject for AI investigations. The decisions are made with uncertainty and incomplete data; multiple, parallel problems may exist; there is a single correct solution; and the clinical judgments required for decision-making are seldom fully defined. The clinical decision-making process, as described by Gorry in 1973, has these properties:

- It is based less on a detailed knowledge of pathophysiology than on chunks of knowledge and experience that are applied heuristically.
- Clinicians know facts, but their knowledge is also largely judgmental. This allows them to form hypotheses rapidly. They apply precise logical or statistical reasoning.
- It is easier for experts to state their rules in response to misconceptions of others than to define them without a context.

He arrived at these conclusions after analyzing experience with an acute renal failure program using decision analysis. The cases of most interest were those in which physicians did well but the programs did not. (These findings are consistent with Elstein's observations presented in Section 9.2.) Gorry concluded that the clinical decision tools were inadequate and that successful systems had to include medical concepts (i.e., "understanding") and support conversational capabilities. Both features are now considered essential in AIM; they imply a major reliance on symbolic reasoning (or inference) as contrasted with numerical computation.

Since most AIM applications are expert systems, we first present a four-component model for such a system. This is shown in Fig. 9.7. The Knowledge Base is a representation of the expert knowledge. It is structured so that (a) it may be searched and (b) it preserves relationships among concepts. It is used for all problems addressed by the system. There is also a Global Database. This contains the data that describe the status of a particular problem. It is composed of both the initial problem statement plus any data derived from the application of knowledge in the Knowledge Base. (Sometimes these are organized as a single database with the Knowledge Base called the static data and the Global Database the dynamic data.)

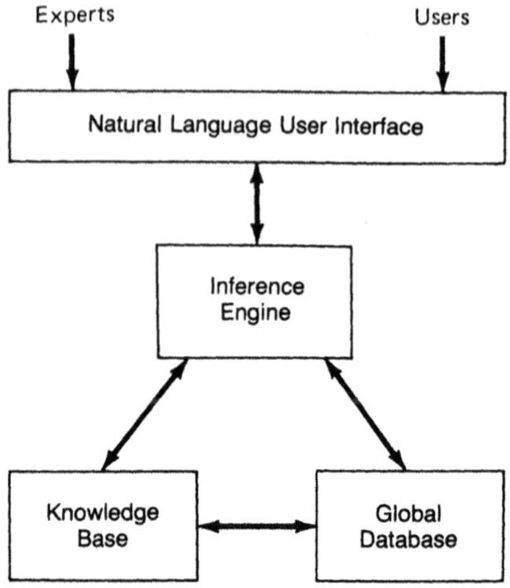

FIGURE 9.7. Sample expert system.

The Inference Engine is the control program that uses the Knowledge Base to create or modify the contents of the Global Database. As its name implies, it uses inference (as opposed to direct retrieval or computation) to search the Knowledge Base and Global Database. The control used to direct the search processing is called a heuristic—it is a "rule of thumb" rather than an algorithm that produces an exact solution. This means that the expert system can use the contents of the Knowledge Base to guide in the search and that inference mechanisms may be used where exact matches do not exist. The final component of an expert system is a natural language interface that is used by the expert to enter new knowledge as text and by the expert system to provide results and explanations using this text. (Ideally, problem queries would also be entered as text; in most cases, however, some structuring of the input data is assumed.)

The examples of the next subsections will clarify this initial description of an expert system. The major issues in creating medical expert systems are:

- *How to represent the medical knowledge*. The knowledge is organized separately from the Inference Engine, and some systems allow the user to apply the same Inference Engine for any knowledge base (i.e., the systems are domain-independent). Most systems are not as general as a DBMS. The representation of medical knowledge is an area of active research.
- *How to build a knowledge base*. Current procedures require 6 months to several years to formulate a baseline; the full knowledge base may take 5 or more years to build. A programmer is required to support this process. This implies that the Knowledge Base and the Inference Engine are closely associated.
- *How to produce a clinically acceptable system*. Problems of efficacy, reliability, responsiveness, acceptability, etc. must be resolved. In a sense, the

expert system is like the CIS of the early 1970s. The supporting technology is not yet mature, and it is difficult to separate the application from its research issues.

The use of AI offers the promise of (a) expert consultations where other techniques fail and (b) the ability to maintain cumulative pools of expert knowledge. The use of AI techniques also is associated with issues of style that emphasize more flexible user environments, explanation of the rationale for a recommendation, ability to deal with incomplete data, the use of inferential techniques, etc.

The following subsections describe some representative examples of AIM applictions. A final section compares these systems with the clinical decision-making tools of the previous section.

9.4.1. Some Rule Based Systems

Rule based expert systems—also called production systems—maintain the knowledge base in the form of IF . . . THEN . . . rules. For example:

IF there is acute abdominal pain, and
the patient has had an appendectomy
THEN rule out appendicitis

At first glance, this may look like the IF . . . THEN . . . ELSE . . . statements of structured programs or the IF . . . THEN <action> statements of RMRS/CARE. The difference is that in a production rule the THEN clause contains statements of fact (the consequents) that will be accepted as true if the preceding IF clauses (the antecedents) are true. On the other hand, the programming and query IF . . . THEN . . . statements are used to define actions to be taken when the IF conditions are satisfied. Moreover, the actions to be taken will depend on the sequence of the statements. That is, for a program with a series of IF . . . THEN . . . ELSE . . . statements, the order of the statements fully defines the order in which they will be used. We say it is highly structured. In the case of the production rules, however, there is no concept of order. Each rule represents a small chunk of knowledge (usually within some restrictive context). This provides a mechanism to manage data that are poorly structured, e.g., in situations where there is uncertainty. The inference engine may chain through the rules; where there are multiple rules affecting the same fact, evidence gathering can be used to determine which should be applied.

Another—and perhaps more important—distinction is that with production rules we are codifying knowledge about facts and not describing actions. Results are gained by searching the rules for desired facts called goals. There are two basic modes for searching in a production system:

- Goal-directed search in which one attempts to satisfy those antecedents which would allow the consequents (or goals) to be validated. In the previous example, one would first examine the Global Database (i.e., the set of known facts for this instance) and see if the patient had acute abdominal pain. If that were not yet known, then the system would make "acute abdominal pain" a subgoal and identify the antecedents of all production rules that could be used to establish whether or not this was true. The process would be repeated in a similar way until it was determined that the patient did or did not exhibit acute abdominal pain. This is also called top-down or backward reasoning.

- Data-driven search in which one collects rules for which all the antecedents are known to be correct and then asserts that their consequents are correct. The Global Database is enlarged to include these consequents and the process repeats. This is also called bottom-up or forward reasoning.

Another search technique, hypothesis directed reasoning, will be discussed in Section 9.4.2.

As can be anticipated, all searching involves iterations—some of which will lead to dead ends. Backtracking is used to recover from situations in which a search path will not lead to a goal. In a blind search, nothing is known about the knowledge base; the larger the knowledge base, the longer the search time. However, when there is some understanding of the knowledge base, it can be used to improve search performance. Such knowledge is implemented as heuristics in the control mechanism, i.e., the Inference Engine. When Fig. 9.7 represents a production rule system, the Inference Engine implements a search strategy with appropriate heuristics, the Knowledge Base is composed of production rules of the form,

IF <antecedents> THEN <consequents>

and the Global Database contains the state (valid facts) for the current problem (instance). Production rule systems are the easiest model of an expert system to explain.

We shall now examine several members of a family of production systems developed at Stanford University. Fig. 9.8 presents a diagram of the family members.[12] There are several generations of systems beginning with DENDRAL (see Chapter 2), but this discussion will be limited to MYCIN, PUFF, and ONCOCIN. It should be noted that the tree includes systems designed to use the knowledge base as an explanation or teaching tool (GUIDON), to acquire knowledge (TEIRESIAS), to build expert systems (EMYCIN), and to manage a respiratory ventilation system (VM). We begin with MYCIN, a key pioneering AIM application which has been influential and widely referenced.

MYCIN, an expert system developed by Shortliffe, Buchanan, and others, specializes in the diagnosis and therapy selection for patients with specific infectious diseases: blood infections and meningitis. The knowledge base uses production rules of the form shown in Fig. 9.9. Each rule is identified by a number and consists of antecedents, consequents, and a rationale, i.e., justification and citations. The system uses a goal-directed search; that is, if it is not known if the infection that requires therapy is meningitis, then this becomes a subgoal to be established by either applying other production rules or interacting

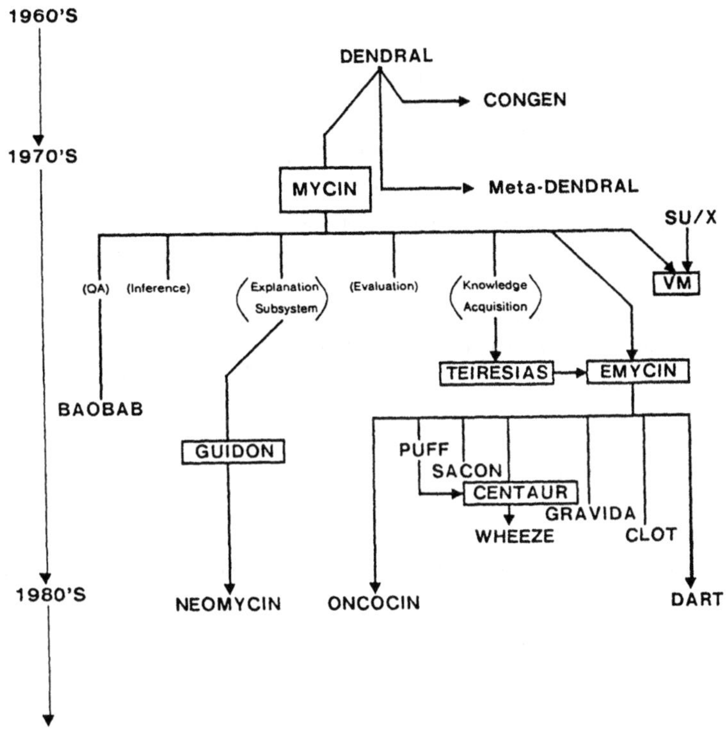

FIGURE 9.8. Stanford programs relating to MYCIN. (from Buchanan BG, Shortliffe EH, *Rule Based Expert Systems*, © 1984, Addison-Wesley, Reading, Massachusetts. Reprinted with permission.)

with the user. As in most AIM applications, one must deal with uncertainty. In the case of MYCIN, each rule is assigned a certainty factor (CF) between -1 and 1. While the numerical range is the same as a correlation, the CF is not a computed statistical value. Rather, it is a number that combines subjective probabilities and utilities to represent the importance of the fact. In the example of Fig. 9.9 the CF is given as (.5) for suggestive evidence.

MYCIN's Inference Engine searches the rules in the Knowledge Base and establishes facts and their certainty. The certainty of antecedents is used to establish the certainty of consequents. For example, the CF of a production rule is the product of the consequent's CF and the lowest CF of all the antecedents, i.e., the product of the certainty of the general rule and that of the least certain antecedent in a conjunction. In this way, when MYCIN arrives at a goal (or subgoal) it has some estimate for the certainty of that goal. It also has an audit trail of how it arrived at this certainty and a description of the rules it used. Through HOW and WHY functions, the system can justify its actions. This

RULE 280

IF:
1) The infection which requires therapy is meningitis, and
2) The type of the infection is fungal, and
3) Organisms were not seen on the stain of the culture, and
4) The patient is not a compromised host, and
5) The patient has been to an area that is endemic for coccidiomycoses, and
6) The race of the patient is one of: black asian indian, and
7) The cryptococcal antigen in the csf was not positive

THEN: There is suggestive evidence (.5) that cryptococcus is not one of the organisms (other than those seen on cultures or smears) which might be causing the infection.

AUTHOR:YU

Justification: Dark-skinned races, especially Filipino, Asian, and Black (in that order) have an increased susceptibility to coccidiomycoses meningitis.

Literature: Stevens, D.A. et al. Miconazole in Coccidiomycosis. Am. J. Med, 60:191-202, Feb 1976.

FIGURE 9.9. Sample rule from MYCIN. (From DA Stevens et al., *American Journal of Medicine,* Feb. 1976. Copyright by Yorke Medical Group, reprinted by permission.)

feature is useful in explaining why a diagnosis or therapeutic recommendation was made; it is also useful to the expert in the testing and evaluation of the knowledge base.

There were three evaluations of MYCIN in the mid-1970s. In each case there was a 75% overall approval of the program's advice. The third study also was able to demonstrate that the system advice "was comparable to that of infectious disease experts and that 75% is in fact *better* than the degree of agreement that could generally be achieved by Stanford faculty being assessed under the same criteria."[13] Yet the system was not used in a routine clinical setting. As its developers explained:

Although we have frequently referred to human engineering issues throughout this book and have considered them from the outset in our design of MYCIN and its descendents, we have also noted that MYCIN was never used routinely in patient-care settings. Yes, the program was able to explain its reasoning, and this seemed likely to heighten its acceptability. And yes we spent much time attending to detail so that (a) user aids were available at any time through the use of HELP and question mark commands, (b) the system automatically corrected spelling errors when it was "obvious" what the user meant, and (c) a physician could enter only the first few characters of a response if what was entered uniquely defined the intended answer. However, there were still significant barriers that prevented us from undertaking the move to formal implementation.[14] (From Buchanan BG, Shortliffe EH, *Rule Based Expert Systems,* © 1984, Addison-Wesley, Reding, Massachusetts. Reprinted with permission.)

The barriers included limitations of the knowledge base, the absence of a perceived need for such a system, and the inability to provide a reliable, convenient and inexpensive computer resource. Thus, in 1978 MYCIN became a static system. Consequently, by the time AAMRSs consistently were meeting Barnett's first criteria of "Will people use it?" expert systems were still unable to pass this first critical test. The next system to be considered, however, is being used routinely for other than experimental purposes. In fact, it also satisfies the second of Barnett's criteria. "Will people pay for it?"

PUFF is an expert system that interprets measurements from respiratory tests administered to patients in the pulmonary (lung) function laboratory. It is in daily operational use at the Pacific Medical Center in San Francisco and, from the installation in 1979 through mid-1982, had been used to interpret the results of over 4,000 cases. Approximately 85% of the reports generated were accepted without modification; a sample is shown in Fig. 9.10.[15] The use of an expert system for pulmonary function interpretation was chosen for several reasons. There was a practical need for tools to support such analyses. The function was not understood well enough for the biomedical researchers to solve it, but it was small enough to suggest that an AI solution was practical. All the data required for decision-making were available in the database and interactive queries were not necessary. There was interest in the AI and biomedical research communities, and a clinical environment anxious to use the system was found.

PUFF was developed using EMYCIN which provides an environment for implementing expert systems. The EMYCIN-PUFF system consisted of 64 production rules using a set of 54 clinical parameters. Because EMYCIN uses INTERLISP, it was not practical to install the system at the Pacific Medical Center. Consequently, the system was reprogrammed in BASIC to run on a PDP-11. The BASIC-PUFF system was enlarged to contain 400 production rules and 75 clinical parameters. Thus, PUFF is an example of:

- An expert system in routine clinical use
- An expert system that interfaces with a clinical database thereby avoiding lengthy interactions
- A knowledge based application that produces very acceptable results for an analysis that had not been solved by traditional paradigms.
- A system that uses AI techniques once they have been developed and demonstrated in an AI environment.

A major reason for the success of PUFF is that, by avoiding physician interaction, it also avoided one of the major difficulties associated with performance and the human interface.

The final of the production systems to be considered, ONCOCIN, is concerned with the problem of physician use of an extent system. It was designed to assist clinical oncologists in the treatment of cancer patients. When chemotherapy is used, protocols normally are followed to define a sequence of therapies with modifications as toxicities (side effects) are identified. We have seen how clinical algorithms have been used to guide this process (p. 303), and in Chapter 10 a more general database approach will be considered. In this section we shall examine how AI techniques can be applied to demonstrate a rule-based consultation system with an explanation capability for use in a busy clinical environment.

ONCOCIN is composed of two major modules: the Interviewer, which interacts with the clinician, and the Reasoner, which applies the production rules of the

PUFF

PRESBYTERIAN HOSPITAL OF PMC
CLAY AND BUCHANAN, BOX 7999
SAN FRANCISCO, CA. 94120
PULMONARY FUNCTION LAB

JAMES
P186455.
DR. WAYBURN

PUL

WT 69.0 KG, HT 182 CM, AGE 66 SEX M
REFERRAL DX-

**TEST DATE 06/28/82

		PREDICTED (+/-SD)	OBSER	(%PRED)	POST DILATION OBSER	(%PRED)
INSPIR VITAL CAP (IVC)	L	4.5(0.6)	3.2	(71)	3.3	(73)
RESIDUAL VOL (RV)	L	2.4(0.4)	2.4	(99)	1.9	(78)
TOTAL LUNG CAP (TLC)	L	6.9(0.7)	5.6	(81)	5.2	(75)
RV/TLC	%	35.	43.		37.	
FORCED EXPIR VOL(FEV1)	L	3.3 (0.5)	2.2	(66)	2.3	(69)
FORCED VITAL CAP (FVC)	L	4.5 (0.6)	3.2	(71)	3.3	(73)
FEV1/FVC	%	76.	69.		70.	
PEAK EXPIR FLOW (PEF)	L/S	9.1 (1.7)	4.1	(45)	4.8	(52)
FORCED EXP FLOW 25-75%	L/S	3.3 (0.8)	1.4	(42)	1.6	(48)
AIRWAY RESIST(RAW) (TLC 5.6)		2.5	3.5		1.2	

DF CAP-HGB= 0.0 (TLC 5.1) 25. 18.1 (72) (56%IF TLC= 6.9)

ARTERIAL BLOOD GASES	PH	PCO2	PO2	SAT%	HCO3	BASEX.
REST ROOM AIR	7.48	40.0	77.0	96.0	30.0	7.0

****

INTERPRETATION: THE REDUCED TLC AND IVC INDICATE A MILD RESTRICTIVE DEFECT. THE FORCED VITAL CAPACITY, FEV1/FVC RATIO AND MID-EXPIRATORY FLOW ARE REDUCED AND THE AIRWAY RESISTANCE IS INCREASED, SUGGESTING MODERATE AIRWAY OBSTRUCTION. FOLLOWING BRONCHODILATION, THE EXPIRED FLOWS SHOW ONLY SLIGHT IMPROVEMENT. HOWEVER, THE DECREASE IN AIRWAY RESISTANCE INDICATES SOME REVERSIBLE COMPONENT. THE LOW DIFFUSING CAPACITY INDICATES A LOSS OF ALVEOLAR CAPILLARY SURFACE, WHICH IS SEVERE.

WHEN CORRECTED FOR AGE, ARTERIAL PO2 AND PCO2 ON ROOM AIR ARE WITHIN NORMAL LIMITS. THE ARTERIAL PH IS SLIGHTLY INCREASED. THIS IS CONSISTENT WITH A MILD METABOLIC ALKALOSIS WITHOUT RESPIRATORY COMPENSATION.

CONCLUSIONS: THE REDUCED DIFFUSING CAPACITY IS CONSISTENT WITH THE COMBINATION OF DISEASES. IN VIEW OF THE RESPONSE TO BRONCHODILATORS, CONTINUED USE WOULD BE RECOMMENDED.

PULMONARY FUNCTION DIAGNOSIS:
1. MODERATE OBSTRUCTIVE AIRWAYS DISEASE.
2. SEVERE DIFFUSION DEFECT.
3. MILD RESTRICTIVE LUNG DISEASE.
4. MILD METABOLIC ALKALOSIS.

ROBERT FALLAT, M.D.

FIGURE 9.10. Sample PUFF pulmonary function report. (From Aikins JS, Kunz JC, Shortliffe EH, Fallat RJ. PUFF: an expert system for interpretation of pulmonary function data. *Comp Biomed Res* 16:203, 1983. Reproduced with permission of Academic Press.)

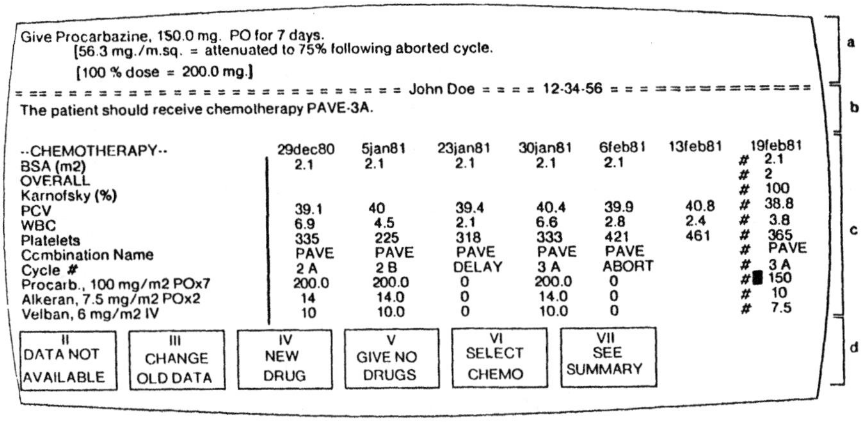

FIGURE 9.11. The clinician enters the data from the current visit in the rightmost column of the Flowsheet Section. This is passed to the Reasoner which makes recommendations. In this case, the explanation section shows the system's justification of the therapy advice corresponding to the user-controlled cursor location (box). The soft key descriptions act as special function keys. All selections can use the mouse; they are managed by the Interviewer. (From Langlotz CP, Shortliffe EH. Adapting a consultation system to critique user plans. *Int J Man-Machine Studies* 19:483, 1983. Reproduced with permission of Academic Press.)

Knowledge Base to make recommendations. The system differs from most medical applications in that the current prototype uses a high-resolution bit map display that supports text, graphics, and the use of a mouse. In this way, management of the user interface is less imposing than the traditional dialog mode. (A sample screen from the system in use since 1981 is shown in Fig. 9.11).[16] The Reasoner also differs from the systems presented earlier in that it does not employ the techniques supported by EMYCIN. Because there is a need to provide links between patient visits to assess temporal trends, ONCOCIN cannot use EMYCIN's data structures. Because the rules (which are similar in format to the MYCIN rule shown in Fig. 9.8) are based on protocol definitions, ONCOCIN does not have to deal with uncertainty. Finally, because of the nature of the Interviewer interactions, a data-directed search mode is required.

Why then does ONCOCIN use AI techniques? Shortliffe and his colleagues answer the question in this way:

Complicated though the chemotherapy protocols may be, they are largely algorithmic, and other groups have been able to encode much of the knowledge using less complex representation techniques. Our reasons for choosing an AI approach for encoding the knowledge of oncology chemotherapy are varied. It should be stressed that all protocols have important loopholes and exceptions: when an aberrant situation arises for a patient being treated, the proper management is typically left unspecified. . . . The protocols often defer to the opinions of the attending physicians without providing guidelines on which they might base their decisions. Hence there is no standardization of responses to unusual problems, and the validity of the protocol analysis in these cases is accordingly subject to question. Our long-term goal is to develop approaches to these more complex problems that characterize the management of patients being treated for cancer. It is when these issues are addressed that the need for AI techniques will be most evident. . . . Even in the short term, however, AI representation and control techniques have permitted us to keep the knowledge base flexible and easily modified. They have also allowed us to develop explanation capabilities and to separate kinds of knowledge explicitly in terms of their semantic categories. (From Shortliffe EH, Scott AC, Bischoff MB, et al. In: ONCOCIN: An Expert System for Oncology Protocol Management, *Seventh International Joint Conference on Artificial Intelligence*, 1981, pp. 876-881. Reprinted with permission, William Kaufman Inc.)

In this section we have reviewed three systems that apply production rules. The first, MYCIN, was a successful research system, the second, PUFF, is in clinical use, and the third, ONCOCIN, is an advanced system for research use. Recent evaluations show that ONCOCIN provides lymphoma treatment advice comparable to the treatment provided in a referral center and also leads to more completeness in the data collected.

Buchanan and Shortliffe believe that the use of production rules provides a simple and modular approach to implementing expert systems. This simplicity, however, can limit the depth of knowledge representation; not all medical problems can be expressed as a set of rules. Where the rule is valid only in a given context, this context must be supplied in the antecedent clauses or in additional rules. Finally, many researchers find that clinicians organize diagnostic knowledge in a descriptive fashion and that the structuring and presenting of this knowledge in the form of production rules is difficult and unnatural. Consequently, other approaches to AIM rely more heavily on cognitive models that evoke the differential diagnosis process as it is currently understood. One such system is the topic of the following subsection.

9.4.2. The INTERNIST/CADUCEUS System

INTERNIST-I is an experimental expert system developed by Myers, Pople, Miller and their colleagues to provide computer-assisted diagnosis in general internal medicine. CADUCEUS is the successor system that implements a richer knowledge structure. Most available documentation refers to information about INTERNIST-I which is probably the largest medical expert system available at present. Its knowledge base contains roughly 70-75% of the major diagnoses in internal medicine. Some expert systems have greater knowledge of narrower fields, but one of the limitations of many expert diagnosis systems is that their knowledge domain is considered to be too narrow to be clinically useful. The ability of one system to contain such a large proportion of the knowledge base of so broad a field is impressive indeed.

TABLE 9.3. Summary of results for major diagnoses in 19 cases used in the INTERNIST-1 evaluation.

Category	Internist-1	No. of instances Clinicians	Discussant
Total possible diagnoses	43	43	43
Definitive, correct	17	23	29
Tentative, correct	8	5	6
Failed to make correct diagnosis	18	15	8
Definitive, incorrect	5	8	11
Tentative, incorrect	6	5	2
Total no. of incorrect diagnoses	11	13	13
Total no. of errors in diagnosis	29	28	21

From Miller AM, Pople HE Jr, Myers JD. Reprinted by permission of *The New England Journal of Medicine* 307: 473, 1982. Copyright 1982 Massachusetts Medical Society, reprinted by permission.

In a recent evaluation, 19 cases were selected from the Case Records of the Massachusetts General Hospital published in *The New England Journal of Medicine*, and a comparison was made between the diagnosis of INTERNIST-I, clinicians at Massachusetts General Hospital and the case discussant. The results are presented in Table 9.3.[17] As can be seen, the system performs well as a computer program, but not yet as well as an expert. Since this was an evaluation of a research system and not a clinical tool, the results should be perceived as positive.

Why did the system not perform better? First there was the problem of missing knowledge. If only 75% of the diagnoses were known and if there were three diagnoses in the case, then the probability that all the knowledge was available would be (.75) × (.75) × (.75) or .42. To minimize this problem, the 19 cases were selected to exclude those where the knowledge base was known to be deficient. Beyond that, there were limitations due to the structure or content of the knowledge. Facts may have been omitted, simplifying assumptions made, or information inadequately conveyed. Finally, there were limitations resulting from deficiencies in the design or implementation of the computer program. Work on CADUCEUS is intended to rectify these problems.

Unlike the production rules described earlier, INTERNIST-I organizes medical knowledge into structures related to a differential diagnosis. That is, for a given diagnosis, it identifies what its manifestations are. There are far too many manifestations to be applied in a production rule, and their complexity does not facilitate their reorganization as a hierarchy of production rules. In fact, there are two competing alternatives for classifying the relationships among diagnosis (i.e., diseases) and manifestations. The first of these is through the use of a "causal graph" such as the one shown in Fig. 9.12.[18] It defines a network of interrelated pathological states (manifestations) that might arise in the course of a disease (diagnosis). This view treats each disease as an individual entity.

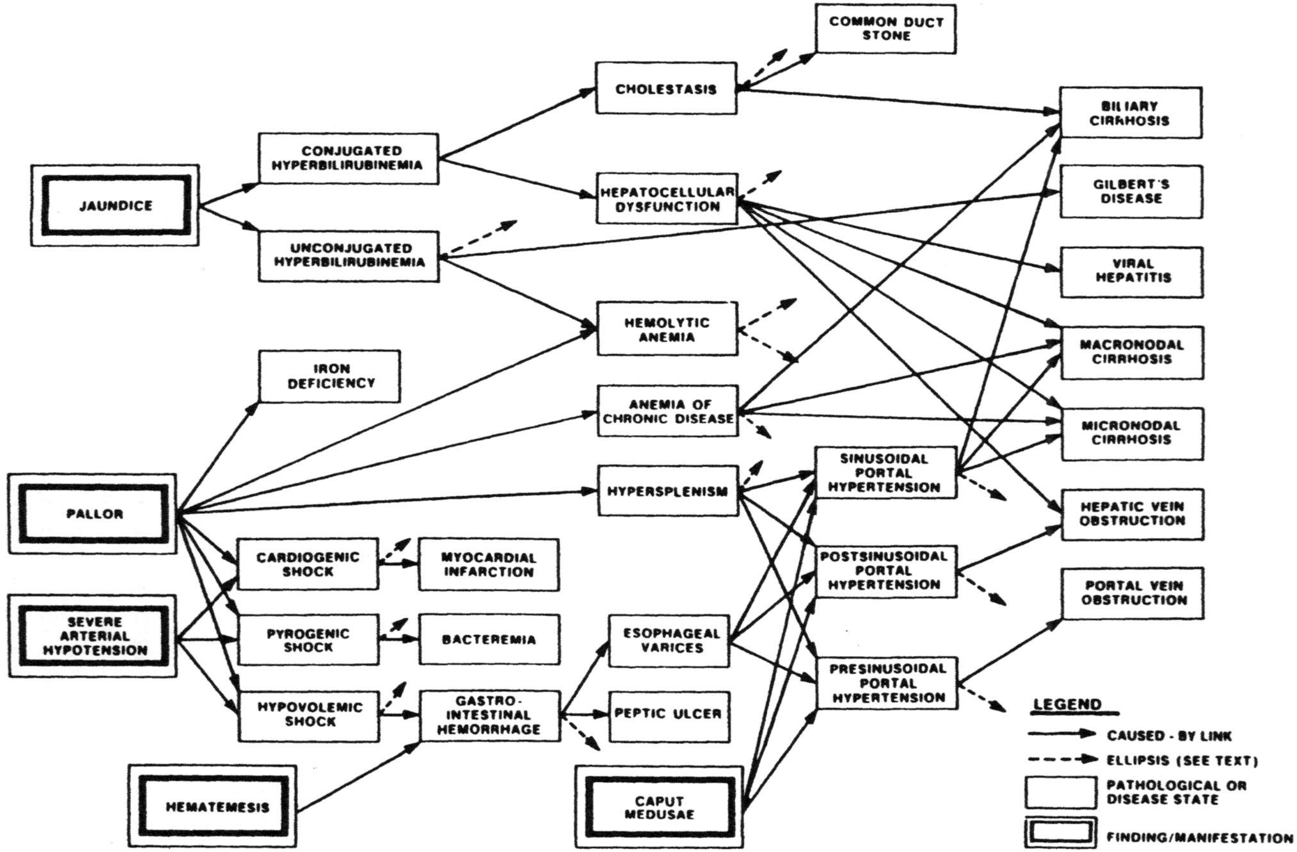

FIGURE 9.12. A portion of a Casual Network. (From Pople HE Jr, In: *Articial Intelligence in Medicine*, 1982, Szolovitz P, ed., p. 152. Reproduced with permission of Westview Press, Boulder, CO.)

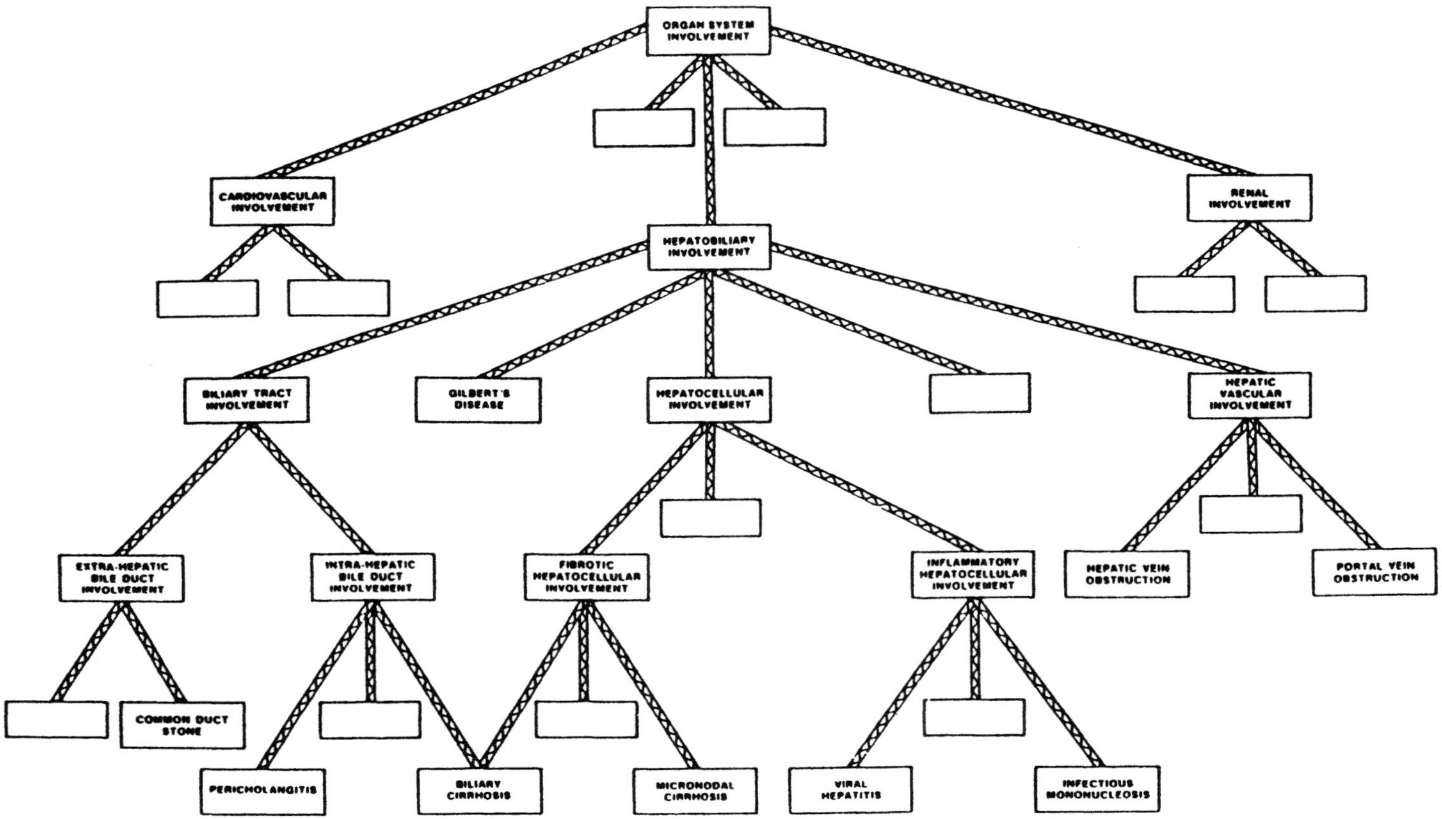

FIGURE 9.13. Portions of the nosologic "tangled hierarchy" of disease categories. (From Pople HE Jr. In: *Artificial Intelligence in Medicine*, 1982, Szolovitz P, ed., p. 157. Reproduced with permission of Westview Press, Boulder, CO.)

However, there is also knowledge about disease entities based on anatomica locus, etiological agent, and other discriminating characteristics. These may best be identified by structuring knowledge in the form of a taxonomy of disease (i.e., nosology) as shown in Fig. 9.13. These views of medical knowledge form the basis of the CADUCEUS design. They were formulated only after considerable experience with the limitations of the constructs used for INTERNIST-I. In what follows, however, we shall consider only the structure of the INTERNIST-I system.

INTERNIST-I uses both of these concepts in organizing its knowledge base. The basic unit is disease organized in a "disease hierarchy" which goes from the general to the specific. For each diagnosis, a disease profile is constructed of manifestations: historical items, symptoms, physical signs, laboratory results, etc. Three numerical variables are assigned to each manifestation; the first two are with respect to the disease and the third is disease-independent.

- An evoking strength that goes from 0 for nonspecific to 5 for pathognomonic for the disease
- A frequency value that goes from 1 for occurs rarely to 5 for occurs in essentially all cases
- Import of the manifestation that goes from 1 for usually unimportant to 5 for absolutely must be explained.

In addition to the disease profiles, the knowledge base also stores relations among the diagnosis and manifestations. The INTERNIST-I knowledge base, when it was described as being 75% complete, contained 500 disease profiles, 3,550 manifestations of disease, 2,600 links among diagnosis, and 6,500 relations among manifestations. A portion of a manifestation list is shown in Table 9.4.

The system operates as follows. The user enters the initial positive (present) and negative (absent) findings. The program uses hypothesis directed reasoning. It first retrieves a complete differential diagnosis from the knowledge base including all diseases that can explain any of the findings. Hypotheses are formed and assigned scores; those falling below a given threshold score are temporarily discarded as unattractive. (They are available for reconsideration.) Diagnostic logic is then applied using a heuristic to identify the most attractive diagnosis. If one diagnosis scores markedly higher than all other diagnoses, it is accepted; otherwise questions will be asked to pursue a probable diagnosis, rule out questionable diagnoses, or discriminate among several diagnoses. The selection of the questions to be asked (i.e., facts to be ascertained) depends upon how a partitioning algorithm has separated the manifestations to support a hypothesis. Whenever a diagnosis is concluded, all of the manifestations associated with it are removed and the process repeats in an attempt to identify other diagnoses. Processing is considered complete when all remaining manifestations have an import of two or less. Table 9.5 contains an extract of a sample dialog with commentary.

TABLE 9.4. Portion of sample manifestations list.

DISPLAY WHICH MANIFESTATION LIST?
ALCOHOLIC HEPATITIS

AGE 16 TO 25. . .0 1
AGE 26 TO 55. . .0 3
AGE GTR THAN 55. . .0 2
ALCOHOL INGESTION RECENT HX. . .2 4
ALCOHOLISM CHRONIC HX. . .2 4
SEX FEMALE. . .0 2
SEX MALE. . .0 4
URINE DARK HX. . .1 3
WEIGHT LOSS GTR THAN 10 PERCENT. . .0 3
ABDOMEN PAIN ACUTE. . .1 2
ABDOMEN PAIN COLICKY. . .1 1
ABDOMEN PAIN EPIGASTRIUM. . .1 2
ABDOMEN PAIN NON COLICKY. . .1 2
ABDOMEN PAIN RIGHT UPPER QUADRANT. . .1 3
ANOREXIA. . .0 4

.
.
.

LIVER BIOPSY FOCAL NECROSIS AND INFLAMMATION. . .2 5
LIVER BIOPSY HEPATOCELLULAR NECROSIS MARKED. . .2 3
LIVER BIOPSY MALLORY BODIES. . .3 3
LIVER BIOPSY PERIPORTAL FIBROSIS MILD. . .1 3
LIVER BIOPSY PERIPORTAL INFILTRATION NEUTROPHIL(S). . .3 5
LIVER BIOPSY PERIPORTAL INFILTRATION ROUND CELL(S). . .1 2
LIVER BIOPSY SMALL BILE DUCT(S) PROMINENT. . .1 2

LINKS FOR ALCOHOLIC HEPATITIS:

Predisposes to	MALLORY WEISS SYNDROME. . .1 1
Causes	SINUSOIDAL OR POSTSINUSOIDAL PORTAL HYPERTENSION. . .1 2
Causes	HEPATIC ENCEPHALOPATHY. . .2 2
Causes	RENAL FAILURE SECONDARY TO LIVER DISEASE <HEPATORENAL SYNDROME>. . .2 2
Coincident with	PANCREATITIS ACUTE. . .2 2
Precedes	MICRONODAL CIRRHOSIS <LAENNECS>. . .2 3

The first number after each manifestation is its evoking strength for the diagnosis; the second is the frequency of the manifestation in the disease.

9.4.3. Some Other Expert Systems

We have just examined two different types of expert systems. In the first, the knowledge base was constructed from small, modular "chunks" of knowledge; in the second, a network was formed that linked the elements in a larger context. Smaller application domains—such as that addressed by PUFF—are well suited to production rules. In many other areas of medical knowledge, such an approach

TABLE 9.5. Extract of a sample INTERNIST-1 dialog.

INTERNIST-1 consultation SUMEX-AIM Version
PLEASE ENTER FINDINGS.

*SEX MALE
*AGE 26 TO 55
*RACE WHITE
*ALCHOLISM CHRONIC HX
*EXPOSURE TO RABBITS OR OTHER SMALL MAMMALS
*FEVER
*MYALGIA
*LEG <S> WEAKNESS BILATERAL
*LEG <S> WEAKNESS PROXIMAL ONLY

Sixteen additional Findings are enterred.

*GO

DISREGARDING: EXPOSURE TO RABBITS OR OTHER SMALL MAMMALS, LEG <S> WEAKNESS PROXIMAL ONLY, PRESSURE ARTERAL ORTHOSTATIC HYPOTENSION, CREATININE BLOOD INCREASED, UREA NITROGEN BLOOD 60 TO 100

CONSIDERING: AGE 26 TO 55, SEX MALE, ANOREXIA, MYALGIA, VOMITING RECENT, FECES LIGHT COLORED, FEVER, JAUNDICE, LIVER ENLARGED SLIGHT, SKIM PALMAR ERYTHEMA, SKIN SPIDER ANGIOMATA, WBC 14000 TO 30000, PLATELETS LESS THAN 50000

RULEOUT: HEPATITIS CHRONIC ACTIVE, ALCOHOLIC HEPATITIS, HEPATIC MILIARY TUBERCULOSIS, MICRONODAL CIRRHOSIS <LAENNECS>, HEPATITIS ACUTE VIRAL

At this point, INTERNIST-1 reports concerning the initial differential diagnosis that will be the focus of problem solving attention. Three lists are displayed, labeled respectively DISREGARDING, CONSIDERING, and RULEOUT. The CONSIDERING list identifies those positive findings whose differential diagnostic tasks were combined in coming to the differential diagnostic focus, which is described by the RULEOUT list. The DISREGARDING list tells what positive findings are not consistent with the differential diagnosis as formulated and are therefore being disregarded for the moment; they will, however, be attended to in due course. The keyword RULEOUT indicates what strategy INTERNIST-1 is going to pursue relative to this task definition.

JAUNDICE INTERMITTENT HX?
NO

WEIGHT LOSS GTR THAN 10 PERCENT?
NO

The program asks a series of questions that have been selected in accordance with its problem solving strategy, then repeats the scoring and partitioning process of the task definition procedure.

DISREGARDING: EXPOSURE TO RABBITS OR OTHER SMALL MAMMALS, LEG<S> WEAKNESS BILATERAL, LEG <S> WEAKNESS PROXIMAL ONLY, PRESSURE

.
.
.

The program continues in this fashion until it has enough information to score one diagnosis as significantly higher than all others.

TRANSFUSION <S> MULTIPLE HX?
NO

DISREGARDING: SKIN SPIDER ANGIOMATA, CREATININE BLOOD INCREASED, UREA NITROGEN BLOOD 60 TO 100

TABLE 9.5. Extract of a sample INTERNIST-1 dialog—*cont'd.*

CONSIDERING: FECES LIGHT COLORED, JAUNDICE, LIVER ENLARGED SLIGHT, ALKALINE PHOSPHATASE BLOOD GTR THAN 2 TIMES NORMAL, SCOT GTR THAN 400, WBC GTR THAN 30000, SGPT 200 TO 600

PURSUING: HEPATIC LEPTOSPIROSIS
CONCLUDE: HEPATIC LEPTOSPIROSIS

DISREGARDING: SKIN SPIDER ANGIOMATA, UREA NITROGEN BLOOD 60 TO 100

CONSIDERING: OLIGURIA HX, CREATININE BLOOD INCREASED

RULEOUT: RENAL LEPTOSPIROSIS, CLOMERULONEPHRITIS ADVANCED CHRONIC, LEAD NEPHROPATHY, GLOMERULONEPHRITIS ACUTE, PYELONEPHRITIS CHRONIC, DIABETIC NEPHROPATHY

Having decided the nature of the hepatic involvement, INTERNIST-1 now turns its attention to the differential diagnosis of renal disease in this patient.

is restrictive. The CASNET and EXPERT systems present another alternative for the organization of medical knowledge.

The CASNET project was initiated in the very early 1970s and—until its completion in 1978—centered on the implementation of a glaucoma consultation program (Kulikowski and Safir). The approach was to develop a causal-associated network (CASNET) based upon descriptive and normative models. The descriptive component consisted of four sets of elements.

- Observations or findings
- Pathophysiological states
- Disease states
- Treatment plans or general classes of therapies.

Fig. 9.14 contains a specific glaucoma example for the first three sets. The normative component consists of decision rules that provide

- inference of a pathophysiological state
- preference for a treatment.

Each rule has associated with it a degree of confidence or expectation that represents a subjective (rather than Bayesian) judgment.

At a 1976 meeting of the American Academy of Opthalmology and Otolaryngology, 44 cases were presented to CASNET and the level of clinical proficiency was considered to be expert in 25% of the cases and very competent in 52% of the cases. Since then, the system has been generalized as a new system called EXPERT (Kulikowski and Weiss). This system is being used in a variety of applications including AI/RHEUM—an expert system for rheumatism. A 1982 retrospective testing of AI/RHEUM with 84 carefully studied cases produced a diagnostic accuracy of 94%. Because one of the key problems in expanding the scope of such systems is the cost and difficulty in building the expert knowledge base, the AI/RHEUM project is also experimenting with natural ways to

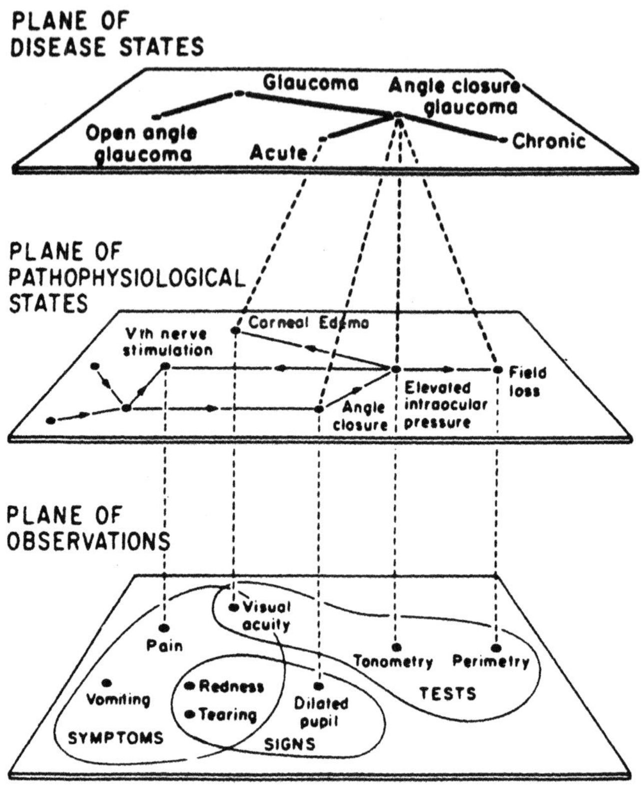

FIGURE 9.14 Example of the three-level description of disease abstracted from the CASNET/glaucoma model. Reprinted by permission of Westview Press, from *Artificial Intelligence in Medicine*, edited by P. Szolovitz, p. 31. © 1982 Westview Press, Boulder, Co.

present medical data to be incorporated into the knowledge base. In the AI/RHEUM disease domain, there is a poor understanding of causality. Thus, it is common for physicians to describe diagnostic rules as a criteria table in the form shown in Fig. 9.15.[19] Such a representation is easily constructed by the experts and readily transformed into rules to be processed by the EXPERT programs. Where the knowledge of causality is stronger, of course, other knowledge representations would be preferred.

Each of the previous systems was developed to provide some decision making advice. Miller has developed the ATTENDING system for a different purpose; it was designed to critique an anesthetist's preoperative plan. When used in this mode, the anesthetist selects or is presented a case. He analyzes the case and enters an outline of his proposed plan. For example, consider the hypothetical case:

A 34-year-old male with a history of asthma requiring several past hospitalizations comes to surgery after an auto accident for repair of a likely fractured spleen. His blood pressure

CRITERIA USED FOR
POLYMYOSITIS/DERMATOMYOSITIS

Major Critera	Minor Criteria
1. Abnormal muscle enzymes, severe	1. Heliotrope eyelids
2. Abnormal muscle biopsy, severe	2. Raynaud's phenomenon OR Esophageal hypomotility
3. Proximal muscle weakness, severe	3. Abnormal muscle enzymes, mild
4. Myopathic EMG	4. Proximal muscle weakness, mild
5. Gottron's papules	5. Abnormal muscle biopsy, mild

DEFINITE	PROBABLE	POSSIBLE
CLINICAL		
A. 3 majors (2 or more from #1, #2, or #3)	A. 2 majors (1 or more from #1, #2, or #3)	A. 1 major from #1, #2, or #3
B. 2 majors (1 or more from #1, #2, or #3) 3 minors	B. 1 major from #1, #2, or #3 2 minors	B. 2 minors
		C. Majors #4 and #5
REQUIRED		
None required	None required	None required
EXCLUSIONS		
Autoimmune hemolytic anemia Anti-RNP +, with ENA over 1:1000 anti-DNA +, 1:160 or greater Diffuse skin sclerosis extending above wrists	Same	Autoimmune hemolytic anemia Anti-RNP +, with ENA over 1:1000 Anti-DNA +, 1:160 or greater

FIGURE 9.15. Disease criteria for Polymyositis/Dermatomyositis. (Copyright 1979, The Institute of Electrical and Electronics Engineers, Inc.)

is 90/50. He recently ate lunch.[20] (From Miller PL, *Anesthesiology* 58:362-369, 1983. Reprinted with permission of JB Lippincott.)

The anesthetist's plan might be (a) induction with thiopental, (b) rapid sequence intubation with succinylcholine, and (c) maintenance with enflurane, curare, nitrous oxide, and oxygen. The physician enters his plan into the computer. It is analyzed and a critique is prepared. This critique is phrased in natural language and is structured to identify positive aspects of the plan before (tactfully) pointing out potential problems. For instance, the following critique might be generated:

There are a number of basic principles involved in this patient's management. First, in a patient with asthma, one must consider the problem of bronchospasm. Second, in the presence of hypovolemia, one must attempt to prevent hypotension. Third, a patient with a full stomach must be protected from aspiration.

Intubation of this patient is clearly important because of a full stomach. Rapid sequence intubation is a reasonable approach. This does, however, have the possible risk of bron-

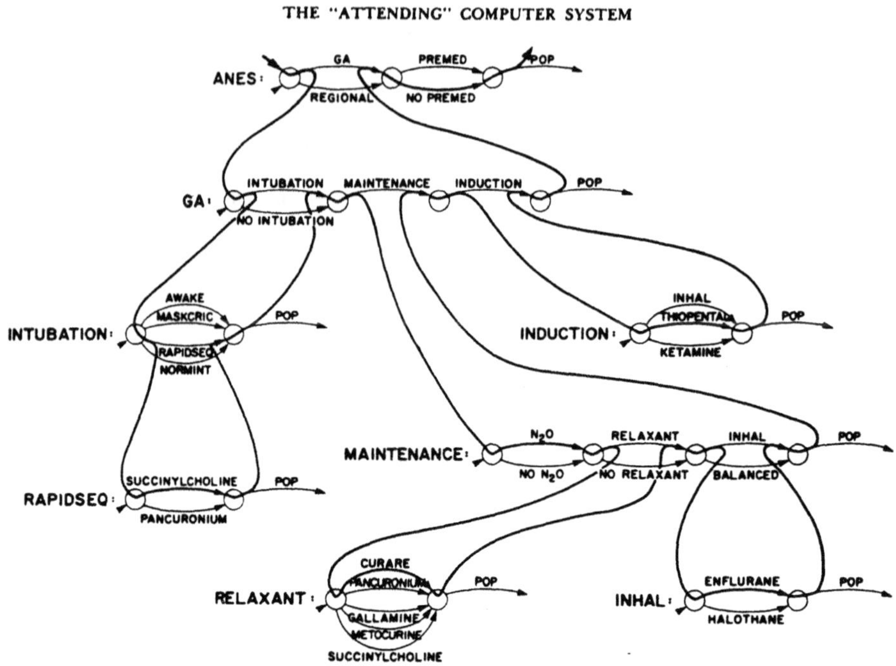

FIGURE 9.16. An Augmented Decision Networks (ADN) path in ATTENDING. (From Miller, Critiquing Anesthetic Management: The ATTENDING Computer System, *Anesthesiology* 58. Copyright 1983 by J.B. Lippincott Co., reprinted by permission.

chospasm. An alternative approach, perhaps, to rapid sequence intubation would be intubation after mask induction with cricoid pressure.

In regard to induction, induction using thiopental could have two possible risks. . . .

ATTENDING is implemented using Augmented Decision Networks (ADN). Fig. 9.16 illustrates the path through the ADN for the above example. This illustrates yet another form for the structuring of medical knowledge.

There are many AIM systems. They range from large-scale pioneering efforts to recent microcomputer applications. Some provide domain-independent environments that facilitate development in many specialties (or even non-medical applications), others are quite rigid in their design. Some are in clinical use, most are teaching or research systems. A few—such as ONCOCIN—are designed to take advantage of new, lower cost AI-oriented hardware. While the largest number of applications continue to rely on large scale research-oriented facilities, it is probably only a matter of time before many are converted to run on workstations. All applications, however, have the following characteristics:

- Each addresses the structuring of medical knowledge
- Each applies heuristics—usually relying on numeric qualifiers—to direct decision making and speed processing.
- Each provides at least a partial solution in a problem domain so vast that no direct solution can be anticipated.
- Each recognizes the importance of natural language and the need for extensive explanation facilities. Of course, the research goals of many systems have limited their involvement in these tools.

9.5. Concluding Remarks

This chapter began with a discussion of the decision-making process and then divided decision-making systems into two groups: those that do not use AI and those that do. This distinction tends to reflect divisions within medical informatics. Researchers in the former category seek well-understood functions and expect precision and repeatability. AI researchers are bolder. They attempt more ambitious projects; their agenda includes both research in AI and research in medicine. The analytic techniques are more mature; as the HELP experience shows, they can be applied on a very large scale in a clinical setting. AIM, on the other hand, is still in the research and prototype stage, but it offers techniques to integrate the complex reasoning logic presented in Table 9.2.

Still, there are many more similarities than differences. Both approaches represent a response to the availability of reliable, inexpensive computational power. Both are directed toward the organization and structuring of medical knowledge. There is a continuum from the CARE queries through the HELP sectors to the INTERNIST-I knowledge base. In each case, the representation of knowledge is sufficient for its objectives. In each case the structuring of knowledge is cumulative and transferrable. The styles of the different techniques are also merging. The use of text messages is commonplace. (Fig. 9.17 contains a report from Bleich's 1969 paper;[21] compare it with Miller's critique.) Help messages and explanations are expected of all systems. Modern workstations are being used with ONCOCIN, are being developed for HELP, and soon will be widespread.

Medical computing has matured. Clinical information systems have demonstrated their utility; they are now ready for the next level of exploitation. Clinical decision-making systems have been built on the CIS. Neither HELP nor PUFF could succeed without the rapid access to their clinical databases. The emphasis next must be on increasing our medical knowledge. Fortunately, we have two paradigms to help in this: statistics and artificial intelligence. They should be seen as complementary and overlapping, and not as competing forces. They share the common goals of building on our knowledge of medicine and developing tools that help imperfectable man to apply this knowledge to patient care.

ACID-BASE EVALUATION MAY 15, 1969 5:46 PM

SERUM ELECTROLYTES (MEQ/L):

NA	=	140
K	=	40
K	=	4.0
CL	=	110
CO2T	=	20

BLOOD PH = 7.19

BLOOD PCO2 = 49.9 (CALCULATED FROM CO2T AND PH)

PATIENT'S WEIGHT (IN POUNDS) = 150

IS THERE EVIDENCE OF PULMONARY CONGESTION OR CONGESTIE HEART FAILURE?
NO

EVALUATION NOTE

THE PH OF 7.19 UNITS IS LOWER THAN CAN BE ACCOUNTED FOR BY THIS DEGREE OF HYPERCAPNIA, AND INDICATES THAT A METABOLIC ACIDOSIS IS SUPERIMPOSED ON THE RESPIRATORY ACIDOSIS.

FURTHERMORE, THE FINDING OF A NORMAL PLASMA CONCENTRATION OF UNMEASURED ANIONS (14.0 MEQ/L) INDICATES THAT THE MOST LIKELY CAUSES OF THE METABOLIC ACIDOSIS ARE:

1) PYELONEPHRITIS WITHOUT GLOMERULAR FAILURE
2) RENAL TUBULAR ACIDOSIS
3) CARBONIC ANHYDRASE INIHIBITION (DIAMOX)
4) AMMONIUM CHLORIDE INGESTION
5) URETEROSI GMOIDOSTOMY
6) MASSIVE DIARRHEA, PANCREATIC DRAINAGE, OR FISTULAE OF THE SMALL INTESTINE.

IN AN EFFORT TO CORRECT THE METABOLIC COMPONENT OF THE ACIDOSIS IT IS SUGGESTED THAT SUFFICIENT ALKALI BE GIVEN TO RAISE PLASMA BICARBONATE CONCENTRATION TO A VALUE THAT WOULD BE MORE IN KEEPING WITH UNCOMPLICATED HYPERCAPNIA.

THE CALCULATED QUANTITY OF BICARBONATE REQUIRED TO ACHIEVE THIS GOAL IS APPROXIMATELY 250 MEQ. IT IS SUGGESTED, HOWEVER, THAT 132 MEQ OF SODIUM BICARBONATE BE GIVEN DURING THE NEXT FEW HOURS, AND THAT SERUM ELECTROLYTES AND BLOOD PM BE MEASURED AGAIN AT THAT TIME.

FINALLY, EVERY EFFORT SHOULD BE MADE TO IMPROVE PULMONARY VENTILATION AND TO MAINTAIN BLOOD PCO2 AT A VALUE OF NO GREATER THAN 45 MM HG.

THANK YOU FOR REFERRING THIS INTERESTING PATIENT TO US.

REFERENCES:

1) BRACKETT, N.C., JR., COHEN, J.J., AND SCHWARTZ, W.B.
CARBON DIOXIDE TITRATION CURVE OF NORMAL MAN.
NEW ENG. J. MED., 272, 6, 1965.

2) BEESON, P.B. AND MCDERMOTT, W.
CECIL-LOEB TEXTBOOK OF MEDICINE
12TH EDITION (1967), P. 763.

<*>

FIGURE 9.17. A 1969 acid-base evaluation report. Underlined information was typed in by the physician. (From Shortliffe et al., Seventh International Joint Conference on AI, 19. Reprinted by permission of William Kaufmann, Inc.)

For Further Reading

There are several collections of papers now available on this topic. J. A. Reggia and S. Tuhrim have edited a two volume series called *Computer-Assisted Medical Decision Making* (Springer-Verlag, 1985). The volume by W. Clancey and E. H. Shortliffe *Readings in Medical Artificial Intelligence: The First Decade*, Addison-Wesley, 1984 is limited primarily to papers in AI. The P. Szolovits (ed) *Artificial Intelligence in Medicine*, Westview, 1982, also presents an excellent overview.

In addition to papers in the references, there are several very good current survey articles. E. H. Shortliffe, B. G. Buchanan and E. A. Feigenbaum, Knowledge Engineering for Medical Decision Making: A Review of Computer-Based Clinical Decision Aids, *IEEE Proc.* (67,9): 1207-1224, 1979; B. Kleinmuntz, Diagnostic Problem Solving by Computer: A Historic Review and the Current State of the Science, *Compt. Biom. Med.* (14,3):255-270, 1984; D. A. Bergman and R. H. Pantell, The Art of Science in Medical Decision Making, *J. Pediatrics*, (104,5): 649-656, 1984; and two survey papers by Reggia and Rada in M. D. Schwartz (ed), *Applications of Computers in Medicine*, IEEE Computer Society, 1982.

References

1. Ledley, R. S. and L. B. Lusted, Reasoning Foundations of Medical Diagnosis, *Science*, 130, July 1959, p. 9.
2. *Ibid*, p. 20.
3. Feinstein, A. R., Clinical Biostatistics XXXIX. The Haze of Bayes, the Aerial Palaces of Decision Analysis, and the Computerized Ouija Board, *Clinical Pharmacology and Therapeutics*, 21 (4) 1977 p. 495.
4. Elstein, A. S., L. S. Shulman, S. A. Sparafka, et al. *Medical Problem Solving*, Harvard University Press, 1978.
5. *Ibid*, p. 281.
6. *Ibid*, p. 247-8.
7. Grimm, R. H., et al., Evaluation of Patient-Care Protocol Use by Various Providers, *NEJ Med.* 292:1975, p. 507.
8. Bleich, H. L., Computer Evaluation of Acid-Base Disorders, *J. Clin. Invest.*, 48 1969, p. 1690.
9. Warner, H., *Computer-Assisted Medical Decision-Making*, Academic Press, 1979, p. 137ff. Examples from HELP which follow are taken from this book and the chapter on HELP in B. I. Blum (ed) *Information Systems in Patient Care*, pp. 109-128.
10. Faught, E., S. Trader and G. Hanna, Cerebral Complications of Angiography for Transient Ischemia and Stroke-Prediction of Risk, *Neurology* 29, ;1979, 4-15.
11. Turing, A. M., Intelligent Machinery (1947), in B. Meltzer and D. Miochie (eds), *Machine Intelligence 5*, Halstead Press, New York, NY 1970.

12. Buchanan, B. G. and E. H. Shortliffe, *Rute Based Expert Systems, The MYCIN Experiments of the Stanford Heuristic Programming Project*, Addison-Wesley, 1984, p573.
13. Buchanan, op. cit. p. 573.
14. *Ibid*, p. 599.
15. Aikins, J. S., J. C. Kunz, E. H. Shortliffe, and R. J. Fallat, PUFF: An Expert System for Interpretation of Pulmonary Function Data, *Comp. Biomed. Res.* 16, 1983, 199-208, p. 203.
16. Langlotz, C. P. and E. H. Shortliffe, Adapting a Consultation System to Critique User Plans, *In. J. Man-Machine Studies* 19, (1983) 479-496, p. 483.
17. Miller, A. M., H. E. Pople, Jr., J. D. Myers, INTERNIST-I, An Experimental Computer-Based Diagnostic Consultant for General Internal Medicine, *NEJ Med.*, 307: 468-476, 1982, p. 473. The extract of the Sample Manifestation List was also taken from this paper.
18. Figures 12 and 13 plus portions of the example are taken from H. E. Pople, Jr., Heuristic Methods for Imposing Structure on Ill-Structured Problems: the Structuring of Medical Diagnosis, in P. Szolovits (ed), *Artificial Intelligence in Medicine*, Westview Press, 1982, pp. 119-190.
19. Kingsland III, L. C., G. C. Sharp, D. R. Kay, S. M. Weiss, G. C. Roeseler, and D. A. B. Lindberg, An Expert Consultant System in Rheumatology: AI/RHEUM, *Sixth Annual Symposium on Computer Applications in Medical Care*, 1982, p 748-752.
20. Miller, P. L., Critiquing Anesthetic Management: the ATTENDING Computer System, *Anesthesiology*, 58:362-369, 1983.
21. Bleich, H. L., Computer Evaluation of Acid-Base Disorders, *J. Clin. Invest.* 48: 1689-1695, 1969, p. 1694.

10
A Case Study

10.1. Introduction

This final chapter differs from the others in that it is filled with details, is narrow in scope, and is primarily of interest to persons who intend to develop a system. The previous chapters provided a general framework and exposed the reader to concepts and the state of the art. This chapter will guide the user through the process of developing a system. It describes one system—the results of some 20 effort years—in sufficient detail to allow the reader to understand how it works. The objective is to provide a case study that (a) draws on the material already presented and (b) illustrates the tradeoffs considered by the implementors.

Throughout this book I have tried to validate the following hypotheses:

- Information system technology is mature and widespread. Data Base Management Systems (DBMS) provide environments to implement database applications; networking provides a tool to link complementary applications.
- Few health care facilities use clinical information systems (CIS) for patient care support; most use information systems for administrative assistance. Yet there is 10 years' experience in how the CIS can improve patient care.
- The exploitation of the CIS experience will come about in one of two ways. New generations of commercial products will integrate expanded CIS functionality for wider dissemination. Alternatively, individual institutions will use the newer technology to implement locally desired features. The commercialization of COSTAR and HELP are examples of the first approach.

One goal of this book has been to raise awareness to create a demand for patient care-oriented tools in the offerings of the marketplace. Response to this demand will take time, and many organizations may prefer to take advantage of the modern development environments to produce tools designed to meet their specific needs. Although this approach is commendable, there is always the danger that developers will not take advantage of previous experience, and—after excessive effort—they will simply reinvent the wheel. (Or, worse yet, they may produce wheels that are elliptical.)

Traditionally, software developers have had difficulty in transferring their work. The transfer of applications is a simple process when standards are used. Compilers can be used with many operating systems; scientific FORTRAN libraries may be used with many different computers. As we have seen with the HIS, however, the larger the system is, the more difficult it will be to have it accommodate local requirements. If one is to implement only part of such a system, how does one capture its essence? There are three ways:

- *Understand the user interfaces.* For example, once one fixes the contents of an automated ambulatory medical record, much of the system design necessarily will follow.
- *Understand the algorithms used.* For example, if the system is to use Bayesian statistical analysis, then a knowledge of the computation and data requirements will suggest a design approach.
- *Understand the data model.* For example, if the database contents and structure are defined, then the system may be reviewed as reports from and updates to the database.

The approach taken for this chapter is to emphasize the data model. The discussion details the database layout and—where appropriate—the rationale for selection among alternatives. It is believed that this type of presentation will ease the transfer of concepts to new applications. Nevertheless, the reader should remember that most of the system implementation process involves "housekeeping" and "special cases;" details that largely are obscured in this chapter.

10.2. The Johns Hopkins Oncology Clinical Information System

In what follows we shall describe the database structure of a system implemented for the Johns Hopkins Oncology Center. The Center was organized in 1976 as part of the National Cancer Program sponsored by the National Cancer Institute. It grew out of a series of separate departmental activities at Johns Hopkins and was designed to bring together a multidisciplinary, focused approach to cancer. Housed in a separate building in The Johns Hopkins Hospital complex, the center has 60 high-technology single-patient beds, an active outpatient clinic capable of seeing 500 patients per week, educational and administrative space, and 36,000 square feet of laboratory research space.

The goals of the Oncology Center are (a) basic and clinical research; (b) education of postgraduate fellows, house staff, medical students, community physicians, nurses, physician's assistants, radiation therapy technicians, and others; and (c) specialized clinical management of patients with cancer. The Oncology Clinical Information System (OCIS) was developed to support these goals. The primary emphasis is the collection and use of clinical information for prospective application in both clinical trials and individual therapy. The focus

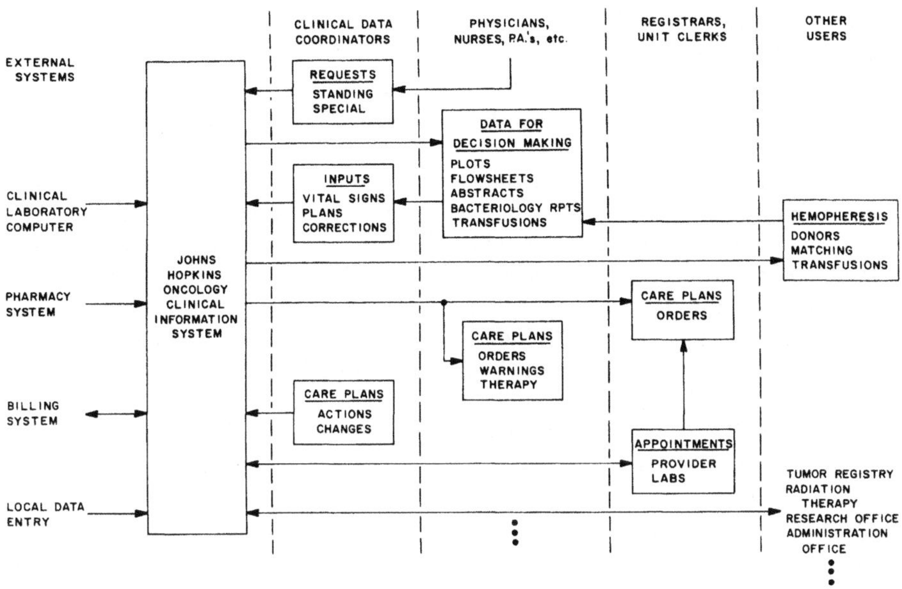

FIGURE 10.1. Overview of the OCIS.

is on the individual patient and the medical provider. All data items collected are oriented toward identifying patient events without regard to where the patient may be treated (inpatient, outpatient). Special tools have been developed to assist in identifying patients on study, displaying summary on-study data, and supporting retrospective analysis. The operation of the system is supported primarily from patient care revenue.

The OCIS contains information on all patients admitted to the Johns Hopkins Oncology Center inpatient or outpatient units. Among the data are the routine demographic information, history of prior therapy, laboratory results such as hematology and chemistry data, and special-purpose data from research laboratories. In addition, quantitative measurements of the patient's status such as the performance level, pertinent symptoms, and physical findings are recorded. This information is collected at each clinic visit for outpatients and daily for patients on the inpatient services. Direct computer-to-computer links are used to capture laboratory results and pharmacy data.

Fig. 10.1 illustrates how the OCIS is integrated into the daily patient care process. It receives machine-sensible inputs from the clinical laboratory computer, the pharmacy system, and the hospital billing system. Current charges are returned to the billing system in the form of magnetic tapes. All other data are received as paper reports and processed by the Center's data entry staff.

The clinical data coordinators act as part of the health care team and translate a need for information into a request. Requests may be periodic (e.g., daily, each outpatient visit, each Friday) or one-time (i.e., special). Outputs include plots, flowsheets, abstracts of diagnosis and therapy, sorted bacteriology reports, and blood transfusion histories. Outputs are delivered to the clinical staff as requested. Clinical data coordinators enter vital signs (temperature, pulse rate, blood pressure) and corrections to the database on line. They also process the protocols and clinical algorithms that define the actions contained in the daily care plans.

The daily care plans are printed in several formats. One is used by providers. It identifies tests and procedures ordered, therapy recommended (including dose computation), a list of significant clinical findings and warning messages (e.g., warning of a 20% weight change over the last 7 days), and a summary of status. Another format is sent to the unit clerks to order the tests. This plan indicates the container, laboratory, and requisition to be used. In the case of serum tests, it computes the total blood to be drawn. The clinical data coordinator inputs to the system any changes or additions to the plan.

Other OCIS functions include the appointment system which is linked to the daily care plan. It schedules each test and provider encounter. The admission system is used to maintain a current census of inpatients, a list of scheduled admissions, and a projected occupancy. The hemopheresis system maintains a blood donor list, matches donors with patients, and reports on the result of each transfusion. Other system users with special requirements and/or a need to share data generated by other applications are the Tumor Registry, Radiation Therapy, the Research Office, and the Administration Office.

The development of the OCIS was begun in the mid-1970s when plans were made to consolidate various oncology activities in a single facility. While there was no funding for a computer or software, the facility architecture and staffing profiles were predicated on the assumption that a computer system would be available. Over 250 wall jacks with cables terminating in a computer room were set into place.

During the period of planning, it was decided to begin the development of a prototype system. At this time, outpatients were being treated in a Johns Hopkins clinic, and inpatients were being treated at the Baltimore City Hospital. In each case, procedures had been established for patient management based on the careful evaluation and monitoring of clinical data. It was recognized that the labor-intensive procedures in use for that small population could not be extrapolated to support a facility with 60 beds and 100 outpatient visits a day. Clearly, computer support was required.

On the basis of the Oncology Center's clinical practices, it was determined that an information system must (a) organize and display the clinical data as an integrated report that combined inpatient and outpatient data in ways that could indicate trends and facilitate decision making; (b) manage the basic patient record functions, including a hospitalwide tumor registry, summary patient abstracts, current census, and appointments; (c) schedule patient care activities and therapies as determined by clinical algorithms (because most cancer therapies involve sequences of actions over long periods of time, the ability of the computer to provide reminders was considered an important tool for dealing with the problem of information overload); and (d) maintain clinical data for retrospective analysis.

TABLE 10.1. Events in the implementation of the OCIS.

Date	Event
July 1975	Begin analysis and prototype system
December 1975	Prototype tumor registry operational
July 1976	Prototype system complete
October 1976	Oncology Center facility opened
August 1977	Computer delivered, start new system
December 1977	Data base moved to new computer
April 1978	Patient data on line
April 1979	Limited daily care plans used, two units
August 1979	Second computer installed
June 1980	Phase I system complete
January 1982	Phase II system in partial use
August 1982	Phase II conversion complete

Consequently, in July 1975, one year before the center was to open, work on a prototype began.

The first task in the development of a prototype was the conversion of an automated tumor registry file into a format that would be expanded to support the needs of the center. The database was transferred, and programs were developed to produce patient abstracts and reports. At the same time, work began in the development of formats that could display clinical data effectively. Flow sheets and printer plots were designed and, after many iterations, the formats presented in the following sections were established.

The prototype system operated on a computer at the Applied Physics Laboratory. The tumor registry was a functional system with a current database. It ran in the batch mode and was used for searches, reports, abstract generation, and quality assurance. The remainder of the prototype system was used on a limited basis. Because of the difficulty in establishing a current database, the display system was most effective for retrospective studies; its primary contribution was the establishment of database format requirements.

In 1976, in part as the result of a gift from the Educational Foundation of America, there were sufficient funds available to purchase a computer and support the development of a system for the Oncology Center. Called the Phase I system, this would convert the prototype to operate as an interactive system on a dedicated computer. A PDP-11 was selected with MUMPS as the development environment. Work on the prototype system stopped, and the development of the new system began.

Table 10.1 contains a brief chronology of the system development activity. As can be seen, the prototype system was converted to an on-line system using the prototype's database in a period of nine months. The reasons for this rapid implementation were (a) the existence of a prototype so that the design requirements were well known, (b) the use of MUMPS with its powerful data access tools and interactive debugging, and (c) the fact that all activity was devoted to development with no effort spent on system maintenance.

Development of the system continued and new functions were added. The success of the OCIS began to limit its effectiveness. The system became saturated at 20 jobs, daily production processing required 20 hours a day, it was difficult to add new functions to the existing system, and during periods of computer downtime there was no automated backup. It was therefore decided to add a second computer, which would expand functionality and provide a backup capability.

The second computer was installed in 1979. At this time Standard MUMPS was available and the previous version of MUMPS was no longer supported. Because the two versions were sufficiently different, it was decided to reprogram the OCIS rather than convert it. This became known as the Phase II system. It also was decided to use a new programming tool, TEDIUM® which would provide database management system functionality and improve system maintainability. Unfortunately, TEDIUM®* was only in its initial stage of development and the development staff was faced with (a) conversion of what was by now a complex system, (b) maintenance of the old MUMPS system, and (c) the use of a new and poorly documented tool. The result was a major slip in the schedule and some user frustration. However, the conversion was successful. Parts of the new system were put into operational use in 1981, and the old MUMPS system was retired in 1982.

As can be seen from this brief discussion, the OCIS was some 7 years in the making. It progressed through a prototype to establish a baseline design, a MUMPS system that worked well, but that also had limited growth capabilities, and a redesigned system using DBMS concepts and program generation. Externally, there are few distinctions between the system of the late 1970s and the version currently in use. The major difference is that many new applications and reports have been added.

In parallel with the software activity was the development of a support staff and the training of users. As shown in Fig. 10.1 there are three users of the system:

- Clinical data coordinators
- Clinical users
- Clerical users.

The clinical data coordinators act as interfaces between the OCIS and the clinical users. They collect, input, and validate data that are not routinely processed; they enter special requests; they train the clinical users; and they participate in all data management activities. While clinical users are free to access any OCIS functions they require, the availability of the clinical data coordinators removes the burden of having to learn how to use the system.

In general, the clinical users are encouraged to use the system cafeteria style. The patient records are intended to supplement their regular sources of information. In the initial years, the data were not always complete and timely. By

---

*TEDIUM® is a registered trademark of Tedious Enterprises, Inc.

the late 1970s, operations were placed on a 7-day a week, 24-hours-a-day setting and the clinical users began to depend on the data system. Attitudes toward the system varied. Some felt it very useful; others saw where it might be helpful for others; a few were outspokenly negative. Informal surveys now find general acceptance high; the responses also show that many of the clinical users do not recognize which daily functions are actually managed by the OCIS. Consequently, the system serves as a clinical tool that always is used, sometimes appreciated, and—in periods of downtime—sorely missed.

For clerical users, the OCIS is a tool that must be used to support their functions. Outpatient registrars use an appointment system and patient registration screens, the records room uses lists of charts to be pulled, the Tumor Registry has screens for preparing and reviewing abstracts, etc. In each case, an attempt was made to customize a set of functions that naturally matched the users' processing flow. Unlike the clinical users, however, the clerical users always have had to use the system.

During the 7 years of development many programs were designed, implemented, tested, and revised; the role of the clinical data coordinators was formulated, revised, and finally established; the clinical users were exposed, acclimated and ultimately convinced; and the clerical users were asked to participate in the development and finally required to use the resultant tools. If one did not have to develop the computer programs, one still would have to train all the users. In what follows we shall present a static review of the system architecture, i.e., a description of the programs. The reader should be aware, however, that the dynamics of local design, iteration, and training require as much (if not more) effort than that allocated to the system implementation process.

10.3. The Data Model

The OCIS was designed using TEDIUM® which contains a program generator that manages a relational data model. It uses high level program specifications to produce MUMPS programs. The OCIS operates on two PDP-11/70s which share a distributed database. On weekdays there are some 60 jobs active at any one time. The system definition consists of some 1,000 relations and 5,000 programs defined. The key relations for the most generally useful functions will be described.

In the standard notation for a relation, each term (i.e., column heading or attribute) that forms the relation is written within a single set of parentheses. Thus, for example, the relation PATIENT which links patient identifier, name, age, and sex might be written

PATIENT (<u>ID</u>,NAME,AGE,SEX)

The term ID is underlined to indicate that it serves as a key for the relation. That is, the values of NAME, AGE, and SEX are functionally dependent on the value of ID. Each tuple (i.e., record) in the relation (i.e., table) will be uniquely identified by the key (i.e., index terms).

For the purpose of this description we shall use the less familiar functional notation:

PATIENT(ID) = NAME,AGE,SEX

The differences are only notational. The functional description, however, has an advantage in the MUMPS environment in that it also implies a hierarchical order. Consider a patient data relation

DATA(ID,DATE,TIME,TEST) = RESULT

This implies a hierarchical structure such that for each patient there may be one or more dates; for a date one or more times; and for a time one or more tests. Thus, the notation represents both the logical relation and its physical organization.

Relational DBMSs do not use this notation; a relation assumes nothing about the order in which the tuples are stored. When implementing systems on small computers, however, it is important to understand how the data are stored; failure to do so may result in unacceptable response times. Moreover, when using a language such as MUMPS, it is best to fit the data model into hierarchical structures that can be efficiently managed. For these reasons, we use the functional notation here. Transformation to the standard relational notation does not modify the model.

In the remainder of this section we shall describe the principle relations in the data model. The presentation shall take the form of:

- *Problem statement*. What functions were to be performed and what design considerations were traded off.
- *Implementation description*. How was the function implemented in the OCIS and how is it used.
- *Data model description*. What are the key relations and procedures used to implement this function.

The objective of the presentation is to illustrate how a DBMS may be used to implement a clinical information system for patient care. As already noted, the success of a system requires an effective data model, a satisfactory user interface, a responsive environment, a trained and motivated staff, and an accurate and timely database. Therefore, a valid data model is a necessary but not sufficient condition for a viable system.

10.3.1. Data Management for Patient Care

The most common way in which clinical information systems support patient care is through the collection and organization of clinical data. In most cases, the display is keyed to panels that are organized by the test or procedure that produced the result. When treating patients where there are many test results or when working with the chronically ill who will be managed over long periods of time, such test-oriented panels are not satisfactory. In such situations, alternative formats are required to present the data for medical decision-making.

Since the database is designed for patient care, it must be organized so that all clinical data are addressable by patient identifier and date ranges. The data should be grouped by format category and use. Because the patient diagnosis, clinical laboratory results, bacteriology reports, and radiology reports are in different formats, each must be treated separately. Presentations of the data should be organized as logically cohesive groups. For example, clinical laboratory data may be grouped by test (SMA-6, SMA-12), by type of test (serum chemistry, hematology), or by organ system (liver function, kidney function). Data may be presented as an individual report, as a flow sheet, or in the form of a plot. Flexibility in designing and requesting outputs is necessary.

In the OCIS three categories of data are maintained:

- The patient abstract which contains the patient demographics, diagnosis, therapy, history, and follow-up information. This contains both coded and textual information. Fig. 10.2 contains a sample abstract.
- The laboratory results which are in the form of time-sequenced numeric or coded values. These are normally presented in the form of a flow sheet or plot (Figs. 10.3-10.5).
- Special tests and procedures, e.g., bacteriology results and transfusion histories. These are displayed in formats designed for each special group of data.

All data are available online. In addition, selected data products are printed for use during morning rounds or at an outpatient visit. To produce these data displays, it is necessary to have two system facilities:

- A general-purpose formatting tool that allows the user to define a plot or flowsheet format for a specific patient, diagnosis, etc.
- A general-purpose request system that will automatically generate specified outputs for selected patients according to a given schedule; e.g., for a given group of patients, print a certain plot every Monday plus specified flowsheets daily.

Finally, we note that access to patient data will be either direct or indirect. Direct patient data access requires a knowledge of either the patient name or identifier. Indirect patient access establishes the patient identifier from some other reference such as a patient locator organized by nursing unit. The description of the data model for data management will assume that the direct mode is used.

In displaying information, the first task is to identify or select the patient. At The Johns Hopkins Hospital, a seven digit patient history number is used as a key to a unified patient medical record. It is called HNO in the OCIS and is defined in the relation

PATID (HNO) = NAME

```
        JOHNS HOPKINS HOSPITAL          HISTORY NO: 002826933
           ONCOLOGY CENTER                    NAME: **********
                                              DATE: 04/12/82
                                                          CLASSONCOLOGY
THURMONT, MD. 21788                                       SEER 021/21788
SOCIAL SECURITY NO
SEX MALE                  RACE CAUCASIAN        MAR. STATUS PEDIATRIC (16 OR UNDER)

:--------------------------------------------------------------------------:
: ADMINISTRATIVE INFORMATION  PRIMARY - 1                                  :
:--------------------------------------------------------------------------:
:ADMISSION DATE:  12/18/81            DISCHARGE DATE:  01/06/82            :
:PRELIMINARY: NO                      REGISTRY REPORTABLE: YES             :
:CCPDS COMPATABILITY FLAG: YES        ACCS NO: 812529                      :
:FIRST REPORTED TO CCPDS:                                                  :
:ABSTRACTOR: GMS                      MICROFILM: N                         :
:FIRST DATA ENTRY ID: JMK             DATE OF INITIAL GENERATION: 01/08/82 :
:LAST DATA ENTRY ID: JMK              DATE OF LAST GENERATION: 04/12/82    :
:--------------------------------------------------------------------------:
: DIAGNOSIS PRIMARY - 1                                                    :
:--------------------------------------------------------------------------:
:                                                                          :
:     JHH DIAGNOSIS        12/22/81  WILM'S TUMOR -STAGE IV (LUNG          :
:                                    METASTASES)                           :
:                                                                          :
:SITE:                     189.0     KIDNEY, NOS                           :
:MORPHOLOGY:               8960/39   NEPHROBLASTOMA, NOS                   :
:GRADE:                    NOT DETERMINED, N/S, N/A                        :
:LATERALITY:               LEFT ORIGIN OF PRIMARY                          :
:EXTENT:                   DISTANT                                         :
:   METASTATIC SITES:          PULMONARY                                   :
:BASIS OF DIAGNOSIS:       HISTOLOGY, X-RAY (CHEST)                        :
:                                                                          :
:REPORT SECTION                                                            :
:                                                                          :
:     8119934 1. LEFT KIDNEY (NEPHRECTOMY): NEPHROBLASTOMA (WILM'S TUMOR   :
:WITH CAPSULAR PENETRATION, EXTENSION TO ADJACENT NORMAL KIDNEY AND CALYCEAL :
:SYSTEM, VASCULAR AND URETERAL MARGINS NEGATIVE FOR TUMOR. 2. URETER:      :
:NEGATIVE FOR TUMOR. 3. RETROPERITONEAL LYMPH NODE: NEGATIVE FOR TUMOR.    :
:NOTE: HISTOLOGY IS FAVORABLE.                                             :
:                                                                          :
:                                                                          :
:SPECIAL NOTES:                                                            :
:                                                                          :
:     12/21/81 CHEST X-RAY SHOWS BILATERAL LUNG METASTASES                 :
:                                                                          :
:                                                                          :
:--------------------------------------------------------------------------:
:--------------------------------------------------------------------------:
: TREATMENT PRIMARY - 1                                                    :
:--------------------------------------------------------------------------:
:  FROM  :    TO   : LOC  : TYPE : DESCRIPTION                             :
:12/20/81:01/28/82: JHH  :  R   : LEFT FLANK AND RENAL BED 2100R X 30 DAYS :
:12/22/81:         : JHH  :  S   : LEFT NEPHRECTOMY (81-19934)             :
:12/28/81:         : JHH  :  C   : TREATMENT DAY #1 POG 8000 REGIMEN J -   :
:        :         :      :      : VINCRISTINE, ACTINOMYCIN D, ADRIAMYCIN, :
:        :         :      :      : CYTOXAN                                 :
:--------------------------------------------------------------------------:
```

```
        JOHNS HOPKINS HOSPITAL          HISTORY NO: 002826933
           ONCOLOGY CENTER                    NAME: **********
                                              DATE: 04/12/82
:--------------------------------------------------------------------------:
: TREATMENT  (CON'T)  PRIMARY - 1                                          :
:--------------------------------------------------------------------------:
:  FROM  :    TO   : LOC  : TYPE : DESCRIPTION                             :
:12/29/81:01/08/82: JHH  :  R   : WHOLE LUNG 1200R X 12 DAYS               :
:--------------------------------------------------------------------------:
: HISTORY                                                                  :
:--------------------------------------------------------------------------:
:ONSET OF SYMPTOMS:        2 - 3 WEEK HISTORY OF DECREASED APPETITE AND FULL :
:                          SENSATION IN ABDOMEN, OCCASIONAL VOMITING AFTER :
:                          MEALS.  TWO DAY HISTORY OF LUQ PAIN.            :
:FAMILY HISTORY:           POSITIVE FOR LEUKEMIA ON PATERNAL SIDE.         :
:MEDICAL HISTORY:          POSITIVE FOR CHICKEN POX, IMMUNIZATIONS UTD     :
:PSYCHIATRIC ILLNESS:      N/S                                             :
:SOCIAL HISTORY:                                                           :
:      TOBACCO:            NEG.                                            :
:      ETOH:               NEG.                                            :
:      DRUGS:              NEG.                                            :
:CONGENITAL DEFECTS:       NEG.                                            :
:ALLERGY:                  NEG.                                            :
:OCCUPATION:               8 YEAR OLD CHILD                                :
:EXPOSURE:                 NEG.                                            :
:COMMENTS:                                                                 :
:--------------------------------------------------------------------------:
: FOLLOW UP                                                                :
:--------------------------------------------------------------------------:
:  DATE   : LST SN  : COND : QUAL : COMMENTS                               :
:04/12/82:03/82    : NED  : SU   : PER PED. ONC. LIST                      :
:--------------------------------------------------------------------------:
:REFERENCE SOURCE                                                          :
:                         REFERRING PHYSICIAN                              :
:                                                                          :
:                 THURMONT, MD 21788                                       :
:                                                                          :
:                             JHOC FACULTY                                 :
:                                                                          :
:                 FREDERICK, MD 21701                                      :
:                                                     662-4599             :
:--------------------------------------------------------------------------:
                           END OF ABSTRACT
```

FIGURE 10.2. Sample patient abstract.

JOHNS HOPKINS ONCOLOGY CENTER

HISTORY NO:
NAME:
DATE: 05/01/82

STANDARD FLOW

J7715		27JUL78 DAY 50	28JUL78 DAY 51	29JUL78 DAY 52	30JUL78 DAY 53	31JUL78 DAY 54	01AUG78 DAY 55	02AUG78 DAY 56
PAT STATUS								
TEMPERATUR	DEG C	36.9	36.9	37	37.1	37.2	37.1	37.2
BODY WT AM	KG	76.5	77.3	77.0		76.8	77.3	78.3
CARE LEVEL		3	3	3	3	3	3	3
TOTL INTAK	ML	1270	1500	2255	1730	2160	2580	2010
TOTL OUT	ML	2600	4050	2900	4000	2300	2700	2575
HEMATOLOGY								
WBC	#/CU	297*	132*	374*	297*	231*	649*	462*
HCT	%	22.0	24.0	26.0	22.5	21.5	21.5	21.5
PLATELETS	/MM3	143000*	173000	152000	161000	180000	161000	160000
POLYMORPHS	%	100*	100*	100*		100*	100*	500*
CHEMISTRY								
SER NA	MEQ/L	141				145		138
SER K	MEQ/L	3.9*				4.2		4.2
SER CL	MEQ/L	108*				107*		106
SER CO2	MEQ/L	26				26		25
SER UR NIT	MG/DL	15				16		14
SER CREAT	MG/DL	1.3				1.4		1.3
SER GLUC	MG/DL	131*				113		120*
TOT SER PT	GM/DL					5.8*		5.8*
SER ALBUMN	GM/DL					4.4		4.3
TOT BILI	MG/DL					0.7		0.7
SGOT	IU/L					8		7
SER ALKPHO	IU/L					65		64
SER CA	MG/DL					8.4*		8.1*
SER PO4	MG/DL					3.3		3.0*
SER PO4	MG/DL							2.6
SER CHOLES	MG/DL					128		124
SER UR ACD	MG/DL					6.8		6.9
SER MAG	MEQ/L							1.4*
DIAG TESTS								
HBS AG						0		
IGG	MG/DL					356		
IGA	MG/DL					5		
IGM	MG/DL					13		
24H URINE	ML		1900		3700		2900	
UR CREAT	MG/DL		53		57		76	
URINE NA	MEQ/L				70			
URINE K	MEQ/L				20			
URINE CL	MEQ/L				61			
UR TTL PRT	MG/24		1994*		3632*		3682*	
URINE MG	MEQ/L				1.5			
CHEMO								
ANTIBIOTIC								
OTHER MEDS								

FIGURE 10.3. Sample flow sheet, horizontal format.

Because patients may have more than one name over time, it is useful to retain a record of these secondary names in

PATSNM(HNO,SNAME) = null

(There are no data elements for PATSNM, thus the data entry is null i.e., a string of zero length.) Finally, for a name index, both the primary and secondary names are merged into

JOHNS HOPKINS ONCOLOGY CENTER - 2N-BAH HISTORY NO:
PROVIDER: NAME:
DATE: 07/31/82

1980	IGA MG/DL	IGM MG/DL	IGG MG/DL	24BJ MG/24	24TP MG/24	SEMC GM/DL	SEAB GM/DL
04/16	42:	30:	4265:	-------:	-------:	4.4:	3.0:
04/22	-------:	-------:	-------:	848:	1484:	-------:	-------:
04/24	36:	20:	3048:	779:	1230:	3.9:	2.9:
05/01	42:	36:	2596:	-------:	-------:	3.0:	3.2:
05/05	42:	44:	2221:	0:	320:	-------:	-------:
05/08	35:	36:	1864:	0:	126:	2.3:	2.9:
05/20	-------:	-------:	-------:	-------:	-------:	1.8:	3.6:
05/21	-------:	-------:	-------:	-------:	102:	-------:	-------:
05/22	40:	25:	1760:	0:	140:	2.1:	4.1:
05/31	47:	34:	1385:	-------:	-------:	-------:	-------:
06/02	-------:	-------:	-------:	-------:	-------:	1.2:	3.5:
06/05	70:	36:	1296:	-------:	54:	1.2:	3.6:
08/12	35:	49:	882:	-------:	-------:	-------:	-------:
08/14	44:	43:	832:	-------:	-------:	-------:	-------:
08/28	54:	45:	1053:	-------:	-------:	-------:	3.9:
08/29	54:	45:	1053:	-------:	-------:	-------:	-------:

FIGURE 10.4. Sample flow sheet, vertical format.

SECFLG is a flag to indicate if the value in NAME is a primary or secondary name. This information is necessary if the HNO value was in error and must be changed or if the patient record is to be deleted.

From these three relations one can access a patient by either the HNO—in which case an exact match is required—or by name—in which case a partial entry can be used to list out all possible matches for the input with a prompt for the user to select the desired patient. Note that there is also enough information to read the secondary name flag (SECFLG), get NAME from PATID, and display the message:

"THIS IS A SECONDARY NAME FOR ",NAME

The two index elements for PATNAM are required to provide a unique index to differentiate among patients with the same name. The OCIS database contains some 40,000 patients, and a phonetic spelling system (such as Soundex) is not considered necessary. For larger databases this may be desirable. To support this, two of the above relations may be expanded and a new relation added for the soundex index:

```
PATID(HNO) = NAME,SOUNDEX
PATSNM(HNO,SNAME) = SOUNDEX
PATSNDX(SOUNDEX,HNO) = SECFLG
```

We next describe the data model for the abstract. All data are indexed by HNO. The data are grouped into logical blocks that either (a) may be reused for

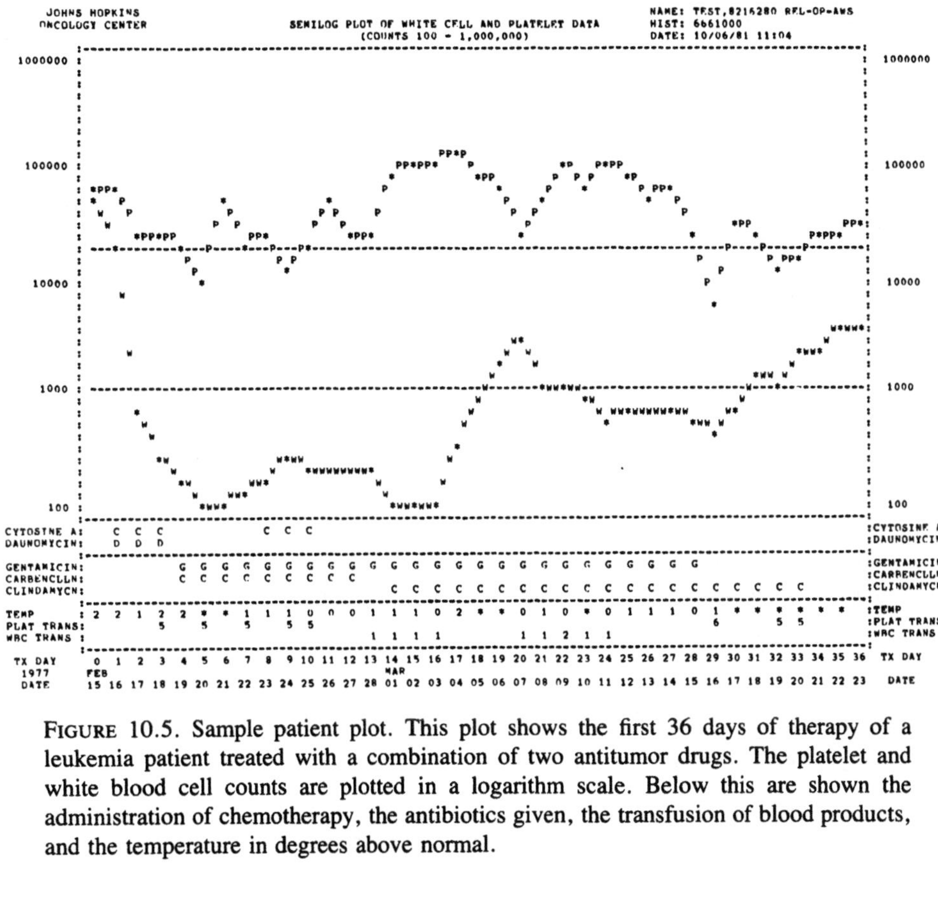

FIGURE 10.5. Sample patient plot. This plot shows the first 36 days of therapy of a leukemia patient treated with a combination of two antitumor drugs. The platelet and white blood cell counts are plotted in a logarithm scale. Below this are shown the administration of chemotherapy, the antibiotics given, the transfusion of blood products, and the temperature in degrees above normal.

different functions or (b) represent a single unit for update purposes. The OCIS uses separate relations for patient demographics and addresses†

PATID1(HNO) = AGE,DATE.OF.BIRTH,RACE,SEX,SPECIAL.CODES
PATADR(HNO) = ADDRESS,CITY,STATE,ZIP,PHONE

In a cancer center, the diagnosis and treatment are organized as independent primary sites. Thus the diagnosis and treatment data are indexed by primary site number (PRIM.NO). The key relations are:

PATDX.ADMINISTRATIVE(HNO,PRIM.NO) = ADM.DATE,
PRELIMINARY,STAFF.IDS

---

†To improve readability we use the period as a valid character in a variable name and impose no limit on the length of names, e.g., DATE.OF.BIRTH. In some cases we also suppress detail by the use of generic elements which may actually be expanded to more than one term, e.g., SPECIAL.CODES

```
PATDX.CODE(HNO,PRIM.NO) = DIAGNOSIS.CODE,SITE,
  MORPHOLOGY,OTHER.CODES
PATDX.DESCR(HNO,PRIM.NO) = REPORT,NOTES
PATTX(HNO,PRIM.NO,FROM) = TO,LOC,TYPE,DESCR
```

Note that the relation for treatment (PATTX) has an added index (FROM date). This allows for multiple entries with different dates. Since the data model used here implies order, all treatments will be automatically retained in chronological order. The relation definition assumes that no more than one treatment entry is entered for any given date; if this is not true, an additional index term will be required. Note that in this data model, elements that are text strings of arbitrary length are supported. For example, the "variable" REPORT actually stands for the extract from the pathology report which, in Fig. 10.2, begins, "811993 1. LEFT KIDNEY . . ." In most systems, such text requires special processing. However, for the purposes of initial design, it is sufficient to abstract such data as a single element.

The history and follow-up relations are quite simple:

```
PAT.HISTORY(HNO,TYPE) = HISTORY
PAT.FOL.UP(HNO,DATE) = LAST.SEEN,CONDITION,QUALITY.
  OF.SURVIVAL,COMMENT
```

There are several different history text types. The variable TYPE acts as a sequencing index; the name of the type is maintained in a separate relation

```
HISTORY(TYPE) = HISTORY.NAME
```

When printing the history block, the name of the text field is taken from HISTORY and the text comment is taken from PAT.HISTORY.

The referring physicians also have their names and addresses in a separate relation

```
MDREF(MD.ID)=MD.NAME,MD.ADDRESS,MD.PHONE
```

The "reference source" in the patient abstract provides a link to that relation:

```
PAT.REF(HNO,SNO) = MD.ID
```

The variable SNO is a sequence number used to order the physicians in the abstract listing. The separation of the physician data from the patient data guarantees that changes made to a physician's address or phone number will be reflected in all appropriate patient abstracts.

In considering the abstract, we have focused upon the relations indexed by patient. It also may be necessary to access these data by other criteria such as diagnosis. To provide this access, we introduce secondary indices (also called inverted indices). In some DBMSs, there is a mechanism to identify a term as a secondary (or alternate) key. In the data model we use, the secondary key is specified in a separate relation. For example, the index to patient by diagnosis is

DXPAT(DIAGNOSIS.CODE,HNO,PRIM.NO) = null

All elements in DXPAT are contained in PATDX.CODE, so DXPAT can be defined as a secondary relation to PATDX.CODE. In the system used, such a definition will cause any changes to PATDX.CODE to be automatically reflected in DXPAT. One may read a secondary relation, but only primary relations can be written into or deleted. PRIM.NO is required to guarantee a one-to-one relationship between the two tables.

The use of secondary relations has an obvious advantage. However, there is a cost in updating, editing, and deleting entries. The designer must always trade off speed of retrieval against update processing time and allocation of file space. Where the index is a secondary relation, the DBMS generally can perform the update automatically. However, in cases where the index is not a proper subset of the primary relation (e.g., the patient name index PATNAM contains SECFLG which is not in the primary relation PATID) then it is the responsibility of the designer to coordinate all file processing among the relations.

The OCIS abstract represents the descriptive portion of the patient record. Although there are some categories of repeating information—such as the treatment summary—most of the abstract is composed of separate fields that are either present or not present. The data model must supply a definition for each such field. In contrast to this structure, the clinical data used to produce the plots and flowsheets provides an example of a large number of data points (about one-half million in the current OCIS database) that can be abstracted in the form of one or two simple relations.

The relation for numeric and coded information that represents patient status, laboratory results, and medication summary is

PDATA(HNO,DATE,ITEM) = VALUE

for items recorded only once a day and

PDATAT(HNO,DATE,ITEM,TIME) = VALUE

for items with more than one entry per day. One would prefer to use a single format for both categories, but for very large files compromises must be made between the simplicity of the data model and the resources allocated. It should be noted, however, that the choice of data model was based, in part, upon the fact that the MUMPS language will not accept a null value for an index; if it did, then the PDATAT definition would be sufficient.‡ This is not a restriction in other DBMSs; thus the data model will always be constrained by the environment in which it is to be implemented.

The PDATA definition given here organizes data first by patient and then by date. This is a convenient structure for creating flowsheets or displaying all

‡Because the MUMPS B-tree manager uses leading character key compression, there is almost no storage overhead for identical high order key term values. Thus repetitions of HNO,DATE in the index require minimal additional file space.

clinical data recorded on a particular date (see Figs. 10.3 and 10.4). It is not effective for producing plots. For a plot, one generally is concerned with a limited number of items over an extended period of time. (The plot shown in Fig. 10.3 contains 10 items over a period of 36 days.) Again, there is a tradeoff between redundancy (i.e., secondary relations) and processing time. Because each day the OCIS must print one or more plots and flows for each of the patients to be treated (some 50 inpatients and 100 outpatients), redundant relations are maintained to improve report processing performance. The plot data relation is

PLOTD(HNO,ITEM,DATE) = VALUE

with entries for only the values of ITEMs used in plots requested for that HNO.

As just seen in the patient data model, all data are stored as independent points. Input from the clinical laboratory, however, is in the form of sets of points organized by group (i.e., test). Processing involves transfer of the clinical laboratory data in small batches, validity tests of the batches, and update of the PDATA/PDATAT relations and any secondary relations. Most data can be processed automatically; some manual processing is required for invalid HNOs, amended reports, and independent entries. Additional relations are defined for an audit trail and to hold data that cannot be processed using one of the automatic procedures.

Several dictionaries also are required. There is a dictionary of valid values for ITEM. This dictionary defines the format, a normal range of values, and the bounds for reasonable (acceptable) values. All entries are checked to first see if the VALUE for the ITEM satisfies the format criteria. If so, numeric data are tested against a reasonable range of values. Unreasonable values are rejected. The next test is against a normal range; values outside the normal range are flagged. The OCIS does not support testing of normal values against multiple criteria (e.g., age or sex plus the ITEM), but this is not considered necessary for the special patient population being treated.

Items within the ITEM dictionary are then grouped by category in two levels. This allows a user to reference generic groups of data such as PATIENT STATUS or VITAL SIGNS (a subset of PATIENT STATUS). All plots and flow sheets are defined by specifying either specific ITEM values or generic groups of items. For example, the plot format (called "WP") shown in Fig. 10.5 has the definition shown in Fig. 10.6. There are three relations: PLOT, which defines the headings, PLOTP which defines the ITEMs to be plotted, and PLOTE, which defines the ITEMs to be listed as events at the base of the plot. Flowsheets are defined in a similar fashion with just two relations: FLOW and FLOW.LIST.

It can be seen from Fig. 10.6 all that is required to print a plot is the patient identifier (HNO), the start date, and the plot format (e.g., "WP"). All information about contents and form are available in other relations. The formatting and printing of the plot, of course, is not the result of a simple query; it requires a sophisticated program. However, all the data necessary to produce it are accessible through simple queries.

The final issue regarding the clinical data plots and flowsheets is the man-

PLOT("WP") = "SEMILOG PLOT . . .", other descriptive data

PLOTP("WP",1) = "WBC", scale information
PLOTP("WP",2) = "PLATELETS", scale information

PLOTE("WP",1) = "CHEMOTHERAPY*"
PLOTE("WP",2) = "ANTIBIOTICS*'
PLOTE("WP",3) = line code
PLOTE("WP",4) = "TEMPERATURE", print as degrees above 38°
PLOTE("WP",5) = "PLATELET TRANSFUSION", print as a number
PLOTE("WP",6) = "WBC TRANSFUSIONS", print as a number

FIGURE 10.6. Example of a plot definition. ITEMs with an asterisk are generic groups. Any ITEMs belonging to that group will be printed if they are found in the patient data for the period being processed. Lower case elements are used here to present a description of the coded data normally stored.

agement of relations that maintain standing orders. The following simple relation is used:

REQUEST(HNO,REQ.NUMBER) = OUTPUT.ID,DATE.RANGE,FREQUENCY

The OUTPUT.ID indicates the plot or flowsheet format (e.g., "WP"). DATE.RANGE indicates if only the most current data or all data within a given date range are to be included. Finally, FREQUENCY specifies when the report should be printed; choices include every day, Mondays only, for each visit, after each update, etc. Every night the request file is queried for all patients to be seen the next day (i.e., all inpatients and all outpatient appointments). Those entries satisfying the frequency criteria are used to initiate a request for the appropriate plots and flowsheets.

The management of other categories of patient data is implemented in a similar fashion. In the case of microbiology data, the structure of the data is somewhat more complex. There are three levels of information:

- The identification of the report.
- Descriptions of the organisms cultured from the specimen.
- Optional list of the antibiotic sensitivities for each organism.

The relations are

PATBAC(HNO,DATE,REPORT.ID) = SPECIMEN.TEST.ORDERED
PATORG(HNO,DATE,REPORT.ID,ORGANISM) = GROWTH,
  PERIOD,DESCRIPTION
PATSEN(HNO,DATE,REPORT.ID,ORGANISM,DRUG) = SENSITIVITY

```
JOHNS HOPKINS ONCOLOGY CENTER                          HISTORY NO: 2129046
                                                             NAME: **********
MICROBIOLOGY DATA (BY DATE)                                  DATE: 01/08/85
------------------------------------------------------------------------------
   10/23/84  BLOOD       BACT CULTURE; NEGATIVE AT 7 DAYS (C704)
             BLOOD       BACT CULTURE; NEGATIVE AT 7 DAYS (C712)
             SPUTUM       BACT MICRO EXAM; TYPE 3:  GOOD SPECIMEN.; MANY POLYMO
                         RPHONUCLEAR CELLS; FEW SQUAMOUS EPITHELIAL CELLS; RARE
                         NORMAL UPPER RESPIRATORY FLORA (J714)
                         STAPHYLOCOCCUS EPIDERMIDIS - BACT CULTURE; POSITIVE AT
                          1 DAY; MODERATE (J714)
                         SUSCEPTIBILITY                      A     B    C     D     E
                            METHICILLIN                (E)  2     4    8     16    16+
                            PENICILLIN                 (E)  0.1   1    4     16    16+
                            ERYTHROMYCIN               (D)  0.5   1    2     -     2+
                            CLINDAMYCIN                (E)  0.5   1    2     8     8+
                            TETRACYCLINE               (B)  1     2    4     16    16+
                            CHLORAMPHENICOL            (C)  2     4    8     16    16+
                            CEPHALOTHIN                (E)  0.5   2    8     32    32+
                            VANCOMYCIN                 (B)  1     2    2.5   4     4+
             THROAT       VIRAL CULTURE; NO VIRUS ISOLATED BY TISSUE CULTURE AS
                          OF 12/14/84; NOV 84 (E747)
             URINE (CLEAN CATCH)       VIRAL CULTURE; NO VIRUS ISOLATED BY TISS
                         UE CULTURE AS OF 12/14/84; NOV 84 (E754)
             SPUTUM       FUNGAL MICRO EXAM    NO FUNGUS SEEN BY POTASSIUM HYDR
                         OXIDE (K454)
                         CANDIDA ALBICANS - FUNGAL CULTURE; POSITIVE AT 7 DAYS
                         (K454)
   10/24/84  BLOOD       BACT CULTURE; NEGATIVE AT 7 DAYS (C815)
             BLOOD       BACT CULTURE; NEGATIVE AT 7 DAYS (C827)
             BLOOD       BACT CULTURE; NEGATIVE AT 7 DAYS (C858)
             TISSUE (OTHER)       BACT MICRO EXAM; NO POLYMORPHONUCLEAR LEUKOCY
                         TES SEEN; NO CELLS SEEN; NO ORGANISM SEEN (P941)
                         BACT AER AND ANA CUL; NEGATIVE AT 7 DAYS (P941)
```

FIGURE 10.7. Sample bacteriology report.

To provide indices to produce patient reports sorted by specimen and organism there are

ORGPAT(HNO,ORGANISM,DATE,REPORT.ID) = null
SPCPAT(HNO,SPECIMEN,DATE,REPORT.ID) = null

Again, there are dictionaries for **ORGANISM** and **SPECIMEN** and entries within **REQUEST** to determine what types of outputs are to be produced for each patient. A sample report is shown in Fig. 10.7.

There are also relations used for the management of transfusions and other patient care processes. In general, each relation follows the general pattern of:

- Primary relation with a key of history number and date
- Inverted index if the data in the relation can be usefully listed or accessed by other parameters
- Dictionaries to ensure entry of only valid data.

10.3.2. Protocol-Directed Care

In the previous section, the ways in which the OCIS collects, stores and displays data were presented. Because the Oncology Center provides tertiary care to cancer patients, it is common to use aggressive therapy and record as many as 100 data items per patient day. The data management system assists the medical decision making process by presenting those data so trends and deviations are readily recognized. However, since the OCIS has an extensive database of clinical events for patients with a limited number of diseases, the OCIS also has been programmed to aid in the daily management of patients. That is the subject of this section.

To understand how an automated system may be used as a therapy planning aid it is necessary to describe the general process of patient care in the Oncology Center. Patients are treated for their cancer as well as for disease or therapy-related medical complications. Much of this therapy follows predefined protocols which may be grouped into four categories.

1. *Research protocols*. These define a set of therapeutic actions to be followed for a specific population to produce a consistent set of data to evaluate a hypothesis. Since each protocol is designed to select among two or more randomly assigned therapies, they must be sufficiently detailed and specific to avoid the introduction of clinical judgments that might invalidate the protocols. A research protocol is typically recorded in the form of a document of up to 60 pages.
2. *Individual therapy*. This involves the use of anti-tumor drugs generally in multi-drug combinations administered using complex time-sequenced relationships. Therapy may extend for months or years. An example is the use of a drug sequence demonstrated to be effective by a previous research protocol.
3. *General support and response to life threatening crisis*. These involve the use of established procedures to deal with reactions and problems associated with the antitumor therapy. In many cases, these actions are anticipated and documented as part of the research protocol. Examples are (a) the use of antibiotic drugs to treat infections when it is known that the antitumor drug will severely lower the white blood cell count and (b) management of fluid balance.
4. *Disease-specific continuing care*. This entails the recommended long- and short-term care and patient monitoring associated with a specific disease independent of the therapy selected. These actions may also be included in the research protocol documentation. Examples are (a) routine 6-month chest x-ray studies for all patients with breast cancer and (b) routine 3-month monitoring of serum protein electropheresis for certain multiple myeloma patients.

At any given time an individual patient may be treated using one or more research protocols (e.g., an antitumor protocol and an antibiotic protocol). These research protocols may be supplemented by other support protocols (e.g., hypercalemia protocol to help manage high levels of serum calcium) and long-term follow-up (e.g., annual battery of tests). The situation is further complicated by the fact that:

1. Protocols may have different branches in which patients are given different doses of the same drug or combinations of different drugs.

2. The Center is a teaching institution and thus subject to housestaff rotation.
3. At any one time there are over 2,000 patients being actively treated by the Center.
4. There are at present more than 125 formal research protocols active in the Center.

There are several ways in which automated assistance can be used in protocol management. As discussed in Chapter 9, one approach is to formulate an algorithm (or flow chart) for the protocol. The algorithm may be used as a document or encoded in the form of a computer program. Such approaches have been demonstrated to improve compliance. The major difficulty, however, is that each algorithm is limited to a single protocol. An alternative technique is to structure the therapy knowledge so that it can be used by an expert system such as ONCOCIN. Here therapy is based upon rules such as:

RULE 075
To determine the current attenuated dose for all drugs in MOPP or for all drugs in PAVE:
If 1) This is the start of the first cycle after a cycle was aborted, and
2) The blood counts do not warrant dose attenuation
Then: Conclude that the current attenuated dose is 75 percent of the previous dose.

However, the use of AI techniques for this type of application is still in the research stage.

A third alternative is the use of a database to structure the decision rules. In this case the data are structured in a manner similar to the way they are organized in ONCOCIN except that (a) the powerful search capabilities of ONCOCIN are not available and (b) the rules are partially coded and not written as text. One may consider this to be a "table-driven" approach. Only general purpose algorithms are used; all protocol definitions and actions are stored in relations and there is no explanation facility.

Fig. 10.8 illustrates the flow used to produce the daily protocol-directed care plans. First a protocol is defined. A summary of the protocol text is entered into the protocol file as a descriptive document; the actions associated with the protocol are documented as treatment sequences. The treatment sequence is a list of actions (e.g., order a test, administer a drug, print a message) combined with criteria for its initiation (e.g., every 3 days, each Monday, until acknowledged). A schema (associated with the protocol) defines the relationships among the treatment sequences within the protocol.

Treatment sequences are assigned to individual patients. Each day, all patients to be treated have their current status matched against their active treatment sequences. The output is a list of recommended orders for each patient. These orders are printed in a variety of formats for use by unit clerks, physicians, faculty, etc. Fig. 10.9 contains a sample daily care plan and Fig. 10.10 illustrates an order guide. The protocol features of the OCIS have been in use since 1979 for all inpatient orders managed by the phlebotomy team; all bone marrow

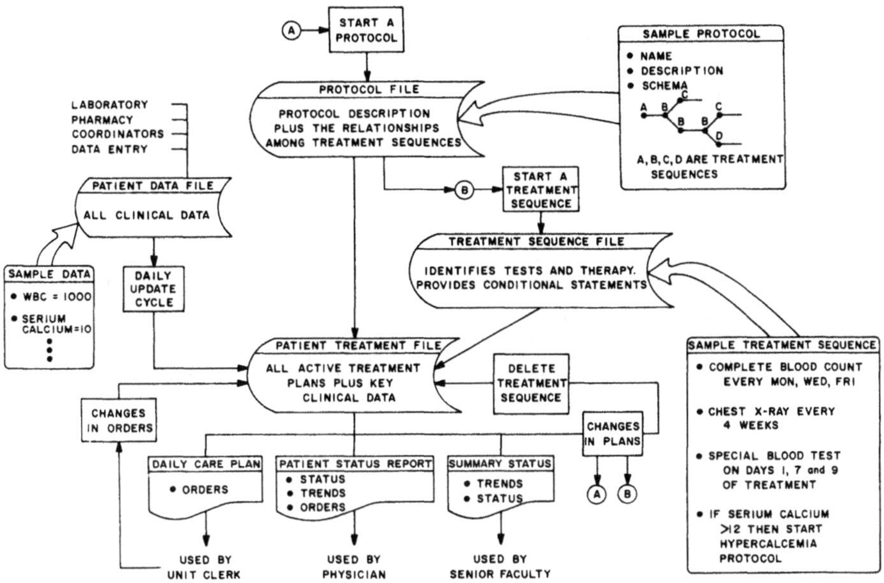

FIGURE 10.8. Processing flow for daily care plans.

transplant patients and leukemia patients have had their protocols managed in this way since 1980.

An overview of the data model is presented in the Entity-Relationship diagram* shown in Fig. 10.11. There are two categories of data. The protocol data, which are independent of any patient, are shown in the left column. All other data are patient specific. Data from the protocol relations are copied over to the patient data relations. In this way they can be edited to meet special patient requirements. The protocol data consists of the following sets of relations.

- *Protocol description.* This is a description of the protocol written in text. The text is structured to allow descriptive sections (attributes) to be extracted for printing or processing. Examples of protocol description attributes are: (a) general description, (b) requirements for entering a patient onto the study, (c) evaluation criteria (outcome measures) and (d) dose modifications in the event of toxicity. It can be shown that all but the first can be structured to allow automatic interactions between protocol rules and the patient's clinical data. When treated as descriptive text, the general form of a relation is

PRODES(PROTOCOL.ID,SECTION.ID) = TEXT

*Ovals in the diagram represent entities (which are implemented as relations). The diamonds are relationships that indicate how the entities interact with each other. Entities are usually described with nouns and relationships are given verbs for names (see Chapter 5).

JOHNS HOPKINS
ONCOLOGY CENTER

GENERAL DAILY CARE PLAN

HISTORY NO:
NAME:
PLAN DATE: 08/06/80
WEDNESDAY

20 W F   HODGKIN'S DISEASE
HT 155   ADM WT 44   BAS 1.4   IDEAL WT 45   WT(08/05/80) 43.2
BLOOD TYPE O+   HLA
PROTOCOL E1475 'BLEO-MOPP-XET   DAY 29   STARTED 07/09/80
SECOND CYCLE - BLEO MOPP 8/6/80

PROVIDER LENHARD, DR R

PROTOCOL GENERATED INSTRUCTIONS

```
****************************************************************************
*  MAX CUMLATIVE DOSE OF BLEOMYCIN IS 36 MG/M2                             *
****************************************************************************
```

ENTER PERFORMANCE STATUS
ENTER TUMOR MEASUREMENTS
MEASURE LONGEST DIAMETER & ITS PERPENDICULAR DIAMETER IN CM
SEE PROTOCOL (SECTION 5.21) FOR CHEMO DOSE MODIFICATION IF WBC < 4000 OR PLTS < 100000
SEE PROTOCOL (SECTION 5.12) FOR DOSE MODIFICATION IF TOTAL BLIL > 1.5

MEASURABLE TUMOR SITES

				INITIAL		LAST	
ID	GRID	O/T	M/METHOD	SIZE (CM)	DATE	SIZE (CM)	DATE
A				9.7 7.4	07/09/80	9.7 7.4	07/09/80
			TOTAL AREA	71.78		71.78	

RECENT CLINICAL FINDINGS

VALUE	DESCRIPTION	LAST FINDING	STARTING	THROUGH
5.6	CUMULATIVE TOTAL BLEOMYCIN	07/16/80	07/09/80	08/07/80
44	INITIAL BODY WT AM	07/09/80	07/09/80	07/09/80
43.2	LAST BODY WT 'AM	08/05/80	07/10/80	08/07/80
97	PERCENT BODY WT AM BASED ON 44	08/05/80	07/10/80	08/07/80
0.7	MAXIMUM SER CREAT	08/04/80	07/09/80	08/07/80
9100	MINIMUM WBC	07/16/80	07/09/80	08/07/80
704000	MINIMUM PLATELETS	07/16/80	07/09/80	08/07/80

CHEMOTHERAPY DRUG HISTORY

NAME	DOSE	GIVEN	% BASELINE
NITR MUST	8.3 MG	07/16/80	100 % OF 6 MG/M2
PROCARB	120 MG	07/22/80	85% OF 140 MG
VINCRIST	1.9 MG	07/16/80	95% OF 2.0 MG
PREDNISONE	56 MG	07/22/80	100% OF 40 MG/M2
BLEOMYCIN	2.8 U	07/16/80	100% OF 2.8 U

DRUGS TO BE ORDERED ON 08/06/80

2.80 MG BLEOMYCIN I.V., BASED ON 1.4 M2 X 2 MG/M2.
8.40 MG NITROGEN MUSTARD I.V., BASED ON 1.4 M2 X 6 MG/M2
1.96 MG VINCRISTINE I.V. MAX SINGLE DOSE 2.0 MG.
BASED ON 1.4 M2 X 1.4 MG/M2.
140 MG PROCARBAZINE P.O., BASED ON 1.4 M2 X 100 MG/M2.

FIGURE 10.9. Sample general daily care plan. This plan is for the first day of the second cycle of therapy. The comment in the box warns the physician that one of the drugs to be administered, Bleomycin, has a maximum cumulative dose. The sections on measurable tumor sites, recent clinical findings and chemotherapy history are automatically updated from the clinical database each day. The actual drug dose is computed on the basis of a body surface area (BSA, see top of plan) of 1.4. The general plan includes a list of all tests and procedures required for the protocol. Twelve tests are to be ordered from this plan. General physician comments are listed at the beginning of the plan. Messages related to a procedure are listed in the procedure ordering section. Most messages tend to be reminders. The next version of the system will be able to generate warning messages based on data trends.

```
              JOHNS HOPKINS                  HISTORY NO:
             ONCOLOGY CENTER                       NAME:
                                             PLAN DATE: 08/06/80
          GENERAL DAILY CARE PLAN                      WEDNESDAY

TESTS AND PROCEDURES WITH DATE LAST PERFORMED (> INDICATES ORDERED 08/06/80,
                                                 * ORDERED STAT 08/06/80)

BLOOD AND SERUM TESTS
    >HCT   HEMATOCRIT      08/05/80          >DIFF  WBC DIFF       08/05/80
    >PLTS  PLT CNT         08/05/80          >WBC   WBC            08/05/80
    >HGB   HEMOGLOBIN      08/05/80           M12   SMA-12         08/01/80
     IGSV  IG SURVEY       07/04/80           SCU   SER COPPER     07/04/80
     M6    SMA-6           08/04/80          >SALK  S ALK PHOS     08/04/80
    >SGOT  SGOT            08/01/80          >SGPT  SGPT           08/01/80
    >TBLI  TOT BILI        08/01/80          >SUN   S UREA NIT     08/04/81
    >SCR   SER CREAT       08/04/80          >SURC  S UR ACID      08/01/80
RADIOLOGY PROCEDURES
     CXR   CHEST XRAY      07/08/80
PHYSICIAN PROCEDURES

    REPEAT ANY X-RAY TO DOCUMENT RESPONSE OR PROGRESSION
P.A. PROCEDURES
     MUMP  MUMPS SKIN      07/04/80           TRIC  TRICH SKIN     07/04/80
     PPD   PPD SKIN        07/04/80
DATA COORDINATOR INSTRUCTIONS

    HAS DISEASE PROGRESSED? CHECK WITH M.D. RE: STOPPING TX SEQUENCES
```

FIGURE 10.9. Sample general daily care plan. (continued)

- *Protocol schema*. This is a set of activities (treatment sequences) and branching criteria that defines the protocol. The activities are abstracted as groups of actions and the schema provides a high level plan for the initiation and termination of each group. The schema may be thought of as a flow chart or program that describes the protocol. The schema is written with one statement to a line in the fashion of a computer program. (At present, the schema is used only for documentation; all treatment sequences are entered and deleted manually.)
- *Treatment sequence*. This is a collection of activities that are referenced by the protocol schema. All actions within the treatment sequence are based upon a schedule relative to the start of the treatment sequence. The general form of a treatment sequence is

  TS(TS.ID,SEQUENCE.NO) = CONDITION,SCHEDULE,ACTION

  CONDITION refers to the value of a clinical finding (see Figure 10.9) such as "LAST WBC < 1000." SCHEDULE indicates when the ACTION should be taken. This may be an absolute criteria (e.g., Monday, Wednesday and Friday) or relative to some previous ACTION (e.g., every four days except on weekends.) ACTION values are defined in a separate dictionary.
- *Clinical actions*. These are the various activities performed in patient care. Examples are: (a) drug therapies; these contain the attributes: drug name, dose, route, etc. (b) procedures; these contain the attributes: name, procedure

```
JOHN HOPKINS                                        HISTORY NO: [redacted]
ONCOLOGY CENTER                                           NAME: [redacted]
                                                     PLAN DATE: 08/23/84
PHYSICIAN ORDER GUIDE                                   THURSDAY   PAGE 1

48 Y.O. W F   L-2/ACUTE LYM LEUK                   HT  162.0 CM   BSA 1.75 M2

  09/18/83 MARKERS REPORTED BACK CALLA+,IA+.
     WEIGHTS:   ADMIN   66.0 KG    IDEAL    KG      CURRENT (08/20/84)   67.5 KG

PROTOCOLS                                          STARTED        DAY
    J8302      ALL/REMISS. INDUCT. & BMT           07/16/84       39
               AC-D-D 12 GRAMS

 BLOOD PROCEDURES
:----------------------------------------------------------------------------:
:  TEST NAME              AMOUNT       TUBE          LAB          SLIP       :
: HEMATOCRIT              3 CC         SM LAVEND(    ONC          ONCOLOGY   :
: WBC                                  SM LAVEND     ONC          ONCOLOGY   :
: PLT CNT                              SM LAVEND     ONC          ONCOLOGY   :
: BLOOD CULT                           BLOOD CULT    BACT         BACT       :
: STAT GLUC               3.00 CC      SM RED        MAIN CHEM    EMERG CHEM :
: STAT M6                 4.00 CC      SM RED        MAIN CHEM    EMERG CHEM :
:                         SEND STAT                                          :
:----------------------------------------------------------------------------:
:                                                                            :
:----------------------------------------------------------------------------:
:                                                                            :
:----------------------------------------------------------------------------:
TOTAL BLOOD TO BE DRAWN:   10CC

 URINE PROCEDURES
:----------------------------------------------------------------------------:
:  TEST NAME                           CONTAINER     LAB          SLIP       :
: 24UR CR,PR              24 HR        24 HR UR      SP CHEM      URINE CHEM :
:                         24 HR URINE FOR CR CL & T. PROTEIN                 :
:----------------------------------------------------------------------------:
:                                                                            :
:----------------------------------------------------------------------------:
:                                                                            :
:----------------------------------------------------------------------------:

 RADIOLOGY PROCEDURES
:----------------------------------------------------------------------------:
:  TEST NAME                                         LAB          SLIP       :
:----------------------------------------------------------------------------:
:                                                                            :
:----------------------------------------------------------------------------:
:                                                                            :
:----------------------------------------------------------------------------:

 OTHER TESTS AND PROCEDURES
:----------------------------------------------------------------------------:
:  TEST NAME                           TUBE/CONT     LAB          SLIP       :
:----------------------------------------------------------------------------:
```

FIGURE 10.10. Sample order guide.

identifier, special instructions, etc.; (c) tests; these contain the attributes: specimen, collection method volume, procedure id, special instructions, etc. (d) messages; these contain the attributes: message, audience, priority, etc. Each different class of action has its own dictionary relation containing the data required in its processing.

The patient data generally contain information copied from the protocol data with HNO added as leading index. In the case of Standing Orders, the data stored in the Treatment Sequence relation are copied. Since it is possible that the same action (e.g., order complete blood count [CBC]) will be recommended

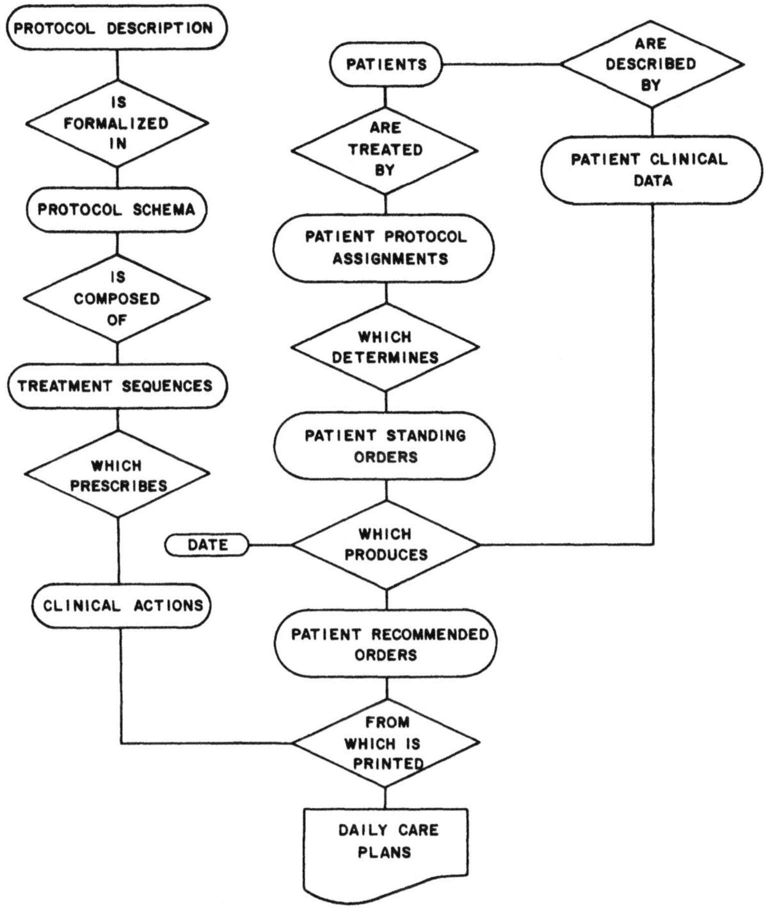

FIGURE 10.11. Entity-relationship diagram for protocol system.

by more than one treatment sequence, the action is used as an index instead of the treatment sequence identifier. Thus we have

PAT.SO(HNO,ACTION,DATE.START,TS.ID) = CONDITION,SCHEDULE

Note that this groups all actions of the same type together. The DATE.START for a treatment sequence allows the same treatment sequence to be assigned on more than one date.

The schedule in PAT.SO may be a function of the last time an action was performed. In some cases, the schedule may represent a complex sequence of actions such as

"Q2D 3 TIMES THEN Q7D" where "Q2D" is every 2 days.

For this reason, a housekeeping relation is added to the standing orders for each action.

PAT.SOA(HNO,ACTION) = LAST.DATE,NUMBER.TIMES,POINTERS

This relation is updated during a verification process in which any deviations from the recommended orders are noted. This implies that the verification process must be completed before the next day's care plans can be generated. The generation of the daily care plans for a patient simply involves the processing of all entries in the Standing Order relations, applying the selection criteria, and if valid, creating an entry in the Recommended Order relation:

PAT.RO(HNO,DATE,ACTION) = OPTIONAL.INSTRUCTIONS

The Recommended Orders are used to print the various care plans; they also serve as a guide for the verification process.

As can be seen, the basic structure of the OCIS Daily Care Plan system is quite straightforward. At the next level of detail, however, some seldom-used algorithms add complexity. For example, some tests are routinely included with other tests (e.g., a WBC count is included with a CBC). Thus, when the second test is performed, the last date for all included tests must be updated. This requires a dictionary relation for all tests which are included as a part of other tests. Nevertheless, it should be clear how the OCIS design has abstracted the problem of protocol directed care so that plans—based on multiple concurrent protocols—can be created easily and used safely.

10.3.3. Administrative Support

Most clinical information systems identify administrative functions that must be supported and then try to append patient care facilities. Because of this initial orientation, they seldom are successful in providing assistance in patient care. The OCIS was developed as a system for patient care. The clinical functions were first designed and implemented. To make these functions operate smoothly, many administrative features such as admissions and appointments had to be added. As these functions were integrated, it was found that purely administrative features such as charge capture and management reporting could be added with only minor programming effort.

Since the OCIS was designed to integrate inpatient and outpatient care, it was necessary to have an appointment system that would indicate which patients would be present on any given day. The appointment system had to be integrated with the care plan system, thus all tests to be scheduled must be indicated. As in the case of any appointment system, multiple clinics must be managed, the schedules of individual providers must be considered, provisions must be made for overbooking, and effective interfaces must be designed for the registrars who use the system.

In a similar way the admitting function (Admission/Discharge/Transfer system

```
JOHNS HOPKINS OCIS                               OUTPATIENT TERMINAL     01/08/85

SCHEDULE OF PATIENTS FOR THE NEXT 7 DAYS

                         DATE           2S    2N    3S    3N    TOTAL    PED

       TUES              01/08/85       15    13    13    14    55       10
       WED               01/09/85       16    13    13    14    56       9
       THUR              01/10/85       14    13    13    15    55       8
       FRI               01/11/85       12    13    13    15    53       8
       SAT               01/12/85       10    13    13    15    51       8
       SUN               01/13/85       9     11    14    15    49       8
       MON               01/14/85       9     10    14    15    48       8
       TUES              01/15/85       7     9     15    16    47       11
<RET> TO CONTINUE: ^
```

FIGURE 10.12. Projected occupancy report. Projections are for the four Center units (2S, 2N, 3S, and 3N) and Pediatric Oncology (PED).

[ADT]) breaks little new ground. There are standard admitting functions, inpatient locator screens, and historic records of admissions. These historic actions are managed by a census system that also integrates protocol starts and outcomes, recent outpatient results, diagnostic indices, etc. A security system is used to deny access to protocol and clinical data from those who are not authorized to view it. The only unusual feature of the OCIS ADT system is that it integrates inpatient and outpatient activities. It is not uncommon to initiate a cycle of treatment as an inpatient, follow the patient as an outpatient, and readmit the patient just as the anticipated toxicities develop. This type of patient management is less expensive and generally more comfortable for the patient. However, such patient management requires a careful coordination of admissions and outpatient visits so that there is neither a risk to the patient nor an unacceptably low occupancy rate for the institution. The OCIS supports this process by scheduling outpatient appointments and readmissions from the inpatient units. Each day the anticipated discharge dates for all inpatients are updated, and a daily report reviews anticipated discharges and scheduled admissions in order to project the occupancy in each unit over of the next 7 days (Fig. 10.12).

Much of the charge capture is managed by hospital systems. Nevertheless, some OCIS processing is required. For example, in the outpatient areas the charge capture is integrated with the appointment and daily care plan processing. For each inpatient a level of care indicator is recorded on a daily basis as an element of clinical data. The original intent was to adjust charges according to the resources required. Such an innovative practice was not approved, and the level of care is used now only to estimate the institutional resources required to manage patients with a given disease or on a given protocol. Each month the level of care data are extracted from the patient data relation (PDATA) to produce detailed and summary reports by nursing unit (Fig. 10.13). These are reviewed by management to assess staffing and patient assignments.

	ADM.	D&D	X-FER	PAT DAYS	DAYS BY CATEGORY I	II	III	IV	V
TOTAL	38	38	0	371	63	55	194	22	37
MAXIMUM	5	4	0	14	4	5	9	2	2
MINIMUM	0	0	0	9	0	0	2	0	0
MEAN	1.22	1.22	0	11.96	2.03	1.77	6.25	0.70	1.19
PERCENT	0	0	0	85	14	12	44	5	8

FIGURE 10.13. Portion of a level of care report. This is a summary of one month's activity in a 14-bed unit. The maximum, minimum, and mean are daily values within the unit.

10.3.4. Special Applications and Research

The OCIS supports a system for managing and administering blood products, an inpatient pharmacy system, a hospital-wide tumor registry (which is integrated with the patient abstract system), and a Research Office system (which coordinates protocol activities). Research is supported by a limited number of online tools. Most analysis is performed on the central mainframe or on local personal computers. Data for analysis generally are copied from the OCIS database. There are tools available to extract data, make magnetic tapes, and support personal computer links.

10.4. System Evaluation

In the previous chapters, individual attributes of a CIS have been evaluated separately. For example, it was shown that timely reminders alter physician behavior. When considering total systems, however, one still tends to rely more heavily upon Barnett's criteria: Will people use it, pay for it, and steal it? At present, the OCIS is installed only at Johns Hopkins and a cancer center in Australia. Nevertheless it is used and is internally funded. In what follows, we briefly examine the OCIS from three perspectives.

- *Utilization*. This is a quantification of how and where the system is used. Clearly, high usage indicates that the system is an integral part of the health care process. Further, high usage levels would suggest that the system is perceived to be beneficial.
- *Cost*. This is a quantification of the cost of the system for both one-time development and operations. It includes all costs that are associated with the information system and is limited to the cost of operation within the facility.
- *Cost benefit*. This is a quantification of the net cost impact of the system, i.e., the difference between the operating costs with the information system and the projected cost of operations if no computer system existed.

TABLE 10.2. OCIS weekly utilization statistics (1981).

	Printed	Online requests
Plots	500	50
Daily clinical data	N/A	1,000
Flow sheets	750	250
Abstracts	275	280
Bacteriology reports	150	25
Other on-line reports		
Searches, queries, special requests	50	N/A

10.4.1. Utilization Measures

The OCIS operates 7 days a week and is the primary support for clinical data displays, clinic scheduling, patient admission, tumor registry operation, the pheresis program and test ordering. Table 10.2 summarizes some weekly utilization statistics based on 1981 operations reports. (This was the last year in which these data were collected routinely.) Another measure of utilization is the catalog of requests for new applications. As is the case of most successful systems, expansion is limited by the size of the programming staff and the computer resources available to support new functions.

10.4.2. System Cost

The cost of the system is divided into one-time costs and ongoing operational costs. The one-time costs include facility preparation, computer equipment, and OCIS software development. The facility preparation cost includes both the planning and cable installation in the original building and the changes made to the original facility such as the cost of supplementary air conditioning. Total facility costs were between $100,000 and $150,000.

Computer equipment costs include two PDP-11/70 computers, four RP-06 disk units (700 M bytes of storage), terminals, and communication equipment. Total equipment costs over a 5-year period are about $600,000.

Software development costs for the OCIS include both initial system development and system maintenance. The Oncology Center's accounting does not differentiate between categories. However, given the current design together with a trained staff, the entire system could be reprogrammed in about 12 man-years of effort. Thus, we have assumed a development cost of $300,000, with all other software costs allocated to system maintenance.

In summary, the total one-time OCIS cost is about $1 million. A large part of that investment was for equipment at prices that prevailed 5 years ago. For example, the total mass storage used by the OCIS can now be replaced by a single unit at about a fourth of the initial price. With the equipment available on the market today, the same computing capability can be purchased at two-thirds the initial cost. If one were willing to assume some technical risk and use prototype database machines, small MUMPS processors, and local area networking, then the equivalent power would be available for about one-fourth the price. And if one is willing to wait 3-5 years, there will be no technical risk associated with such an inexpensive configuration.

Operational cost for the OCIS includes (a) computer operations with operators and data entry, (b) software maintenance including OCIS enhancement, and (c) clinical data coordinators who act as an interface between the information center and the users of the system. In 1982, the Oncology Center employed a faculty of 80 and a staff of 500. The Information Center staff supported one faculty member and a staff of 20. Ten of the staff were clinical data coordinators assigned to the clinical units.

Support for the Information Center is taken from different cost centers within the Oncology Center. With the exception of some separately funded research activities, all operating costs are derived from patient care revenues. The Information Center assessment is based on a guideline of 3% of the charges for the services supported. (The 3% figure includes a 5-year write-off of the capital investment.) Units supporting the Information Center include Medical Oncology, Pediatric Oncology, Radiation Oncology, the Pheresis Center, the Oncology Pharmacy, and the Administrative Offices.

10.4.3. Cost Benefit

In evaluating the OCIS, it should be clear that no manual system could provide the functionality of the automated system. Thus, a cost-benefit analysis would be comparing unlike capabilities.

Moreover, it must be recognized that the traditional methods for cost-benefit analysis consider only those items appearing in the institution's budget. Cost savings to other segments of the economy are not tabulated. Yet some of the most dramatic cost savings that result from the OCIS involve cost savings to patients and third-party payors that may have a negative cost impact on the Oncology Center. Two examples will suffice.

In the discussion of the ADT system, reference was made to the fact that care is taken to coordinate inpatient and outpatient treatment to minimize discomfort and risk. It was pointed out that a patient may be admitted as an inpatient so that antitumor drugs may be administered and, following a day of monitoring, discharged for several days. When the patient begins to have a toxic reaction, he is readmitted for treatment as an inpatient. The plot in Fig. 10.5 illustrates the delay between the start of chemotherapy and a corresponding drop in the white blood cell count. For the protocol followed in this plot, continuous admission is required; for other protocols, however, there is no medical need to retain the patient as an inpatient. The economic impact of that temporary discharge benefits the patient and any third-party payors, but not necessarily the treating institution.

A second example can be found in use of the OCIS to assist in the management

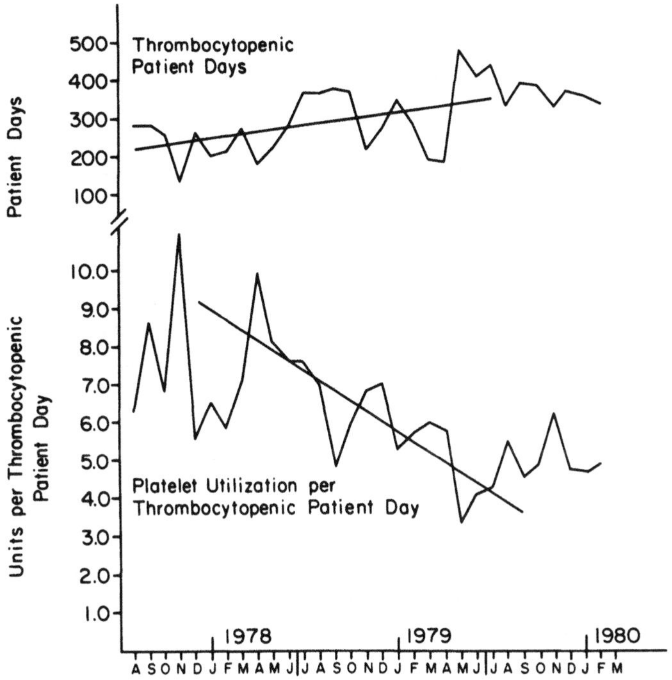

FIGURE 10.14. Johns Hopkins Oncology Center platelet utilization trends.

of platelet transfusions. To evaluate the impact of the new system, platelet transfusion practices over a 3-year period were reviewed. The clinical requirement for platelet transfusion was estimated by determining the total number of days each month that patients manifested platelet counts less than 20,000/mm^3. Over the study period the total need for transfusion doubled from approximately 200 patient days/month to 400 patient days/month (Fig. 10.14). This is consistent with the expanding census of the center as patient referral increased. The rate of utilization of platelets was determined by dividing actual platelet use per month by patient days of platelet counts below 20,000/mm^3. Results indicated that during the study period there was a 50% decrease in the number of units transfused per thrombocytopenic patient day. Throughout the study period it had been recommended that 5 units of platelets be transfused on every day that the patient's platelet count was less than 20,000/mm^3. Thus, the daily rate of 7–11 units noted during 1978 was an inappropriate or ineffective use of the blood products. The average use of five units/thrombocytopenia day experienced in 1980 is more consistent with recommended care. If product utilization in 1980 had continued at 1978 rates, 1,000 additional units of platelets per month at a cost of $20/unit would have been needed. This would indicate a current cost avoidance of $250,000/year. As in the case of the previous example, this cost avoidance provided no cost benefit to the Oncology Center.

In conclusion, one must recognize that it is unrealistic to establish a cost benefit for the OCIS. First, the benefits are not keyed to the computer system but to how the system is used. Patient management using inpatient/outpatient care is possible without a computer system. Yet, without a computer system it is difficult to recognize the toxicity patterns and manage a large number of patients in this way. A platelet transfusion system also is possible without a computer system. In fact, the computer is a very small part of the total system. Any allocation of costs and benefits among the automated and nonautomated aspects of a system will be arbitrary and subjective. Moreoever—even if one could assign proper values—it is not clear that the benefits are always to the using organization's own economic interests. (Of course, this may change with the new emphasis on prospective payments.) Therefore, we can only make the weakest of evaluation statements: the OCIS is used and paid for.

10.5. Concluding Remarks

The OCIS is an information system designed to support medical decision-making in a tertiary care setting. Most of its processing is associated with management of the medical record and supporting communications within the Center. The system does not have an ad hoc query language; neither does it support statistical or AI decision making tools. However, it does produce protocol directed care plans. Perhaps the most important feature of the OCIS is the fact that it runs on minicomputers, is highly modular, and was implemented primarily using internal funding. In this context, the OCIS serves as an existence proof that the CIS technology is sufficiently mature to produce low cost modules designed to assist in paient care. Although the OCIS may be too specialized for general use, its availability should provide an incentive to commercial vendors to include some of its features in their products. Finally, for those institutions that elect to implement their own systems or modules, it is hoped that this description of the OCIS data model will help in the transfer of concepts.

For Further Reading

The following papers contain further information about the OCIS:

1. Lenhard, R. E., B. I. Blum, J. M. Sunderland, H. G. Braine and R. Saral, The Johns Hopkins Oncology Clinical Information System *J. Med. Sys.* 1983, 7:147-174.
2. Lenhard, R. E. and B. I. Blum, Practical Applications of OCIS, A Clinical Information System for Oncology. *Comp. Biol. Med.* 1984, 14:15-23.
3. Blum, B. I. and R. E. Lenhard, Displaying Clinical Data for Decision Making, *J. Clin. Eng*. 1983, 8:61-68.
4. Lenhard, R. E., B. I. Blum and E. E. McColligan, An Information System for Oncology, in B. I. Blum (ed) *Information Systems for Patient Care*, Springer-Verlag, 1984 385-403.

5. McColligan, E. E., B. I. Blum, R. E. Lenhard, M. B. Johnson, The Human Element in Computer Generated Patient Management Plans, *J. Med. Sys.* 1982, 6:265-276.
6. Blum, B. I., A Data Model for Patient Management, J. H. van Bemmel, M. J. Ball and O. Wigertz (ed), MEDINFO 83, 1983 748—751.
7. Blum, B. I. and C. W. Brunn, Implementing an Appointment System with TEDIUM, *Proc. Fifth Annual Symposium on Computer Applications in Medical Care*, 1981 172-181.
8. Blum, B. I. and R. E. Lenhard, Jr., Privacy and Security in an Oncology Information System, *Proc. Second Annual Symposium on Computer Applications in Medical Care* 1978 500-508.

Epilogue

In conclusion, it is of interest to recall that when Copernicus proved that the earth was not the center of the universe, but rather a tiny speck, he injured man's pride. When Darwin suggested that we are not specially created, but rather an extension of the animal world, he salted this wounded pride. When Freud taught that we are not the master of our own house, but that we must be content with tiny vignettes of what goes on in our minds, he seared our salted wound. Finally, in a paper entitled "The Fourth Discontinuity," Mazlish suggests that the computer constitutes yet another blow to man's ego, for in a sense it places him on a continuous spectrum with the machines that he builds. If so, let us now swallow our pride like those who preceded us, comfort ourselves if need be with the reminder that it is we who can always pull out the plug, and set about the task of developing humanitarian uses for these inanimate machines.

Howard Bleich, 1971[1]

In 1977 Friedman and Gustafson prepared a guest editorial for *Computers and Biomedical Research* entitled Computers in Clinical Medicine, A Critical Review.[2] They identified six impediments to a more universal application of computers to medicine (not restricted to clinical information systems). These were:

I. We have not successfully accomplished the patient-computer and/or physician-computer interaction.

II. The physician has not been provided with computer-based medical applications that exceed his own capabilities.

III. A major impediment of the successful utilization of computer technology in medicine and health care has been our inability to prove a significant positive impact on patient care.

IV. We have not produced applications that are easily transferred from one institution to another.

V. We have not conducted research in a manner that is change oriented. (Successful change, in the authors' view, is characterized by clearly understanding the problem first and then finally working out the best solution to that problem. Computer research, they stated, has been characterized by people skilled in one solution (computers) searching for a problem to fit their solution.)

VI. We have not learned from previous mistakes.

A few years later, there was a report on the attitudes of medical personnel toward computers. The abstract follows:

Attitudes toward computers held by various personnel in a medical center were surveyed to determine if recent developments bringing the public into closer regular contact with computers and related devices have resulted in any attitudinal changes since an earlier similar study reported in the literature in 1972. While some differences were found, the overall similarity of results in the two studies seems to indicate that, though people are still favorably disposed toward the use of computers in the health care field, their value is still regarded as unproven.[3]

An interesting question is "What, if anything, has changed since then, and why?" I think that, regrettably, the description of barriers cited by Friedman and Gustafson is almost as valid today as it was when it was written eight years ago. However, attitudes toward computers have changed. This is the result of the personal computer revolution. Computers are more powerful and flexible; users are less intimidated; display terminals are an accepted part of our work environments. The novelty has worn off, and computer tools are accepted whenever they perform useful functions.

A second major change is occurring in the health care industry. Until recently, medical care was reimbursed on the basis of cost, and there were few tools to aid the clinician in either his or her decision-making or commitment of resources. Costs were keyed to expendables (e.g., drugs, supplies) and labor (e.g., professional fees, clerical support). Computer systems initially were designed to reduce or control labor costs. (Their greatest impact, however, came in their ability to enable new functions such as managing large numbers of laboratory tests and supporting new imaging techniques.) The high cost of medical care has led to a revision of the way health care is supported. Groups now provide comprehensive care on a prepayment basis. There is also prospective payment for hospital care based on diagnosis related groups (DRG). Cost incentives are becoming linked to the quality of care and the early identification, management, and treatment of disease. Labor reduction is a secondary issue.

Finally, a third change since the critique was written is that we have more experience. Although we are still in a "prescientific phase," there now is a sizable body of knowledge on which one can build. As has been clearly demonstrated in Part III, the CIS is an effective tool for managing clinical information for the purposes of communication, access, surveillance, and decision-making. We have seen how decision-making tools and the structuring of medical knowledge can be integrated with the CIS; we have also shown how the CIS can alter physician behavior and help manage the complexities of modern medical care; moreover, we have suggested how expert systems may be integrated with the CIS to provide more comprehensive environments.

Most of the costs for medical care are associated with the management of diagnosed diseases and complications related to this therapy. All the tools necessary to support this process have been demonstrated. Although few commercial systems exist, the cost to develop them is continually falling. One goal of this book has been to arouse an awareness of the potential benefit of the CIS to create a demand that would stimulate the development of new products.

As to the future of the CIS, I believe that the necessary computer technology exists; the emphasis must be placed on the medical context in which the tools are used. If we build on our experience (impediment VI), select problems that have a potential for changing the process (impediment V), and concern ourselves with issues of transportability (impediment IV) and evaluation (impediment III), then we will produce useful tools that are used (impediments I and II).

The accomplishment of these ends requires both medical knowledge and an understanding of computing. It combines research with good engineering practices. Clearly, I am biased in my views, but I believe that the greatest computer-related improvement in health care in this century will be related to the management of clinical data. The reader may not agree, but if you have read this far you at least understand the reasons for my optimism.

References

1. Reprinted by permission from Bleich HL, The computer as consultant, *N Engl J Med* (284,3):146, 1971.
2. Friedman RB, Gustafson DH, Computers in clinical medicine, a critical review, *Comp Bio Res* 10:199-204, 1977.
3. Melhorn JM, Legler WK, Clark GM, Current attitudes of medical personnel toward computers, *Comp Bio Res.*, 12:327-334, 1979.

A Computer Glossary

Accumulator A class of register in the CPU that supports the production of an arithmetic or logic result.

Ada This is a new DoD standard programming language designed specifically to support the development and maintenance of real-time embedded mission critical applications. The language was specified by an international committee of computer scientists and contains many of the features generally accepted as being beneficial to this class of application. The language is just entering the production stage. It is named after Ada, Countess of Lovelace, Lord Byron's only daughter, associate of Babbage, and credited as being the world's first programmer. Ada is a trademark of the Department of Defense.

Address The location of a word in memory; all memory is accessed by address.

ALGOL ALGOrithm Language, this was the first of the block structured computer languages. Long used as a standard for documentation of algorithums, it has had a profound effect on the development of languages such as Pascal, PL/1, and Ada.

ALU (Arithmetic Logic Unit) That portion of the CPU that supports the basic arithmetic and logic operations such as adding, shifting, comparing, and setting status flags.

APL (A Programming Language) A high-order language initially intended for interactive mathematical applications. It operates on arrays (e.g., vectors and matrices) and uses a very compact syntax with a special character set. Many installations use APL for commercial/data processing applications.

Application Software That software designed primarily by users in support of an application. A tool that helps the user in his work.

Application Tools Software systems that provide a desired set of features in a user-friendly manner. Examples are a word processor, automated spread sheet and personal calendar.

Applicative Programming Languages See Functional Programming.

Artificial Intelligence (AI) A field of computer science that has received considerable attention lately. There are various definitions, but a key characteristic seems to be the ability to make decisions using inference with a symbolic knowledge base.

ASCII (American Standard Code for Information Interchange) A standard set of 7-bit codes used by computers to represent printing and control characters. The code is generally padded with a leading bit to produce an 8-bit code that is stored as a byte.

Assembler The system software tool used to translate an assembly language program into processible code.

Assembly Language A programming language in which the language instructions set is very similar to the machine instruction set. Also called symbolic assembly language.

Asynchronous Transmission A technique for transmitting data in which one character is sent at a time with variable intervals of time between character transmissions. Compare with synchronous transmission.

Backup The saving of programs and data to retain a recent version in the event of the destruction of the current version.

Baseband A technology used in computer resource networking in which there is no frequency modulation of the signal; that is, the transmission frequency is the same (base) as the original frequency. Baseband transmission is well suited to computer data transfer since it requires no analog to digital conversion. It is generally used with the Time Division Multiplexing.

BASIC (Beginner's All-Purpose Symbolic Instruction Code) A high-order language used primarily for interactive programming. Very common on microcomputers. Originally designed as a tool for teaching programming, it is now used for system development as well.

Baud The unit of measure for transmission of data. It measures the number of state changes; in a binary system where each state change is a bit, it is the same as bits per second. Common values include 110, 300, 1200, 2400, 4800, and 9600.

Benchmark A program that executes a representative set of functions and whose performance can be quantified. Benchmarks are frequently used to compare performance of different systems. When used with database or multiprogrammed systems, benchmarks may not reflect operational responses.

Binary A number system to the base 2 in which all digits are either 0 or 1. The digits in the binary system are called bits for *bi*nary digi*ts*.

Bit A binary integer. The smallest unit of information in a digital computer. It takes on the values 1 and 0.

Block The unit of information normally transmitted to and from a disk or other secondary storage device. In the case of a random access device, access is to a block that contains a group of words, records or characters.

Boolean Logic A class of processing named after George Boole (1815-1864), who developed an algebra with logical operations. Common computer operations include AND an OR comparisons of bit configurations.

Bootstrap A sequence of starting instructions that, in turn, initiates a sequence of instructions to start a process. Derived from the concept of lifting oneself off the ground by pulling at one's bootstraps, except it works with computers.

Broadband A technology used in computer resource networking in which a carrier is used to carry many signals, each modulated to a unique frequency. The broadband carrier is normally coaxial cable designed originally for "Cable TV" service. This technology facilitates the intermixing of video, voice, and digital data; it is normally used with Frequency Division Multiplexing.

Bubble Memory A form of memory in which information are recorded as bubbles of magnetism. Currently of limited use, this technology has the potential for producing large, inexpensive mass storage.

Bucket A set of one or more blocks that contain one or more records. Many file access methods provide access only to the level of a bucket; a serial search of the bucket follows.

Buffer A generic term for a portion of memory used to retain data temporarily. A buffer may be limited to a single character or it may contain 512 or more characters depending on its use.

Bug An error in a computer program. Bugs are a natural byproduct of programming; they are removed by debugging. When not removed, they are called defects.

Bus A path for transferring electrical signals. In some microcomputers there is a single bus used to interface modules. The S-100 bus is a 100-line bus that has become standard for many microcomputers.

Byte A single set of 8 bits used to contain either a binary number or a single character. This is the most common unit of measurement for mass storage e.g., a 5M hard disk has 5M bytes, 5M characters, or 5 × 1,048, 576 × 8 bits.

C A programming language frequently used in the UNIX operating system (a trade mark of Bell Laboratories). UNIX is written in C. The language supports block structures, and assembly language sequences can be inserted into C programs.

Central Processing Unit (CPU) That component of a computer in which the computation or processing is performed.

Character Any printable single element such as a letter, digit, or punctuation mark.

Chip A slice of semiconductor material, usually silicon, upon which is printed an integrated circuit.

CMOS (Complementary MOS) A technology to produce memories which use very little power and are faster than MOS (Metallic Oxide Semiconductor). CMOS is not well suited to very large scale integration (VLSI).

COBOL (COmmon Business Oriented Language) A high-order language used primarily for business applications. Very common on larger computers. This is the most widely used of all mainframe languages.

Compiler The system software tool used to translate a high-order language program into processible instructions. The output of a compiler is object code that can be loaded and executed. Compare with Interpretor.

Computer That section of the computer system that contains the processor and memory. In a microcomputer system, this is generally the least expensive portion. The other components are called peripherals.

Console An interactive terminal tied to a computer and assigned specific functions, e.g., the computer operator's terminal. With many military systems, the console may include additional functions, e.g., a radar operator's console.

Control Language A system language used to provide information about the job to be run. Sometimes called Job Control Language (JCL).

Control Unit That part of the CPU that manages the step by step processing performed within the CPU. It is programmed in microcode.

Controller A device used to manage the interfacing of a peripheral device to the computer.

Core Memory An older technology for memory in which information was recorded on small magnetic cores. Although the technology is no longer used, memory still is occasionally called core when the contents are not lost with power outage.

CPS (Characters Per Second) A measure for printing speed.

CRT (Cathode Ray Tube) A technology used for video terminals and television. Sometimes used as a generic term that includes the keyboard and electronics associated with the tube.

Cursor A special display character on a video terminal that indicates where the next character will be displayed.

Cycle Time The period of time between clock pulses that synchronize the actions within the CPU. Each CPU step requires a single cycle; a single instruction may require more than one cycle. The unit of measure is the megahertz (MHz). Processing speeds for the computer are measured in millions of instructions per second (MIPS).

Daisy Wheel A device used in a letter quality printer in which each letter is on a spoke from a central hub. Daisy wheels are available in many fonts.

Data Counter A class of register in the CPU that contains the address of the data to be processed.

Data Type A form assigned to a class of data fields that defines characteristics of size, use, etc. Examples are; integer, floating point (or real), character string. The ability to define data types implies that the program will implicitly test to see that the rules associated with the data type are not violated. Languages with many such features are sometimes said to have strong data typing.

DBMS (Data Base Management System) An application tool that allows the user to define an integrated data base and then store, retrieve, and query the data base. A DBMS is generally associated with the form it uses in the definition of its data model (or schema). The three basic types are network, hierarchical (or tree), and relational. Compare with File Management System.

Debug To remove errors from a program. Errors are bugs before system release; after that they are defects. The term is said to have originated in the early days of very large computers when a machine failure was traced to the presence of insects.

Decision Support Systems (DSS) These are Management Information Systems (MIS) to which modeling tools have been added. The modeling tools range in complexity from electronic spread sheets to linear programming or statistical analysis systems. DSS is also used as a generic title for information support environments.

Defect In software, a failure on the part of a completed system to perform as specified (advertised). The use of this term reflects an attempt on the part of the software community to establish methods for achieving zero defect products.

Development The process in which an initial statement of needs is transformed into a tested, operational application.

Diagnostics A sequence of test cases designed to determine if any errors exist. Diagnostics is generally reserved for hardware faults; test case is the more common term for certifying software.

Disk A generic name for a storage device in which a thin, flat base is covered with a magnetic media upon which data are stored. The disk spins rapidly and a head reads or writes information from or onto the magnetic media. Any portion of the disk may be read, that is, directly accessed. For different kinds of disks see hard disk, floppy disk, and Winchester disk.

Disk Drive Unit The unit that contains the disk. In some cases the disk (or floppy disk) is removable, and the unit is that piece of hardware designed to accept and process the disk.

DMA (Direct Memory Access) A technique for interfacing a high speed I/O device to the computer so that data can be read from or written to memory without any CPU action. The use of DMA is sometimes called cycle stealing.

Documentation Descriptive information about the hardware and software. Includes user manuals, tutorials, reference manuals, and design information.

Dump The listing of the contents of computer memory to show its state at a point in time, e.g., when a failure occurred.

EBCDIC (Extended Binary Coded Decimal Interchange Code) A standard set of 8 bit codes used to represent characters and control characters. It is generally used with larger computers; the ASCII set is more common for microcomputer equipment.

Emulation A program or system that causes the current system to behave as some target system. The current system is said to emulate the target system. For example, a computer program that interperts and executes the instruction set of another computer emulates the second computer. Emulation may involve a processing penalty but is frequently useful in test and conversion applications.

EPROM (Erasable Programmed Read Only Memory) Functionally the equivalent of the Read Only Memory (ROM), this type of memory can be both written onto and erased for reuse of the chip.

Evolution This is a more positive name for the post release modification of a system. Such modification generally represents over half the total system cost and absorbs the efforts of some half the programming staff. It is generally recognized that most systems evolve, that the evolution destroys the structure of the system, and at some point in time it is less expensive to discard the system than to correct it. The fact that so many programmers are assigned to maintaining existing systems leads to shortages in programmers for developing new systems, which in turn results in backlogs for both new development and modification.

Execute To run a task or job.

Exponent In common use, the exponent represents the number of times a base number is used as a factor. In the floating point representation, the exponent is a power of 2 which is to be multiplied by the mantissa. The floating point exponent is also called the characteristic.

Fault Tolerance In hardware, the concept of reliability is tied to the probability that a component will fail, i.e., wear out. In software, on the other hand, bits do not wear and reliability is tied to the probability that all errors have been found. Since software is very complex, this probability is nonzero. Thus, fault tolerance refers to the concept of system design in which failures and errors are anticipated and tolerated, i.e., recovery is part of the system design.

Field An element of a record. The field is the smallest unit in a database. Examples are weight, name, and date.

Fifth Generation Computer A Japanese activity has been given this name. Its goal is to produce a new generation of computer by the 1990s that will incorporate VLSI and parallelism to support applications implemented by use of artificial intelligence paradigms. The previous generations were vacuum tube, transistor replacement of vacuum tubes, LSI, and VLSI. The first four generations of computers are based on the von Neumann model with a single processor and a serial program that sequences program steps and data to the processor. The Fifth Generation Computer is one of many alternatives to the von Neumann architecture.

File A collection of data, generally stored on some secondary storage media, that contains data organized in a predefined format. The unit stored in a file is called a record; a record is made up of fields or data elements.

File Management System This provides one or more access methods to retrieve records from files. Common access methods are sequential (can access only the first or next record), random (can access only individual records), and index sequential (can access random records or the next record after a previous access).

Fixed Point An internal representation for binary numbers in which a binary point is assumed to be to the right of the rightmost bit. Also called integers; fixed point numbers may be 1 or more bytes in length and may or may not have a sign bit. The most common use is 2 bytes with a sign bit.

Floating Point An internal representation for large fractional numbers that stores the information in a binary form of scientific notation. There is a mantissa and an exponent; usually 4 bytes in length. Double precision adds four more bytes to the mantissa; there is also triple-precision floating point.

Floppy Disk A form of disk that records the information on a plastic base housed in a rigid envelope. Standard sizes are 5¼- and 8-inch with some 3½-inch disk units now being introduced.

FORTH A stack-oriented language that supports efficient programs in a microcomputer environment. The name was chosen to imply that this was a new– or fourth–generation of computer language. Unfortunately, the early implementation limited labels to a length of 5 characters, hence the name FORTH.

FORTRAN (FORmula TRANslation System) A high-order language used primarily for scientific and engineering applications. The large investment in program libraries has made it a de facto standard for such applications. Djkstra has said that we don't know what the language of the 21st century will look like, but we do know that it will be called FORTRAN.

Fourth Generation Languages There is a class of proprietary product (or tool) which is advertised as a fourth generation language (4GL). The tools generally provide some nonprocedural query language, a report generator, and other data processing tools. The name is derived from the concept that the first three generations were machine code (1s and 0s), assembly languages, and high order languages (HOL).

Frequency Division Multiplexing (FDM) A form of multiplexing in which a carrier is used to carry many signals in parallel. Each signal is assigned a unique frequency range and a modulator demodulator (modem) is used to convert to and from the base frequency. Compare with Time Division Multiplexing.

Function Keys Special-purpose keys on a keyboard. Each has a special meaning to the hardware or software, none of which is normally found on a standard typewriter.

Functional Programming Language (Also called applicative programming language) This is a class of programming languages that uses function application as the only control structure. The languages are typically interactive, implemented as interpretive systems, with a limited concept of assignment. Examples are LISP and APL. Compare with Imperative Programming Languages.

Garbage Collection A process managed by the operating system to reclaim storage space allocated dynamically and that is no longer in use. Garbage collection is normally initiated without any action on the part of the application program.

Generators A software tool that transposes a set of statements into an executable program. Also called program generators and application generators depending upon the technique used.

Gigabyte (GB) One billion bytes, or—to be more accurate—1024M bytes.

Graphics This is the drawing of data representations using only lines and blocks of continuous tone or color. Graphics were first, as the name implies, simply line graphs. With advances in technology, color, shades of gray and lines of various formats are also used. Compare with Image Processing.

Hard Disk A disk made of rigid material as opposed to the plastic base of the floppy disk. Hard disks have more capacity than a floppy disk. Frequently, hard disks are configured in stacks, jukebox fashion.

Hardware The equipment that includes the computer and the associated peripherals that comprise the computer system. The hardware does not include the software that is the set of instructions used to make the hardware perform a desired task.

Hash For databases, a technique in which a record key is translated into a physical address for random access of the record. The transformation uses a hash function.

Hexadecimal A number system to the base 16 using the characters 0,1,2,. . .,9,A,B,C,D,E,F. The advantage of this system is that each digit corresponds to a four bit pattern. The bits in a byte can be written as two hexadecimal digits.

High-Order Languages (HOL) Programming languages that use application oriented statements to describe a function to be performed, e.g., Let X = Y + 2. Contrasted with assembly language.

I/O Port The physical and logical interconnection between the computer and its input/output (I/O) peripherals.

Image Processing This is the processing of continuous tone displays. Images may be black and white or color. Resolution is a function of the number of pixels (picture elements) used. Images may use representative colors or tones or may use color as an additional dimension of information, e.g., false color for remote sensing.

Imperative Programming Languages This is a class of programming language that is built upon executable (imperative) statements that are designed to take maximum advantage of the knowledge of where and how data are stored. The languages are typically compiled and rely on the concept of assignment. Examples are FORTRAN, COBOL, and Pascal. Compare with Functional Programming Languages.

Index For databases, an index is a key used to locate a record in a file. An index file is a file of indexes that provides links to the location of the associated records.

Index Sequential A file access method in which one can read, write, or delete a record with a given index. Once a record has been accessed, one can process the next record without prior knowledge of its index.

Ink Jet Printer A nonimpact printer that forms output by spraying ink from a small jet. High-resolution, color outputs can be achieved with this technology.

Input/Output (I/O) Those processing functions that involve input to or output from the computer, e.g., printing or writing data to be stored on disc.

Instruction Register A register in the CPU that contains the code for the instruction to be processed.

Interface Logical: The data passed between two components or modules. Physical: The equipment or standards used to define how data are to be passed between two components.

Interpreter A software tool that executes a program on a line-by-line basis without going through a preliminary computation step. The advantage of an interpretive language is that it allows access to all variables throughout the testing process; a compiled program, however, will execute more efficiently.

Inverted Index An index to a file by some variable. Also called a secondary index. The term comes from the library card catalog where the subject index is created by inverting (reordering) the title index.

JCL (Job Control Language) See Control Language.

Job One or more tasks to be executed.

K The abbreviation for that power of 2 that is closest to 1,000, i.e., 2^{10} or 1,024.

Key A value associated with a record that provides an index to locate it.

Keyboard An input device that is configured like the typical typewriter keyboard.

Kilobytes "Thousands" of bytes where thousands is the power of 2 closest to 1,000, i.e., 2^{10} or K or 1,024.

Library A collection of programs available for reuse in other applications. Also program library.

Life Cycle The software life cycle describes the process of software development. There are several life cycle models, the most popular of which is the hardware based model of: Software Requirements, Top Level Design, Detailed Design, Code and Debug, Test and Accept, Operations and Maintenance. This life cycle is generally depicted as a sequence of stages drawn waterfall fashion. The distribution of effort frequently follows a 40-20-40 rule for pre-code activities, code and debug, and test and accept. Postacceptance costs range from 50% to as high as 80% of the total life cycle cost. About two thirds of the maintenance costs are for enhancement (see Evolution.)

LISP (LISt Processing language) This language was developed around 1960 to support research in artificial intelligence and it remains a de facto standard for AI in the United States. An alternative language, PROLOG, is used for the Fifth Generation Computers.

LOGO A programming language developed primarily to teach young children computer concepts.

LSI (Large Scale Integration) Electronic component parts in which up to 100,000 electrical elements are combined in one chip.

M The abbreviation for that power of 2 that is closest to 1,000,000, i.e., 2^{20} or 1,048,576.

Magnetic Tape A media used to store digital information. Data must be read sequentially. Compare with the disk's direct access.

Magnetic Tape Unit A unit interfaced with the computer that processes magnetic tape.

Mainframe Computer A large computer generally costing $500,000 or more. Compare with Minicomputer and note the range of uncertainty.

Maintenance The modification of a software system once it becomes operational. This includes removal of defects and the introduction of new functions. See also Evolution.

Mantissa That part of a floating point number that represents the value to be multiplied by the power of 2 recorded in the exponent.

Mass Storage Secondary memory that resides on an external device. Mass storage is used to retain data and programs that are too voluminous to be stored in memory. Data and programs are copied from mass storage to memory to be processed, and from memory to mass storage in order to be saved. Mass storage is also called permanent storage; examples are disc, magnetic tape and floppy discs.

Matrix Printer A printer in which printed characters are made up of individual dots. The printing head moves across the line with pins used to produce the dots which form the letters. Through use of multiple passes, some matrix printers now provide letter quality output.

Megabytes "Millions" of bytes where millions is the power of 2 closest to 1,000,000, i.e., 2^{20} or M or 1,048,576.

Megahertz Millions of cycles per second (MHz). This is the basic unit for cycle time. Values from 1 to 12 MHz are common for microcomputers.

Memory That portion of the computer that stores instructions and data for use by the central processing unit (CPU). Sometimes also called working storage. Memory is always accessible by the CPU; contrast this to mass storage which must be read into memory to be processed.

Microcode The low-level sequence of elementary instructions processed by the CPU to produce a machine language instruction. Also called microinstruction.

Microcomputer A small computer using a microprocessor chip. The microcomputer is usually packaged with a keyboard. In personal computer systems there is generally also a floppy disk unit and a display. A microcomputer system may offer multiuser support comparable to that of a small minicomputer.

Microsecond A millionth of a second.

Milisecond A thousandth of a second.

Minicomputer A smaller computer generally costing $150,000 or less. Normally multiuser with mass storage.

MIPS (Millions of Instructions Per Second) This is a measure of the processing power of a computer. Since each instruction may require more than one machine cycle, it is a better measure of throughput than the cycle time. For parallel processors used with AI applications, MIPS stands for Millions of Inferences per Second.

MIS The term MIS (for Management Information System) became popular in the early 1970s to describe systems that used database technology to extract and organize enterprise information for management decision making. By the 1980s it was recognized that simple information retrieval was insufficient, and modeling tools were added to produce Decision Support Systems (DSS).

MODEM (MOdulator-DEModulator) This device is used to link a computer or terminal to and from a telephone line. It converts a digital signal to an audio signal and vice versa.

Monitor A display unit, generally a cathode ray tube (CRT). Integrated with a keyboard and electronics, it is a video display terminal (VDT).

MOS (Metallic Oxide Semiconductor) A technology commonly used for producing memory in large scale integration (LSI). MOS memories have the property of losing their information when power is removed.

Multiplexing The process of interleaving or transmitting two or more different sets of signals using the same bus or communication facility.

Multiprogramming The organization of a system to allow concurrent execution of more than one separate task. All multiuser systems and time-sharing systems use multiprogramming.

Multiuser System A computer system designed for use by more than one user or task at the same time. Most moderate to large interactive systems are multiuser systems.

MUMPS (Massachusetts General Hospital Utility Multiuser Programming System) A high-order language used primarily for interactive data base applications on medium to small computers. Started by the medical computing community, many nonmedical applications have been developed in MUMPS.

Nanosecond A billionth of a second.

Network The term network is usually used to describe the linking of computers and devices by means of communications. Long-haul networks link nodes (computers) between great distances. Local Area Networks (LAN) link computers in a limited geographic area, e.g., within a building complex. The term network is also used to describe the organization of data in a DBMS.

Non-Procedural Languages This is a class of language in which statements describe what is to be done without specifying how (i.e., in what sequence) the activities are to be carried out. Examples are database query languages, some Fourth Generation Languages, and some functional languages. Nonprocedural, however, is a relative term and many so called non procedural languages allow for procedural statements. Compare with Procedural Languages.

Object Code Any code produced by a compiler in a form that may be loaded into a computer ready for execution is called object code. The programming language input to the compiler is called source code.

Octal A number system based on 8 digits; 0,1,2,3,4,5,6,7. This was popular in the early days of computing when computer words were frequently represented in groups of 6 bits (which could be represented as 2 octal digits.) Hexadecimal is now the more common system for representing bit patterns.

Ones Complement A string of bits is said to be the ones complement of another string of bits if for every 1 in the first string there is a 0 in the second and vice versa. For example, 1001 and 0110 are ones complements of each other. Compare with twos complement.

Operating System That portion of the system software that acts as an interface between the programs and the hardware. It allows the equipment to perform the tasks desired by the applications. It also supports application development. Common operating systems are MVS for IBM mainframes, UNIX (a trademark of Bell Laboratories) for medium-sized computers, and CP/M and MS-DOS for single user microcomputers.

Operations The use and running of tested, correct programs, applications, and tools.

Paging The treatment of program memory as a sequence of smaller memory segments called pages. Pages within a program need not be located in sequential memory locations. In fact, the concept of virtual memory allows the user to think of the program's memory space as being much larger than the amount of physical memory available; it does this by keeping in working storage only those pages currently in use.

Parallel I/O An interfacing technique used for input/output devices in which all the bits in a byte or word are transmitted together. Parallel interfaces require at least as many lines as there are bits to be transmitted. Compare with serial I/O.

Parser A program or algorithm that breaks a sentence into its syntactic parts. For a compiler, the parser decodes statements and their expressions.

PASCAL A high order language that combines many of the more advanced features of block-structured languages. General purpose and complete, it is available on both large and personal computers. First designed for teaching applications, the basic syntax has been encorporated in a more complete language called MODULA-2.

PC Board (Printed Circuit Board) A board designed to support electronic circuits. Printed circuit implies that some conductive circuits have been applied to the board.

Peripherals That equipment that is used as an adjunct to the computer to produce the final computer system. For example, input/output equipment.

Personal Computer This term is undergoing change. It first referred to a single-user standalone microcomputer system applied to personal applications such as word processing. One may now have personal computer functionality with a terminal tied to a multiprocessor or network.

PL/1 A high order language first introduced in the late 1960s for use on the IBM third-generation computers. It combines the functionality of FORTRAN and COBOL in a block structured language similar to ALGOL.

Private Branch Exchange (PBX) A device used to switch telephone calls within a business site. Newer units now incorporate digital switching and microcomputer control. They are use to carry data as well as voice.

Privileged Mode Some instructions are normally reserved for use by the operating system program because inadvertent use can result in system failure. These are called privileged instructions and can be used only by programs in the privileged mode.

Procedural Languages This is a class of language in which the program explicitly defines the sequence of actions to be taken. Examples are FORTRAN, COBOL, and Pascal. Compare with Non-Procedural Languages.

Program A collection of instructions that defines how a task should be performed. The program must be translatable into machine instructions that will perform the desired task.

Program Counter A class of register in the CPU that contains the address of the next instruction to be processed.

Programming The process of transferring design concepts into a language that can be translated into machine instructions. The writing of computer programs.

Programming Languages A true language that translates knowledge about a task to be performed into instructions that can be processed by a computer.

PROLOG A language for PROgramming in LOGic, it is used for artificial intelligence applications. It combines a relational data base with pattern matching to implement a predicate calculus.

PROM (Programmable Read-Only Memory) Read only memory that will allow programs to be stored through the use of special equipment. The end user cannot differentiate between PROM and ROM.

Queue A data structure in which data are entered at the beginning and many be removed only from the end. It is also called a First In, First Out (FIFO) structure. Compare with a Stack.

RAM (Random Access Memory) Memory that can be both read from and written into. Selection of the word is by address, hence random access. This type of memory is used by programs loaded from mass storage.

Real-Time Clock A I/O device that provides an external source of time. It is used to compute time of day and processing intervals. It is different from the clock which produces the CPU cycle time signal.

Record A logical grouping of fields (or data elements) that are written to or read from a secondary storage media. Records are physically stored in blocks; records are logically organized as files.

Register A high speed memory location within the CPU used to store temporarily or manipulate values.

Relation This is a mathematical term that defines the membership of a set, e.g., (Mary, Jane) in the "mother of" relation or (3, 9) in the "square" relation. Databases can be organized as relations (two-dimensional arrays or tables). The advantages of relational databases are their simple structure, well-defined mathematical behavior, and normal forms.

Report Generators An application tool that facilitates the preparation of programs that print reports.

Requirements The statement of needs. Tells what a proposed application must do.

ROM (Read Only Memory) Memory that can be read from but not written to. This memory is generally used for system software. The read only property assures that it will not be accidently destroyed. It is also random access.

Routine An alternative term for program.

RPG See Report Generators; also a specific language for report generation.

Sector The physical unit of the disk recording surface that contains a block of data. The location of sectors is specified either through recording special bit patterns through a process called formatting or through the use of a physical mark on the disk. The former is called soft sectored, the latter hard sectored.

Serial I/O An interfacing technique used for input/output devices in which the bits in a byte or word are transmitted one after the other, one at a time. Serial interfaces may require only 4 lines for the data and control signals. It is an economical approach to low data rate transmissions; compare with parallel I/O.

Shifting The process of moving a string of bits either to the left or right. The shifting process may set vacant bits to 0s; in this case shifting is equivalent to multiplying or dividing by powers of 2.

Simulation A program that models part of a real-world system to test or understand aspects of its behavior. There are languages designed to support the creation of simulations. The form of a simulation is independent of the system it models. Compare with emulation.

Single-User System A computer system designed for use by only one user at a time. Most personal computers are single user systems.

Software The information used by a computer to determine what it should do. By extension, software includes the documentation about this information. Some software (system software) is supplied with the computer equipment, other software (application software) is purchased or developed to meet the needs of a user.

Source Code Any code that is written in the form of the programming language is called source code. For compiled HOLs this is input to a compiler, and the translated output is called object code.

Stack A data structure in which data may be entered into and removed from the top. It is also called Last In, First Out (LIFO) structure. Compare with a Queue.

Structured A descriptive term applied to a methodology to imply the absence of non-structuredness. Examples are: Structured Analysis, Structured Design, Structured Programming.

Structured Programming A method of programming that restricts the code to sequences plus the two basic constructs of iteration (e.g., do while) and selection (e.g., if. . .then. . .else). It usually implies the absence of go tos, indentation of the program text, and short programs — generally limited to one or two pages in length.

Subroutine An alternative term for program. Implies that it will be used by other programs.

Supercomputer This class of computer is designed for large-scale computational problems. They frequently are supported by vector processors that allow parallel computation for certain classes of problem.

Synchronous Transmission A technique for transmitting data in which a continuous string of characters is transmitted. Compare with asynchronous transmission. Synchronous transmission is very fast; it requires more complex protocols.

Systems Software That software designed primarily for use by the hardware and the developers of applications. Compare with applications software.

Task A set of functions to be performed by the execution of a sequence of computer programs.

Test The process by which the developers verify that the product (1) has no errors and (2) performs all the necessary functions correctly.

Text Processing An application tool that facilitates the input, management, and printing of textual information. Compare with word processor. Many text processors are now similar to word processors.

Time Division Multiplexing (TDM) A form of multiplexing in which a carrier is used to carry multiple signals with each signal having full use of the carrier for a very small time slot. A synchronous TDM (also called statistical multiplexing) allots time slots only for active channels whereas Synchronous TDM allots time for a channel even in the absence of data. Compare with Frequency Division Multiplexing.

Time Sharing The use of a large multiprogrammed computer system in which each user typically requires only a small portion of the total resource. Commercially, time sharing involves the sale of computer resources as a utility.

Track The portion of the disk surface that can be read without changing the position of the read/write head.

Twos Complement A string of bits is said to be the twos complement of another string if the sum of the two strings is a power of 2. The twos complement is constructed by adding 1 to the ones complement. For example, 1001 and 0111 are twos complements of each other; their sum is 10000 or 2^4. Many computers use this representation for negative numbers. Compare with ones complement.

UNIX A popular operating system; UNIX is a proprietary product and a trademark of Bell Laboratories.

User One who uses the system. For system software the user is frequently perceived to be a programmer. For application software the user should be considered to be a nonprogrammer.

User-Friendly A label applied to all software by the seller. In some cases, it is an accurate code word for a software application that is easy to use and not intimidating.

Video Terminal An output device with a nonpermanent display. Usually a cathode ray tube (CRT), but other technologies are also used. Also video display terminal (VDT).

Virtual A descriptive term used to distinguish the logical content from the physical media. For example, virtual memory provides program access to memory space that may exceed the physical memory space available.

VLSI (Very-Large-Scale Integration) Electronic component parts in which over 100,000 electrical elements are combined in one chip.

von Neumann Bottleneck John von Neumann was one of the pioneers of digital computing. He is generally recognized as the father of the stored program used with a binary digital computer. In his analysis of organisms and automata, he believed that living organisms required redundancy and parallelism, whereas machines—which were faster—should be serial. This serial path between the memory and processor is sometimes called the von Neumann bottleneck because it limits throughput to the performance of a single processor. Parallelism bypasses the bottleneck.

Winchester Disk A specific technology for a hard disk. It usually contains a nonremovable disk in a sealed unit. Because of its relatively low price to manufacture, it is the technology generally used for microcomputer hard disk systems.

Windowing A method by which an interactive output display is divided into windows each of which may be written to independently. With some of the new high-resolution devices, windows can temporarily be superimposed on existing displays in order to respond to a query.

Word Processor A fixed system designed to manage the input, modification, and printing of textual information. Compare with the application tool (set of programs) that provides general-purpose computers a text processing capability.

Words A unit of memory that can be directly read. Generally measured in bits or bytes, e.g., 16-bit words.

Working Storage Memory that is used by programs. The information in working storage is discarded at the completion of the job.

Selected Readings

Achabal, D.D., H. Moellering, J.P. Osleeb, R.W. Swann, Designing and Evaluating a Health Care Delivery System Through the Use of Interactive Computer Graphics, *Soc. Sci. & Med.*, 12:1-6, 1978.

Aikins, J.S., J.C. Kunz, E.H. Shortliffe and R.J. Fallat, PUFF: An Expert System for Interpretation of Pulmonary Function Data, *Comp. Biomed. Res.*, 16:199-208, 1983.

Allegaert, P. et al., A Computer-Assisted Radiology Reporting and Retrieval System, *Medical Informatics,* 7:267-273, 1982.

Arenson, R.L. and J.W. London, Radiology Operations Management Computer System, Hospital of the University of Pennsylvania, in *Proceedings of the American College of Radiology Sixth Conference on Computer Applications in Radiology,* March 1979.

Austin, Charles J., Planning and Selecting an Information System. Hospitals, *J.A.H.A.*, 51:95-101, 1977.

Automation of a Problem-Oriented Medical Record, NTIS Report No. PB 263578, 1977.

Ball, M.J. and S.E. Jacobs, Information Systems: The Status of Level 1, *Hospitals,* pp. 179-186, June 16, 1980.

Ball, Marion J, Kathyrn J. Hanna and James D. Browne, *Using Computers in Nursing*. Reston Pub. Co., Reston, Va., 1984.

Barnett, G.O., Computer-Stored Ambulatory Record (COSTAR), *Research Digest Series,* National Center for Health Services Research, DHEW Publication No. (HRA) 76-3145, 1976.

Barnett, G.O., R. Winickoff, J.L. Dorsey, M.M. Morgan and R.S. Lurie, Quality Assurance Through Automated Monitoring and Concurrent Feedback Using a Computer-Based Medical Information System, *Med Care,* 16:962-968, 1978.

Barnett, G.O., N.S. Justice, M.E. Somand, J.B. Adams, B.D. Waxman, P.D. Beaman, M.S. Parent, F.R. Van Deusen, and J.K. Greenlie, COSTAR—A computer-Based Medical Information System for Ambulatory Care, *Proc. IEEE,* 67:1226-1237, 1979.

Barnett, G.O., The Application of Computer-Based Medical Record Systems in Ambulatory Practice, *New Eng. J. Med.*, 310:1643-1650, 1984.

Barnoon, S., H. Wolfe, *Measuring the Effectiveness of Medical Decisions,* Springfield, Ill., Charles C. Thomas, 1972.

Barrett, J.P., P.L. Hersch and R.J. Caswell, Evaluation of the Implementation of the Technicon Medical Information System at El Camino Hospital, Part II, *Economic Trend Analysis,* Columbus, Ohio: Battelle, May 14, 1979.

Bartone, J.C., *Computers in Medicine: Current Medical Subject Analysis and Research Directory with Bibliography,* ABBE Publishers Association, Washington, D.C., 1983.
Bartone, M.R., *Computer Assisted Instruction and Education: Medical Applications and Subject Analysis with Bibliography.* Washington, D.C.: ABBE Publishers Association of Washington, D.C., 1984.
Baskin, A. and A. Levy, MEDIKAS—an Interactive Knowledge Acquisition System, *Proc. Second Symp. Comp. Appl. Med. Care,* F. Orthner, pp.344-350, 1978.
Battelle Memorial Institute, Evaluation of the Implementation of a Medical Information System in a General Community Hospital, *Evaluation Studies and Analyses,* NTIS PB-232 785, September 30, 1973.
Beckett, R., History of Coding Nomenclature in a General Hospital Medical Records Department, *Pathologist,* 21:395-397, 1977.
Ben-Bassat, M., R. Carlson, V. Puri, M. Davenport, et al., Pattern-Based Interactive Diagnosis of Multiple Disorders—the MEDAS System, *IEEE Trans. Pat. Anal. Machine Intell.,* 2:148-160, 1980.
Bergman, D.A. and R.H. Pantell, The Art and Science of Medical Decision Making, *J. Ped.,* 104:649-656, 1984.
Bernstein, L., E. Siegel and W. Ford, The Hepatitis Knowledge Base Prototype, *Proc. Second Symp. Comp. Appl. Med. Care,* 366-367, 1978.
Bernstein, L.M., E.R. Siegel, and C.M. Goldstein, The Hepatitis Knowledge Base—A Prototype Information Transfer System, *Ann Internal Med,* 93: (Part 2) 169-181, 1980.
Bill, J., R. Anderson, J. O'Fallon, A. Silvers, Development of a Computerized Cancer Data Management System at the Mayo Clinic, *Int. J. Bio-Medical Computing,* 9:477-492, 1978.
Bleich, H.L., Computer Evaluation of Acid-Base Disorders, *J. of Clin. Investigation,* 48:1689-1695, 1969.
Bleich, H.L., Computer-Based Consultation, *Am. J. Med,* 53:285-291, 1972.
Bleich, H.L., The Computer as Consultant, *New Eng. J. Med.* 223:308-312, 1973.
Bloch, D.M., Computer-Generated Management Tools for the Clinical Pathology Lab II. Computer-Generated Graphic Work Flow, *J. Med. Sys,* 6:305-310, 1982.
Blois, M.S., *Information and Medicine: The Nature of Medical Descriptions.* University of California Press, Berkeley, 1984.
Blum, B.I., C.J. Johns, E.E. McColligan, C.R. Smith, D.M. Steinwachs, Low Cost Ambulatory Medical Information Systems, *J. Clin. Eng.* 4,4:372-377, 1979.
Blum, B.I. and R.E. Lenhard, Jr., An Oncology Clinical Information System, *Computer Magazine,* pp.42-50, November 1979.
Blum, B.I., R.E. Lenhard, Jr., and E.E. McColligan, Protocol Directed Patient Care Using A Computer, *Proc. Fourth Symp. Comp. Appl. Med. Care,* pp.753-761, 1980.
Blum, B.I. (ed), *Information Systems for Patient Care,* Springer-Verlag, 1984.
Blum, B.I., A Framework for Medical Information Science, Editor's Introduction, *Medical Informatics* 9:167-172, 1984.
Blum, B.I., Artificial Intelligence and Medical Informatics, *Medical Informatics* (10,4), 1985.
Blum, R.L., Studying Hypotheses on a Time-Oriented Clinical Database, An Overview of the RX Project, *Proc. Sixth Symp. Comp. Appl. Med. Care,* pp.712-715, 1982.
Blum, R.L., Discovery, Confirmation, and Incorporation of Causal Relationships from a Large Time-Oriented Clinical Database: The RX Project, *Comp. Biomed. Res.,* 15:164-187, 1982.
Bouchard, V.E., J.E. Bell, H.R. Freedy, and M.G. Duffy, A Computerized System for

Screening Drug Interactions and Interferences, *Am. J. Hosp. Pharm.*, 29:564-569, 1972.

Braustein, M.L., S.H. Schuman, H.B. Curry, An On-Line Clinical Information System in Family Practice, *J. of Fam. Pract.*, 5:617-625, 1977.

Braustein, M.L., J.D. James, The emerging role of the computer in community pharmacy, *J. Fam. Pract.*, 7:1231-1232, 1979.

Bronzino, J.D., *Technology for Patient Care*, C.V. Mosby St. Louis, 1977.

Bronzino, J.D., *Computer Applications for Patient Care*, Addison-Wesley, Reading, MA, 1982.

Buchanan, B.G. and E.H. Shortliffe, *Rule Based Expert Systems, The MYCIN Experiments of the Stanford Heuristic Programming Project*, Addison-Wesley, Reading, MA, 1984.

Bulpit, C.J., L.J. Beilin, E.C. Coles, C.T. Dollery, B.F. Johnson, Randomised Controlled Trial of Computer-Held Medical Records in Hypertensive Patients, *Br. Med. J.*, 1:677-679, 1976.

Caceres, C.A. and A.L. Weiher, Information Science Applications in Medicine, *Annual Review of Information Science and Technology*, V.6, 1971.

Caceres, C.A., Present Status of Computer Interpretation of the Electrocardiogram: A 20 Year Overview, *Am. J. of Cardiology*, 41:121-125, 1978.

Cannon, S.R. and R.M. Gardner, Experience with a Computerized Interactive Protocol System Using HELP, *Comp. Biomed. Res.*, 13:399-409, 1980.

Card, W.I., M. Nicholson, G.P. Crean, et al., A Comparison of Doctor and Computer Interrogation of Patients, *Int. J. Biomed. Comp.*, 5:175-187, 1974.

Carr, A.C., and A. Ghosh, Accuracy of Behavioural Assessment by Computer, *Brit. J. Psychiat.*, p.141, 1982.

Clancey, W., E. Shortliffe and B. Buchanan, Intelligent Computer-Aided Instruction for Medical Diagnosis, *Proc. Third Symp. Comp. Appl. Med. Care*, pp.117-122, 1979.

Clancey, W. and E. Shortliffe, *Readings in Medical Artificial Intelligence—The First Decade*, Reading MA, Addison-Wesley, Reading, MA, 1984.

Clayton, P.D., D.B. Ostler, J.L. Gennaro, S.S. Beatty and P.R. Frederick, A Radiology Reporting System Based on Most Likely Diagnoses, *Comp. Biomed Res.*, 13:258-270, 1980.

Coffey, R.M., How a Medical Information System Affects Hospital Costs: The El Camino Hospital Experience, *Research Summary Series*, National Center for Health Services Research, DHEW Publication No. (PHS) 80-3265, March 1980.

Collen, M.F., (ed) *Hospital Computer Systems*, John Wiley & Sons, NY, 1974.

Collen, M.F., (ed.), *Multiphasic Health Services*, John Wiley & Sons, N.Y., 1978.

Collen, M.F., S.R. Garfield, R.H. Richart, et al., Cost Analyses of Alternative Health Examination Modes, *Arch. Intern. Med*, 137:73-79, 1977.

Cook, M. and W. McDowell, Changing to an automated information system, *J. Nurs*, 75:46-51, 1975.

COSTAR (*CO*mputer-*ST*ored *A*mbulatory *R*ecord), Laboratory of Computer Science, Massachusetts General Hospital, Harvard Community Health Plan, National Center for Health Services Research, Nat. Tech. Inform. Service (PB-248 314), U.S. Dep. of Commerce, 1975.

COSTAR (*CO*mputer-*ST*ored *A*mbulatory *R*ecord), Functional Specifications (Version 5.5), Laboratory of Computer Science (Massachusetts General Hospital), 1978.

Cote, R.A., Systematized Nomenclature of Medicine, 1st ed. Skokie, Ill., College of American Pathologists, 1977.

Covvey, H.D., N.H. McAlister, E.D. Wigle, Computer-Assisted Medicine: the Limitations of Technology, *CMA Journal,* 118:1315-1319, 1978.

Covvey, H.D. and N.H. McAilster *Computers in the Practice of Medicine,* 2 volumes (Addison-Wesley, Reading, MA, 1980).

Crull, J.E., et al., Demonstration and Evaluation of a Total Hospital Information System, NTIS Publication No. 262106, 1975.

Davis, R., B. Buchanan and E. Shortliffe, Production Rules as a Representation for a Knowledge-Based Consultation Program, *Artificial Intelligence,* 8:15-45, 1977.

deDombal, F.T., D.J. Leaper, J.R. Staniland, et al., Computer-Aided Diagnosis of Acute Abdominal Pain, *Brit. Med. J.,* 2:9-13, 1972.

deDombal, F.T., D.J. Leaper, J.C. Horrocks et al., Human and Computer-Aided Diagnosis of Abdominal Pain: Further Report with Emphasis on Performance of Clinicians, *Brit. Med. J.,* 1:376-380, 1974.

deDombal, F.T. and F. Gremy (eds), *Decision Making and Medical Care: Can Information Science Help?* Amsterdam, North-Holland, 1976.

Derewicz, H.J. and D.D. Zellers, The Computer-Based Unit Dose System in the Johns Hopkins Hospital, *Amer. J. Hosp. Pharm.,* 30:206-212, 1973.

Drazen, E.L., R. Feeley, J. Metzger and H. Wolfe, Methods for Evaluating Cost of Automated Hospital Information Systems, Report by Arthur D. Little, Inc. to National Center for Health Services Research NTIS PB-80-178-593, March 1980.

Drazen, E. and J. Metzger, Methods for Evaluating Costs of Automated Hospital Information Systems, *Research Summary Series,* National Center for Health Services Research, DHHS Publication No. (PHS) 81-3283, July 1981.

Elstein, A., L. Shulman and S. Sprafka, *Medical Problem Solving,* Harvard Univ. Press, 1978.

Emlet, H.E., Jr., et al., Measures and Indicators for Evaluation of Innovations to the Health Care System, Health Systems Division Note HSDN 77-2, AD B019833, 1977.

Epstein, M. and E. Kaplan, Criteria for Clinical Decision Making, *Computational Linguistics in Medicine,* Schneider/Sagvall Hein (eds), Amsterdam, North-Holland, pp.35-44, 1977.

Esterhay, R.J., Jr. and E.S. Walton, Cancer Treatment Research Protocols and PROMIS, *Proc. Fourth Symp. Comp. Appl.Med. Care,* 762-770, November 1980.

Estrin, T. and R.C. Uzagalis, Information Systems for Patient Care, *Computer,* 12:4-7, 1979.

Fagan, L., J. Kunz, E. Feigenbaum and J. Osborn, A Symbolic Processing Approach to Measurement Interpretation in the Intensive Care Unit, *Proc. Third Symp. Comp. Appl. Med. Care,* pp.30-33, 1979.

Farlee, C., The Computer as a Focus of Organizational Change in the Hospital, *J. of Nursing Adm,* pp.20-26, February 1978.

Faught, E., S. Trader and G. Hanna, Cerebral Complications of Angiography for Transient Ischemia and Stroke-Prediction of Risk, *Neurology,* 29:4-15, 1979.

Feinstein, A.R., An Analysis of Diagnostic Reasoning. I. The Domains and Disorders of Clinical Macrobiology, *Yale J. of Biomed.,* 46:212-232, 1973.

Feinstein, A.R., An Analysis of Diagnostic Reasoning. II. The Strategy of Intermediate Decisions, *Yale J. of Bio. and Med.,* 46:264-283, 1973.

Feinstein, A.R., An Analysis of Diagnostic Reasoning. III. The Construction of Clinical Algorithms, *Yale J. of Bio. and Med.,* 47:5-32, 1974.

Feinstein, A., Clinical Biostatistics (XXXIX. The Haze of Bayes, the Aerial Palaces of

Decision Analysis, and the Computerized Ouija Board), *Clin. Pharm. and Therapy,* 21:482-496, 1977.

Fiddleman, R.H., Survey of COSTAR Installations and Vendors, MITRE Technical Report MTR-81W122, The MITRE Corporation, June 1981.

Flagle, C.C., Operations Research with Hospital Computer Systems, in M.F. Collen (ed), *Hospital Computer Systems,* New York: Wiley, 1974.

Fletcher, R.H., et al., Auditing Problem-Oriented Records: A Controlled Comparison of Speed, Accuracy, and Identification of Errors in Medical Care, *New Eng. J. Med.,* 290:829, 1974.

Fox, J., Medical Computing and the User, *Int. J. Man-Mach. Stud.,* 9:669-686, 1977.

Fox. J., D. Barber and K. Bardhan, Alternative to Bayes? A Quantitative Comparison with Rule-Based Diagnostic Inference, *Meth. Inform. Med.,* 19:210-215, 1980.

Friedman, R. and D. Gustafson, Computers in Clinical Medicine, a Critical Review, *Comput. Biomed. Res.,* 10:199-204, 1977.

Friedman, R., J. Horowitz, et al., Issues in Automation of Cancer Treatment Protocols, *Proc. Fourth Symp. Comp. Appl. Med. Care,* pp.200-205, 1980.

Friedman, R.B., S.M. Entine, G.M. Murray, D. Holladay, and C. Steinhart, An Integrated Protocol Management System, *Proc. Third Symp. Comp. Appl. Med. Care,* pp.81-84, 1979.

Freiherr, G., *The Seeds of Artificial Intelligence,* SUMEX-AIM, DHHD, NIN Pub 80-2079, Dec. 1979.

Fries, B.E., C.E. Gutkin, A.S. Ginsberg, Emergency Room Utilization: Data Reconstruction Using a Deterministic Simulation Model, *Comput. Biomed. Res.,* 18:153-163, 1977.

Fries, J.F., Time-Oriented Patient Records and a Computer Databank, *JAMA,* 222:1536-1542, 1972.

Fries, J.F., Alternatives in Medical Record Formats, *Medical Care,* 12:871-881, 1974.

Frost, D.A., F.G. Yanowitz and T.A. Pryor, Evaluation of a Computerized Arrhythmia Alarm System, *Am. J. Card.,* 39:583-587, 1977.

Fryback, D., Bayes Theorem and Conditional Non-independence of Data in Medical Diagnosis, *Comput. Biomed. Res.,* 11:423-434, 1978.

Gall, J.E., et al., Demonstration and Evaluation of a Total Hospital Information System, National Center for Health Services Research, NTIS PB 262 106, 1975.

Gall, J.E., Jr. Computerized Hospital Information Systems Cost Effectiveness—A Case Study, J. van Egmond, P.F. deVries Robbe and A.H. Levy (eds), *Information Systems for Patient Care: Review, Analysis and Evaluation,* Amsterdam, North-Holland, 1976.

Gantner, G.E., History of Coding, *Pathologist,* 21:398-401, 1977.

Gardner, R.M., T.P. Clemmer, Computerized Protocols Applied to Acute Care, *Emergency Medical Services,* 7:90-93, November 1978.

Gardner, R.M., R.O. Crapo and A.H. Morris, Computerized Decision-Making in the Pulmonary Function Laboratory, *Respiratory Care,* 27:799-808, 1982.

Garrett, L.E., W.W. Stead, W.E. Hammond. Effect of Automated Records on Provider Efficiency. *Clin Res.* 30:299, 1982.

Garrett, L.E., *Hosptial Computer Systems,* Vol. 1 Accounting System, Vol. 2 Medical Systems, Petrueolli, 1976.

General Accounting Office, Computerized Hospital Medical Information Systems Need Further Evaluation to Ensure Benefits from Huge Investments, AFMD-81-3, November 1980.

Giebink, G.A. and L.L. Hurst, *Computer Projects in Health Care,* Health Administration Press, Ann Arbor, 1975.

Gill, P.W., D.J. Leaper, P.J. Guillou, et al., Observer Variation in Clinical Diagnosis: A Computer-Aided Assessment of its Magnitude and Importance, *Meth. Inform. Med.,* 12:108-113, 1973.

Given, C.W., L. Simoni, R.S. Gatlin and R.J. Sprafka, The Use of Computer Generated Patient Profiles to Evaluate Resident Performance in Patient Care, *The J. of Fam. Prac.,* 5:831-840, 1977.

Glantz, S.A., Computers in Clinical Medicine: A Critique, *Computer,* pp.68-77, 1978.

Gorry, G., and G. Barnett, Experience With a Model of Sequential Diagnosis, *Comput. Biomed. Res.,* 1:490-507, 1968.

Gorry, G., J. Kassirer, A. Essig and W. Schwartz, Decision Analysis as the Basis for Computer-Aided Management of Acute Renal Failure, *Am. J. Med.,* 55:473-484, 1973.

Gorry, G., H. Silverman and S. Pauker, Capturing Clinical Expertise—A Computer Program that Considers Clinical Responses to Digitalis, *Am. J. Med.,* 64:452-460, 1978.

Greenes, R. A Goal Directed Model for Investigation of Thresholds for Medical Action, *Proc. Third Symp. Comp. Appl. Med. Care,* pp.47-51, 1979.

Greenes, R.A., G.O. Barnett, S.W. Klein, et al., Recording, Retrieval, and Review of Medical Data by Physician-Computer Interaction, *New Eng. J. Med.,* 282:307-315, 1970.

Greenlaw, C.W. and D.D. Zellers, Computerized Drug-Drug Interaction Screening System, *Am. J. Hosp. Pharm.,* 35:567-570, May 1978.

Greist, J.H., L.J. Van Cura, N.P. Kneppreth, A Computer Interview for Emergency Room Patients, *Comput. Biomed. Res.,* 6:257-265, 1973.

Greist, J.H., M.H. Klein, L.J. Van Cura, and J. Faulkner, Computer Applications in Psychiatry at the University of Wisconsin: Current Status, *Curr. Con. Psychiatry,* 3:13-16, 1977.

Greist, J.H., M.H. Klein, H.P. Erdman and J.W. Jefferson, Clinical Computer Applications in Mental Health, *J. Med. Sys.,* 7,2:175-185, 1983.

Griesser, G. (ed), *Realization of Data Protection in Health Information Systems,* Amsterdam, North Holland, 1977.

Grimm, R.H., Shimoni, W.R. Harlan, and E.H. Estes, Evaluation of patient-care protocol use by various providers, *New Eng. J. Med.,* 292:507-511, 1975.

Grousse, W.L., Computer System for Unit Dose Drug Distribution, *Am. J. Hosp. Pharm.* 35:711-714, 1978.

Gustafson, D., J. Griest, F. Stauss, H. Erdman and T. Laughren, A Probabilistic System for Identifying Suicide Attemptors, *Comput. Biomed. Res.,* 10:83-89, 1977.

Haessler, H.A., E. Holland and L.E. Erroll, Evolution of an Automated Database History, *Archives of Int. Med.,* 134:586-591, 1974.

Halse, R.K., S.J. Clark, J.C. Jackson, H.R. Warner and R.M. Gardner, Computerized Medication Monitoring System, *Am. J. Hosp. Pharm.,* 13:1061-1064, 1976.

Haring, O.M., Improving Patient Care by Automated Record Summaries: Final Report, National Center for Health Services Research, pp.77-141, May 1976.

Harrell, F.E., R.M. Califf, D.B. Pryor, K.L. Lee, R.A. Rosati, Evaluating the Yield of Medical Tests, *JAMA* 247:2543-2546, 1982.

Harrell, F.E., Jr., K.L. Lee, R.M. Califf, D.B. Pryor, R.A. Rosati, Regression Modeling Strategies for Improved Prognostic Prediction. *Stat Med.,* 3:143-152, 1984.

Heard, M.R. and J.C. Thomas, A Hospital Information System, Its Impact on Costs,

Personnel and Patients in One Department, *Cost Containment, Caps and Consumerism with the Health Care Delivery System,* vol. 2, Chicago: Center for Hospital Management Engineering of the American Hospital Association, 1978.

Hedlund, J.L., B.W. Vieweg, D.W. Cho, et al., Mental Health Information Systems: A State-of-the-art Report, Health Services Research Center/Health Care Technology Center, University of Missouri, Columbia, 1979.

Henley, R., G. Wiederhold, J. Dervin, M. Jenkin, I. Kuhn, E. Mesel, D. Ramsey-Klee and J. Rodnick, An Analysis of Automated Ambulatory Medical Record Systems, Technical Report #13, Office of Medical Information Systems, University of California, San Francisco Medical Center, NTIS #PB 254 234, June 1975.

Hoffer, E.P., K.D. Marble, P.M. Yurchakard and G.O. Barnett, A Computer-Based Information System for Managing Patients in Long-Term Oral Anticoagulants, *Comput. Biomed. Res.,* 8:573-579, 1975.

Horowitz, G.L. and H.L. Bleich, PAPERCHASE: A computer program to search the medical literature, *New Eng. J. Med.,* 305:924-930, 1981

Horowitz, J.H., H. Thompson, R.H. Friedman, T. Concannon, J.G. Krikorian, and P.M. Gertman, Computer-Assisted Patient Care Management in Medical Oncology, *Proc. Fourth Symp. Comp. Appl. Med. Care,* pp.771-787, 1980.

Horrocks, J.C., A.P. McCann, J.R. Staniland et al., Computer-aided Diagnosis: Description of an Adaptable System, and Operational Experience with 2,034 cases, *Brit. Med. J.,* 2:5-9, 1972.

Horrocks, J.C. and F.T. deDombal, Computer-Aided Diagnosis of Dyspepsia, *Amer. J. Diges. Dis.,* 20:397-406, 1975.

Howard, R.A. (ed), Special Issue on Decision Analysis, *IEEE Trans. Syst. Sci. Cybern.,* vol. SSC-4, September 1968.

Jacinto, M.S., K. Kleinmann and J. Margolin, Pharmacist-Monitored, Computerized Drug Usage Review, *Am. J. Hosp. Phar.,* 31:508-512, 1974.

Jacobson B. and J.G. Webster, *Medical and Clinical Engineering,* Prentice Hall, Englewood Cliffs, NJ, 1977.

Johns, C.J., D.W. Simborg, B.I. Blum and B.H. Starfield, A. Minirecord: An Aid to Continuity of Care, *Johns Hopkins Med. J.,* 140:277-284, 1977.

Johns, R.J. and B.I. Blum, The Use of Clinical Information Systems to Control Cost as Well as to Improve Care, *Trans. of Am. Clin. and Climatological Assoc.,* 90:140-152, 1978.

Johnson, D.C. and G.O. Barnett, MEDINFO—A Medical Information System, *Comp. Prog. Biomed.,* 7:191-201, 1977.

Johnson, D., S.J. Ranzenberger, R.D. Herbert, R.M. Gardner and T.P. Clemmer, Computerized Alarm System for Acutely Ill Patients, *J. Nurse Admin.,* 10:26-35, 1980.

Johnson, J.H., T.A. Williams, R.A. Giannette, D.E. Klingler, and S.R. Nakashima, Organizational Preparedness for Change: Staff Acceptance of an On-Line Computer-Assisted Assessment System, *Behav. Res. Methods Instrum.,* 10:186-190, 1978.

Jonas, S. (ed), *Health Care Delivery in the U.S.,* Springer-Verlag, NY, 1977.

Jysdstrup, R.A. and M.J. Gross, Cost of Information Handling in Hospitals, *Health Services Research,* pp. 235-271, Winter 1966.

Karpinski, R.H.S. and H.L. Bleich, MISAR: A Miniature Information Storage and Retrieval System, *Comput. Biomed. Res.,* 4:655-660, 1971.

Kassirer, J. and G. Gorry, Clinical Problem Solving—A Behavioral Analysis, *Ann. Int. Med.,* 89:245-255, 1978.

Kastner, J.K., S.M. Weiss, C.A. Kulikowski and C.R. Dawson, Therapy Selection in an Expert Medical Consultation System for Ocular Herpes Simplex, *Comp. Bio. Med.*, 14:285-302, 1984.

Kerlin, B. and W. Rappaport, Computer-Based Health Information Systems for Rural Areas: An Analysis of Demonstration Potential, Metrek Division of the MITRE Corporation, MITRE Tech. Rep. MTR-7804, July 1978.

Kingsland, L.C., III, G.C. Sharp, D.R. Kay, S.M. Weiss, G.C. Roeseler, and D.A.B. Lindberg, An Expert Consultant System in Rheumatology: AI/RHEUM, *Proc. Sixth Symp. Comp. Appl. Med. Care*, pp.748-752, 1982.

Kjerulff, K.H., M.A. Counte, Jeffrey C. Salloway, B.C. Campbell and D.E. Noskin, Medical Information System Training: An Analysis of the Reactions of Hospital Employees, *Comput. Biomed. Res.*, 17:303-310, 1984.

Klarman, H.E., Application of Cost-Benefit Analysis to Health Systems Technology, *J. Occupational Med.*, 15, No. 3 pp.172-186, 1974.

Kleinmuntz, B., Diagnostic Problem Solving by Computer: a Historical Review and the Current State of the Science, *Comp. Bio Med.*, 14:255-270, 1984.

Klobernick, S.D., and G.H. Mandell, Implementing a Laboratory Computer System A Case History, *A.J.C.P.*, 61:122-134, 1973.

Komaroff, A.L., W.L. Black, M. Flatley, et al., Protocols for Physician Assistants: Management of Diabetes and Hypertension, *New Eng. J. Med.*, 290:307-312, 1974.

Komaroff, A.L., The Variability and Inaccuracy of Medical Data, *Proc. IEEE*, 67:1196-1207, 1979.

Kuhn, I.M., Looking at Outpatient Medical Record Systems, *Hospitals, J.A.H.A.*, pp.145-152, October 16, 1977.

Kulikowski, C., Artificial Intelligence Approaches to Medical Consultation, *Proc. 4th Illinois Conf. Med. Info.*, 1979.

Kulikowski, C., Artificial Intelligence Methods and Systems for Medical Consultation, *IEEE Trans. on Pattern Anal. and Machine Intel.*, 2:464-476, 1980.

Langill, G. and E. Finch, A Computer Assisted Nursing Adult Program, *Nursing*, 3:36-37, March 1978.

Langlotz, C.P. and E.H. Shortlife, Adapting a Consultation System to Critique User Plans, *In. J. Man-Machine Studies* 19:479-496, 1983.

Laska, E.M., C. Siegel and R. Bank, Management Information Systems in Mental Health, in J.B. Sidowski, J.H. Johnson and T.A. Williams (eds) *Tech. in Mental Health Care Delivery Systems*, N.J.: Ablex Publishing Corporation, pp.27-42, 1980.

Leaper, D., J. Horrocks, J. Staniland and F. deDombal, Computer-Assisted Diagnosis of Abdominal Pain Using Estimates Provided by Clinicians, *Brit. Med. J.*, 4:350-354, 1972.

Leaverton, P.E., and Louis Masse (ed). *Health Information Systems*. New York: Praeger, 1984.

Ledley, R.S. and L.B. Lusted, Reasoning Foundation of Medical Diagnosis: Symbolic Logic, Probability and Value Theory Aid Our Understanding of How Physicians Reason, *Science 130*, 9:9-12, 1959.

Lenhard, R.E., B.I. Blum, J.M. Sunderland, H.G. Braine and R. Saral, The Johns Hopkins Oncology Clinical Information System, *J. Med. Sys.*, 7:147-174, 1983.

Lenhard, R.E. and B.I. Blum, Practical Applications of OCIS, A Clinical Information System for Oncology, *Comp. Biolog. and Med.*, 14:15-23, 1984.

Leveille, A.S. et al., Bayes Theorem in Opthalmologic Computer Diagnosis, *Journal of Pediatric Ophthalmology and Strabismus*, 19:94-96, 1981.

Levenson, D. (ed), *Computer Applications in Clinical Practice: An Overview*, Macmillan, 1985.
Levy, A.H., Is Informatics a Basic Medical Science?, *MEDINFO 77*, pp.979-981, 1977.
Levy, A.H. and A.B. Baskin, Clinical Computing—1977: A Selective Review and Perspective, *J. Med. Sys.*, 1:361-374, 1978.
Lincoln, T.L., Computers in the Clinical Laboratory: What We have Learned, *Med. Instr.* 12:233-236, 1978.
Lincoln, T.L. and R.A. Korpman, Computers, Health Care, and Medical Information Science, *Science*, 210:257-263, 1980.
Lindberg, D.A.B., Diffusion of Medical Information Systems Technology in the United States, *J. Med. Sys.*, 6:219-228, 1982.
Lindberg, D.A.B., *The Growth of Medical Information Systems in the United States*, Lexington Books, 1975.
Lindberg, D.A.B., M.F. Collen and E.E. Van Brunt (eds), *Computer Applications in Medical Care*, Masson Publishing, 1982.
Lucas, R.W., A Study of Patients' Attitudes to Computer Interrogation, *Int. J. Man-Mach. Stud.*, 9:69-86.
Luedtke, P. and R. Luedtke, *Computers for Medical Offices*, Harcourt Brace Jovanovish, 1984.
Martin, J.B., Towards Effective Computer-Aided Medical Care Evaluation Studies, *Inquiry* XV:129-141, June 1978.
McColligan, E.E., B.I. Blum, R.E. Lenhard, M.B. Johnson, The Human Element in Computer-Generated Patient Management Plans, *J. Med. Sys.*, 6:265-276, 1982.
McColligan, E.E., and B.I. Blum, Evaluating an Automated Core Medical Record System for Ambulatory Care, *Proc. AAMSI*, 1982.
McColligan, E.E. Core Record System, in B.I. Blum (ed) *Information Systems for Patient Care*, Springer-Verlag, NY, 1984.
McDonald, C.J., Use of a Computer to Detect and Respond to Clinical Events: Its Effect on Clinician Behavior, *Annals of Interal Med.*, 84:162-167, 1976.
McDonald, C.J., Protocol-Based Computer Reminders, the Quality of Care and the Non-Perfectability of Man, *New Eng. J. of Med.*, 295, 24:1351-1355, 1976.
McDonald, C.J., G.A. Wilson and G.P. McCabe, Physician Response to Computer Reminders, *JAMA*, 244:1579-1580, 1980.
McDonald, C.J., L. Blevins, T. Glazener, J. Haas, L. Lemon and J. Meeks-Johnson, Data Base Managment, Feedback Control, and the Regenstrief Medical Record, *J. Med. Sys.*, 7:111-126, 1983.
McDonald, C.J., *Action-Oriented Decisions in Ambulatory Medicine*, Year Book Medical Publishers, Chicago, 1981.
McDonald, C.J., S.L. Hui, D.M. Smith, W.M. Tierney, S.J. Cohen, M. Weinberger, G.P. McCabe, Reminders to Physicians from an Introspective Computer Medical Record. A Two-Year Randomized Trial. *Ann Intern Med.*, 100:130-8, 1984.
McNeil, B., E. Keeler and S. Adelstein, Primer on Certain Elements of Medical Decision Making, *New Eng. J. Med.*, 293:211-215, 1975.
McNeil, B.J. and S.J. Adelstein, Determining the Value of Diagnostic and Screening Tests, *J. Nucl. Med.*, 17:439-448, 1977.
Menn, S.J., G.O. Barnett, D. Schmechel, et al., A Computer Program to Assist in the Care of Acute Respiratory Failure, *J. Amer. Med. Assoc.*, 223:308-312, 1973.
Mesel, E., D.D. Wirtschafter, J.T. Carpenter, et al., Clinical Algorithms for Cancer

Chemotherapy—systems for community-based Consultant-Extenders and Oncology Centers, *Meth. Inform. Med.*, 15:168-173, 1976.

Mesel, E. and D.D. Wirstshafter, Automating Ambulatory Medical Records: A Claims-Based Medical Profile, *Comput. Biomed. Res.*, 9:89-91, 1976.

Mezzich, J.E., J.T. Dow and G.A. Coffman, Developing an Efficient Clinical Information System for a Comprehensive Psychiatric Institute: I. Principles, Design, and Organization, *Behavior Res. Meth. & Instrumentation,* 13:459-463, 1981.

Miller, R.A., H.E. Pople and J.D. Myers, INTERNIST-I, an Experimental Computer-Based Diagnostic Consultant for General Internal Medicine, *New Eng. J. of Med.*, 307:468-476, 1982.

Miller, P.L., Critiquing Anesthetic Management: The ATTENDING Computer System, *Anesthesiology,* 58:362-369, 1983.

Miller, P.L., ATTENDING: Critiquing a Physician's Management Plan. *IEEE Trans. PAMI* PAMI-5:449-461, 1983.

Miller, P.L. and H.R. Black, Medical Plan-Analysis by Computer: Critiquing the Pharamacologic Management of Essential Hypertension. *Computers and Biomedical Research,* 17:38-54, 1984.

Mitchell, M.M., Automated Anesthesia Data Management and Record Keeping, *Medical Instrumentation,* 16:279-282, 1982.

Mittal, S., B. Chandrasekaran and J. Smith, Overview of MDX—A System for Medical Diagnosis, *Proc. Third Symp. Comp. Appl. Med. Care,* pp.34-46, 1979.

Monson, R.A. and C.A. Bond, The Accuracy of the Medical Record as an Index of Outpatient Drug Therapy, *JAMA* 240, 10:2182-2184, 1978.

Morgan, M.M., D.R. Studney, G.O. Barnett, et al., Automated Quality Assurance in Prenatal Care, *Qual. Rev. Bul.*, 4:33-36, 1978.

Murphy, E., *The Logic of Medicine,* Johns Hopkins Univ. Press, 1976.

Myers, J. and H. Pople, INTERNIST: a Consultative Diagnostic Program in Internal Medicine, *Proc. First Symp. Comp. Appl. Med. Care,* 1977.

Myers, J.D., H.E. Pople and R.A. Miller, CADUCEUS: A Computerized Diagnostic Consultation System in Internal Medicine, *Proc. Sixth Ann. Symp. Comp. Appl. Med. Care,* pp.44-47, 1982.

Nau, D., Expert Computer Systems, *Computer,* IEEE, pp.63-85, February 1983.

Norusis, M. and J. Jacquez, Diagnositc Models Based on Attribute Clusters—A Proposal and Comparisons, *Comput. Biomed. Res.*, 8:173-188, 1975.

Norwood, D.D., R.E. Hawkins and J.E. Crull, Jr., Information System Benefits Hospital, Improves Patient Care, *Hospitals,* Vol. 50, September 16, 1976.

Policy Implications of Medical Information Systems, Office of Technology Assessment, U.S. Congress, Government Printing Office, Stock No. 052-003-00496-8, Washington, D.C., 1977.

Oberst, B.B. and R.A. Reid (eds), *Computer Applications to Private Office Practice,* Springer-Verlag, NY, 1984.

Okada, M., N. Maruyama, T. Kanda, K. Shirakawa and T. Katagiri, Medical Data Base Systems with an Ability of Automated Diagnosis, *Comput. Pgm. Biomed.*, 7:163-170, 1977.

Okada, M. and M. Okada, The Pursuit of a Total Data Processing System Free of Language and Programming, *Comput. Biomed. Res.*, 17:193-207, 1984.

O'Kane, K.C. and M.K. Vaneier, A Review of Medical Information Processing Systems, *Journal of Clinical Computing,* 4:339-356, 1975.

Palley, N.A. and G.F. Groner, A Survey of Clinical Investigations and Their Information Processing Activities, Rand Corp., R-1539-NIH, July 1974.

Pass, T.M., H. Sherman and A.L. Komaroff, Clinical Algorithms and Decision Analysis, *Fourth Illinois Con. Am. Med. Info. Sys.*, 1978, pp.1-18.

Patrick, E.A., F.P. Stelmack and L.Y.L. Shen, Review of Pattern Recognition in Medical Diagnosis and Consulting Relative to a New System Model, *IEEE Trans. Sys. Man. and Cyb.*, Vol. 4, 1974.

Patrick, E.A., Pattern Recognition in Medicine, *Syst. Man. Cybern. Rev.*, Vol. 6, 1977.

Pauker, S.G. and J.P. Kassirer, Therapeutic Decision Making: A Cost-Benefit Analysis, *New Eng. J. Med.*, 293:229-234, 1975.

Pauker, S.G., A. Gorry, J.P. Kassirer and W.B. Schwartz, Towards the Simulation of Clinical Cognition: Taking a Present Illness by Computer, *Amer. J. Med.*, 60:981-996, 1976.

Pauker, S.G., The Practical Use of Decision Analysis in Patient Care, *Proc. First Symp. Comp. Appl. Med. Care*, 1977.

Pople, H., The Formation of Composite Hypotheses in Diagnositc Problem Solving: An Exercise in Synthetic Reasoning, *Proc. 5th Joint Conf. Artific. Intell.*, Cambridge, MA, 1030-1037, 1977.

Pople, H., INTERNIST—Methods for Structuring the Medical Problem List, *Proc. 6th Illinois Conf. Med. Inf. Sys.*, 1980.

PROMIS Laboratory, "Representation of Medical Knowledge" and PROMIS, *Proc. Second Symp. Comp. Appl. Med. Care*, 368-400, 1978.

Pryor, T.A. and F.G. Yanowitz, Computer Applications to Exercise Stress Testing, *Computers in Cardiology*, J. Cos and P. Hugenholtz (ed), St. Louis: October 1976.

Pryor, T.A., R.M. Gardner, P.D. Clayton and H.R. Warner, The HELP System, *J. Med. Sys.*, 7:87-102, 1983.

Rada, R. and L. Ackerman, Expert System for Interpretation of Computerized Axial Tomograms of the Brain, *Conf. on Art. Intell.*, Oakland Univ., pp.233-241, 1983.

Radin, S. and H.M. Greenberg, *Computer in the Doctor's Office*, Praeger, 1984.

Reggia, J., T. Pula, T. Price and B. Perricone, Towards an Intelligent Textbook of Neurology, *Proc. Fourth Symp. Comp. Appl. Med. Care*, pp.190-199, 1980.

Reggia, J., D. Nau and P. Wang, Diagnositc Expert Systems Based on Set Covering Model, *Int. J. Man-Machine Studies*, 19:437-460, 1983.

Reggia, J. and B. Perricone, Answer Justification in Medical Decision Support Systems Based on Bayesian Classification, *Comp. Biol. Med.*, (in press).

Reggia, J.A., B.T. Perricone, D.S. Nau, and Y. Peng, Answer To Justification In Diagnostic Expert Systems Part One: Abductive Inference and Its Justification, Part Two: Supporting Plausible Justifications, *IEEE Trans Biomed Eng* (BME-32, 1985).

Reggia, J.A. and S. Tuhrim (eds) *Computer-Assisted Medical Decision Making* (2 volumes), Springer-Verlag, 1985.

Richart, R., Evaluation of a medical data system, *Comp. Biomed.*, 3:417, 1976.

Rockart, J.F., E.R. McLean, P.I. Hershberg and G.O. Bell, An Automated Medical History System: Experience of the Lahey Clinic Foundation with Computer-Processed Medical Histories, *Archives of Int. Med.*, 132:348-358, 1973.

Rodnick, J.E., The Use of Automated Ambulatory Medical Records, *J. of Family Practice*, 5:253-264, 1977.

Rogers, W., B. Ryack and G. Moeller, Computer-Aided Medical Diagnosis—Literature Review, *Int. J. Biomed. Comp.*, 10:267-289, 1979.

Rogers, J.L., O.M. Haring and R.A. Watson, Automating the Medical Record: Emerging Issues, *Proc. Fourth Symp. Comp. Appl. Med. Care,* pp.255-263, 1980.

Rosati, R.A., A.G. Wallace and E.A. Stead, The Way of the Future, *Arch. Intern. Med.,* 131:285-287, 1973.

Rosati, R.A., J.F. McNeer, C.F. Starner, et al., A New Information System for Medical Practice, *Arch. Intern. Med.,* 135:1017-1024, 1975.

Rosati, R.A., Estimating the Likelihood of Significant Coronary Artery Disease. *Am. J. Med.,* 75:771-801, 1983.

Rubin, M. (ed) *Computerization and Automation in Health Facilities,* CRC Press, Boca Raton, FL, 1984.

Ryan, K.J., Computer Systems in Clinical Microbiology, *Clin. Lab. Med.,* 3:101-110, 1983.

Safran, C., P.N. Tsichlis, A.Z. Bluming and J.F. Desforges, Diagnositc Planning Using Computer-Assisted Decision Making for Patients with Hodgkins Disease, *Cancer,* 39:2426-2434, 1977.

Safran, C.H., et al., Decision Analysis Applied to Lymphangiography in Hodgkin's Disease, *New Eng. J. Med.,* 296:1088-1092, 1977.

Salamon, R., M. Bernadet, M. Samson, C. Derouesne and F. Gremy, Bayesian Method Applied to Decision Making in Neurology—Methodological Considerations, *Meth. Inform. Med.,* 15:174-179.

Schmidt, E.C., D.W. Schall and C.C. Morrison, Computerized Problem Oriented Medical Record for Ambulatory Practice, *Med. Care,* 12:316-327, 1974.

Schmid, W., et al., A Comparative Study of PSE/CATEGO and DiaSiKa: Two Psychiatric Computer Diagnostic Systems, *Brit. J. Psychiatry,* 141:292-295, 1982.

Schoolman, H. and L. Berstein, Computer Use in Diagnosis, Prognosis, and Therapy, *Science,* 200:926-931, 1978.

Schultz, M.D. and L. Davis, The Technology of PROMIS, *Proc. IEEE,* 67:1237-1245, 1979.

Schwartz, W.B., Medicine and the Computer: The Promise and Problems of Change, *New Eng. J. Med.,* 283:1257-1264, 1970.

Schwartz, W.B., G.A. Gorry, J.P. Kassirer and A. Essig, Decision Analysis and Clinical Judgment, *Am. J. Med.,* 5:459-472, 1973.

Schwartz, W.B., Decision Analysis. A Look at the Chief Complaints, *New Eng. J. Med.,* 300:556-559, 1979.

Schwartz, M.D. (ed), *Applications of Computers in Medicine,* IEEE Computer Society, 1982.

Schwartz, M.D. (ed), *Using Computers in Clinical Practice. Psychotherapy and Mental Health Application,* Haworth Press, 1984.

Shapiro, A.R., The SCAMP System for Patient and Practice Management, *J. Med. Sys.,* 7,2:127-136, 1983.

Shapiro, A., The Evaluation of Clinical Predictions, *New Eng. J. Med.,* 296:1509-1514, 1977.

Sheppard, L.C., The Computer in the Care of Critically Ill Patients, *Proc. IEEE,* 67:1300-1307, 1979.

Shortliffe, E.H., *Computer-Based Medical Consultations: MYCIN,* Elsevier/North Holland, Amsterdam, 1976.

Shortliffe, E., B. Buchannan and E. Feigenbaum, Knowledge Engineering for Medical Decision Making, *Proc. IEEE,* 67:1207-1224, 1979.

Shortliffe, E., Medical Computing: Another Basic Science?, *Proc. Fourth Symp. Comp. Appl. Med. Care,* 490-492, 1980.
Shortliffe, E.H., A.C. Scott, M.B. Bischoff, A.B. Campbell, W. Van Melle, and C.D. Jacobs, ONCOCIN: An Expert System for Oncology Protocol Management, *7th Inter. Joint. Conf. on AI,* pp.876-881, 1981.
Shortliffe, E.H., The Science of Bimedical Computing, J. Anderson, F. Gremy, A. Levy, and J.C. Pages (eds), *Information Science and Medical Education,* North Holland, 1984. Reprinted in *Medical Informatics,* 1984 9(3/4).
Shortliffe, E., G. Weiderhold and L. Fagan (eds), *An Introduction to Medical Information Science,* (In Preparation).
Simborg, D.W., L.K. MacDonald, J.S. Liebimon and P. Musco, Ward Information-Management System—An Evaluation, *Comput. Biomed. Res.,* 6:484-497, 1972.
Simborg, D.W. and H.J. Derewicz, A Highly Automated Hospital Medication System Five Years' Experience and Evaluation, *Annals of Int. Med.,* 83:342-345, 1975.
Simborg, D.W., Medication Prescribing on a University Medical Service—The Incidence of Drug Combinations with Potential Adverse Interactions, *The Johns Hopkins Med. J.,* 139:23-26, 1976.
Simborg, D.W., M. Chadwick, Q.E. Whiting-O'Keefe, S.G. Tolchin, S.A. Kahn and E.S. Bergan, Local Area Networks and the Hospital, *Comp. Biomed. Res.,* 16:247-259, 1983.
Simborg, D.W. and Q.E. Whiting-O'Keefe, Summary Time Oriented Record—A Progress Report, *Proc. Fifth Symp. Comp. Appl. Med. Care,* pp.100-104, 1981.
Simborg, D.W., Technology in Hospitals—the Effect of Prospective Reimbursement, *Proc. Seventh Symp. Comp. Appl. Med. Care,* pp.19-22, 1983.
Slack, W.V., D. Porter, J. Witschi, M.J. Sullivan, R. Buxbaum, F.J. Stare, Dietary Interviewing by Computer, *J. Am. Diet Assoc.,* 69:514-517, 1976.
Slack, W.V., G.P. Hicks, C.E. Reed and L.J. Van Cura, A Computer Based Medical History System, *New Eng. J. Med.,* 274:194-198, 1976.
Slack, W.V., L.J. Van Cura and J.H. Griest, Computers and Doctors: Use and Consequences, *Comp. Biomed. Res.,* 3:521-527, 1970.
Slack, W.V., Computer Based Interviewing System Dealing with Nonverbal Behavior as well as Keyboard Responses, *Science,* 171:84-87, 1971.
Slamecka, V., H. Camp and A. Badre, MARIS—A Knowledge System for Internal Medicine, *Inf. Proc. Mgmt.,* 13:273-276, 1977.
Sneider, R.M., R.E. Boyce and C.A. Tapella, The MATRIX Data Base Management System, *Computer,* 12:28-33, 1978.
Snyder, T.L., G.H. Schaeffer (authors). T.L. Synder and C.J. Felmeister (eds), *Personalized Guide to Computers and Your Dental Practice,* CV Mosby, St. Louis, 1984.
Solomon, M., *Using Computers in the Practice of Medicine: Professional and Clinical Guidelines for Managing Your Practice and Improving Patient Care,* Prentice-Hall, Englewood Cliffs, NJ, 1985.
Sondak, V., H. Schwartz and N. Sondak (eds), *Computers and Medicine,* Artech House Inc., 1979.
Sondak, N. and F. Kavaler (eds), *Computers in Medical Administration,* Artech House Inc., 1980.
Starfield, B.H., D.W. Simborg, S.D. Horn and S.A. Yourtee, Continuity and Coordination in Primary Care: Their Achievement and Utility, *Medical Care,* XIV, 7:625-636, 1976.

Starfield, B., D. Simborg, C. Johns, et al., Coordination of Care and its Relationship to Continuity and Medical Records, *Med. Care,* 15:929-938, 1977.

Starmer, C.F. and K.L. Lee, A Mathematical Approach to Medical Decisions: Application of Bayes' Rule to a Mixture of Continuous and Discrete Clinical Variables, *Comput. Biomed. Res.,* 9:531-541, 1976.

Starmer, C.F. and R.A. Rosati, A DSS for Management of Patients with a Chronic Illness, *SIGBDP,* 8(3), 1977.

Startsman, T. and R. Robinson, The Attitudes of Medical and Paramedical Personnel Toward Computers, *Comput. Biomed. Res.,* 5:218,227, 1972.

Stead, W.W., R.G. Brame, W.E. Hammond, et al., A Computerized Obstetric Medical Record, *Obstet. Syn.,* 49:502-509, 1977.

Stead, W.W., W.E. Hammond and M.J. Straube, A Chartless Record—Is it Adequate?, *J. Med. Sys.,* 7,2:103-110, 1983.

Stead, W.W., L.E. Garrett, W.E. Hammond, Practicing Nephrology with a Computerized Medical Record. *Kidney Int.,* 24:446-54, 1983.

Steel, K., et al., Iatrogenic Illness on a General Medical Service at a University Hosptial, *New Engl. J. of Med.,* 304:638-642, 1981.

Steinwachs, D.M. and Turner Bledsoe, Minimal Data Set for Ambulatory Care: Application of a Computerized System for Management and Quality Assurance, *An Examination of Case Studies in Hospital Information Systems,* American Hospital Association, Chicago, 1977.

Stratman, W.C., A Demonstration of PROMIS, *Research Summary Series,* National Center for Health Services Research, DHEW Publication No. (PHS) 79-3247, September 1979.

Studney, D.R., J.B. Adams, A. Gorbach, S. Guenthner, M.M. Morgan and G.O. Barnett, A Computerized Prenatal Record, *Obstetrics and Gynecology,* 50:82-87, 1977.

Szolovitz, P. and S.G. Pauker, Computers and Clinical Decision Making: Whether, How, and For Whom?, *Proc. IEEE* 67:1224-1226, 1979.

Szolovitz, P., Artificial Intelligence Methods for Medical Expert Systems, *Computer Applications in Medical Care,* Masson Publishing, Paris, NY, pp.298-294, 1982.

Szolovitz, P. (ed.), *Artificial Intelligence in Medicine,* Westview Press, CO, 1982.

Taylor, T.R., Clinical Decision Analysis, *Meth. Inform. Med.,* 15:216-224, 1976.

Teach, R.L. and E.H. Shortliffe, An Analysis of Physicians Attitudes Regarding Computer-Based Clinical Consultation Systems, *Comput. Biomed. Res.,* 14:542-558, 1981.

Technicon, Medical Information Systems, Corp., Cost-Benefit Analysis of the Technicon Medical Information System (MIS) for (unnamed hospital), December 1975.

Tversky, A. and D. Kahneman, Judgment Under Uncertainty: Heuristics and Biases, *Science* 85:1124-1131, 1974.

Tversky, A. and D. Kahnemann, The Framing of Decisions and the Rationality of Choice, *Science,* 211:453, 1981.

Vallbona, C., et al., The Health-Illness Profile: An Essential Component of the Ambulatory Medical Record, *Medical Care,* 11:117-124, 1973.

Vallbona, C., et al., Computer Support for a Neighborhood Health Clinic: Design and Implementation, *IEEE Trans. Biomed. Eng.* BME-20:180-184, 1973.

Van Egmond, J., P.F. DeVries Robbé and A.H. Levy (eds), *Information Systems for Patient Care,* North Holland, New York, 1976.

Vanker, A.D. and W. Van Stoecker, An Expert Diagnostic Program for Dermatology, *Comput. Biomed. Res.,* 17:241-247, 1984.

Wagner, G., P. Tautu and U. Wolber, Problems of Medical Diagnosis—A Bibliography, *Meth. Inform. Med.*, 17:54-74, 1978.
Waki, R., P.D. Clayton, F.L. Jensen, F.G. Yanowitz and H.V. Liddle, HELP Based Decision Analysis Applied to Coronary Artery Disease, *Comput. Biomed. Res.*, 15:188-202, 1982.
Wardle, A. and L. Wardle, Computer Aided Diagnosis—A Review of Research, *Meth. Inform. Med.*, 17:15-28, 1978.
Warner, D.M., Scheduling Nursing Personnel According to Nursing Preference: A Mathematical Programming Approval, *OR 24*, 5:842-856, Sept-Oct. 1976.
Warner, H.R., A.F. Toronto, V.G. Stephenson, A Mathematical Approach to Medical Diagnosis. Application to Congenital Heart Diseases, *JAMA*, 177:177-183, 1961.
Warner, H.R., C.M. Olmsted and B.D. Rutherford, HELP—A Program for Medical Decision-Making, *Comput. Biomed. Res.*, 5:65-74, 1972.
Warner, H.R., B.D. Rutherford and B. Houtchens, A Sequential Approach to History Taking and Diagnosis, *Comput. Biomed. Res.*, 5:256-262, 1972.
Warner, H.R., *Computer-Assisted Medical Decision-Making*, Academic Press, 1979.
Watson, R.J., How the Technicon Medical Information System Helps Physicians, *Advances in Auto. Analy.*, Tarrytown, N.Y.: Technicon International Congress Medical, Inc., 1:396-398, 1976.
Watson, R.J., A Large-Scale Professionally Oriented Medical Information System—Five Years Later, *J. Med. Sys.*, (3-21) 1977.
Weed, L.L., Medical Records that Guide and Teach, *New Eng.J. Med.*, 278:593, 1968 and 278:652, 1968.
Weed, L.L., *Medical Records, Medical Education, and Patient Care: The Problem Oriented Record as a Basic Tool*, Case-Western Reserve University Press, 1969.
Weed, L.L., Quality Control and the Medical Record, *Arch. Int. Med.*, 127:101, 1971.
Weed, L.L., Problem-Oriented Content Specific Medical Knowledge in Weinstein, M. and H. Fineberg (eds), *Clinical Decision Analysis*, W.B. Saunders: Philadelphia, 1980.
Weinstein, M.C. and H.V. Fineberg (eds), *Clinical Decision Analysis*, Philadelphia, W.B. Saunders and Co., 1980.
Weiss, S.M., C.A. Kulikowski, S. Amarel and A. Safir, A Model-Base Method for Computer-Aided Medical Decision-Making, *Artific. Intel.*, 11:145-172, 1978.
Weiss, S., C. Kulikowski and A. Safir, Glaucoma Consultation by Computer, *Comp. in Biol. Med.*, 8:25-40, 1978.
Weiss, S. and C. Kulikowski, EXPERT—A System for Developing Consultation Models, *Proc. Sixth Int. Joint. Conf. on Artif., Intell.*, 942-947, 1979.
Weyl, S., J. Fries, G. Wiederhold and F. Germano, A Modular Self-Describing Clinical Databank System, *Comput. Biomed. Res.*, 8:279-293, 1975.
Wheeler, P.S. and D.W. Simborg, The Johns Hopkins Radiology Computer Reporting System, *Electromedica*, 2-3/75 pp.104-108, 1975.
Whitcomb, C.C., C.P. Vogt and N.M. Wilbur, Clinical Laboratory Data Processing with a Central Hospital Computer, *Comput. Biol. Med.*, 8:197-206, 1978.
Whiting-O'Keefe, D.W. Simborg and W.V. Epstein, A Controlled Experiment to Evaluate the Use of a Time-Oriented Summary Medical Record, *Medical Care*, (18,8) 1980 pp.842-852, 1980.
Wiederhold, G., *Databases for Health Care*, Springer-Verlag, NY, 1981.
Wingert, F., *Medical Informatics*, Springer-Verlag, NY, 1979.

Wirtschafter, D., J.T. Carpenter and E. Mesel, A Consultant-Extender System for Breast Cancer Adjuvant Chemotherapy, *Annals of Intern. Med.*, 90:396-401, 1979.

Wirtschafter, D.D., M. Scalise, C. Henke and R.A. Gams, Do Information Systems Improve the Quality of Clinical Research? Results of a Randomized Trial in a Cooperative Multi-Institutional Cancer Group, *Comp. and Biomed. Res.*, 14:78-90, 1981.

Wirtshafter, D.D., et al., A County-Wide Obstetrical Automated Medical Record System, *J. Med. Sys.*, 6:277-290, 1982.

Worthley, J.A. (ed) *Managing Computers in Health Care,* AUPHA Press, 1982.

Young, D.W., Doctors' Attitudes to a Computer-Based Clinical Information System, *Methods of Infor. in Med.*, 20:196-199, 1981.

Yu, V.L., B.G. Buchanan, E.H. Shortliffe, et al., An Evaluation of the Performance of a Computer-Based Consultant, *Comput. Prog. Biomed,* 9:95-102, 1979.

Yu, V., L. Fagan, S. Wraith, et al., Antimicrobial Selection by a Computer—A Blinded Evaluation by Infectious Disease Experts, *JAMA,* 42:1279-1282, 1979.

Zagoria, R. and J. Reggia, Transferability of Medical Decision Support Systems Based on Bayesian Classification, *Med. Decis. Making,* 3:501,509, 1983.

Zielsturff, R.D., et al., Experience with a Computer-Based Medical Record for Nurse Practitioners in Ambulatory Care, *Comput. Biomed. Res.* 10:61-74, 1977.

Zimmerman, J. and A. Rector, *Computers for the Physician's Office,* Research Studies Press, 1978.

Ziportyn, T., Computer-Assisted Medical Decision Making: Interest Growing, *JAMA,* 248:913, 1982.

Zoltie, N., J. Horrocks and F. deDombal, Computer-Assisted Diagnosis of Dyspepsia—Report on Transferability of a System, with Emphasis on Early Diagnosis of Gastric Cancer, *Meth. Inform. Med.*, 16:89-92, 1977.

Index

GPSR Compliance

The European Union's (EU) General Product Safety Regulation (GPSR) is a set of rules that requires consumer products to be safe and our obligations to ensure this.

If you have any concerns about our products, you can contact us on ProductSafety@springernature.com

In case Publisher is established outside the EU, the EU authorized representative is:

Springer Nature Customer Service Center GmbH
Europaplatz 3
69115 Heidelberg, Germany

Batch number: 10682323

Printed by Printforce, the Netherlands